T0228697

Theory and Concepts
of Drug Carrier Systems

Theory and Concepts of Drug Carrier Systems

Edited by **Erica Helmer**

New Jersey

Published by Foster Academics,
61 Van Reypen Street,
Jersey City, NJ 07306, USA
www.fosteracademics.com

Theory and Concepts of Drug Carrier Systems
Edited by Erica Helmer

© 2015 Foster Academics

International Standard Book Number: 978-1-63242-397-9 (Hardback)

Printed in the United States of America.

Theory and Concepts of Drug Carrier Systems

Edited by **Erica Helmer**

New Jersey

Published by Foster Academics,
61 Van Reypen Street,
Jersey City, NJ 07306, USA
www.fosteracademics.com

Theory and Concepts of Drug Carrier Systems
Edited by Erica Helmer

© 2015 Foster Academics

International Standard Book Number: 978-1-63242-397-9 (Hardback)

Printed in the United States of America.

Contents

Preface

This book compiles contributions of prominent experts and researchers in the multidisciplinary arena of novel drug delivery systems. It gives insights into the ongoing and recent potentialities of various drug delivery systems. Emergence of analytical approaches and capabilities to determine particle sizes in nanometer ranges has focused interest towards nanoparticles for more effective methods of drug delivery. The book focuses on various aspects of drug delivery systems such as developments in the optimization, design and adaptation of gene delivery systems for treatment of infectious, genetic, cardiovascular diseases and cancer. The book assesses and reviews procedures under two sections: Powder Technology in Drug Delivery and Nano carriers in Drug Delivery.

All of the data presented henceforth, was collaborated in the wake of recent advancements in the field. The aim of this book is to present the diversified developments from across the globe in a comprehensible manner. The opinions expressed in each chapter belong solely to the contributing authors. Their interpretations of the topics are the integral part of this book, which I have carefully compiled for a better understanding of the readers.

At the end, I would like to thank all those who dedicated their time and efforts for the successful completion of this book. I also wish to convey my gratitude towards my friends and family who supported me at every step.

Editor

Powder Technology in Drug Delivery

Development and Investigation of Dry Powder Inhalers for Cystic Fibrosis

Paola Russo, Antonietta Santoro, Lucia Prota, Mariateresa Stigliani and Rita P. Aquino

Additional information is available at the end of the chapter

1. Introduction

Cystic Fibrosis (CF) is the most common lethal monogenic disorder in Caucasians, estimated to affect one *per* 2500-4000 newborns. CF is caused by mutations in the gene encoding the CF transmembrane conductance regulator (CFTR) [1, 2]. CFTR acts mainly as a chloride channel and has other regulatory roles, including inhibition of sodium transport through the epithelial sodium channel, regulation of ATP channels and intracellular vesicle transport, acidification of intracellular organelles and inhibition of endogenous calcium- activated chloride channels [3-5]. CFTR is also involved in bicarbonate-chloride exchange [6]. In the airways, loss of functional CFTR promotes increase of oxidation status, tissue injury, modification of intracellular signaling pathways, cell apoptosis and inflammatory processes.

Clinically, the reduced volume of the epithelial lining fluid and the increased viscoelasticity of the mucus lead to a dysfunction of the mucociliary clearance, and as a consequence, patients suffer from recurrent and chronic infections caused mainly by bacteria such as *Staphylococcus aureus*, *Haemophilus influenzae*, *Burkholderia cepacia*, and especially *Pseudomonas aeruginosa*. Moreover, the chronic *P. aeruginosa* lung infection causes a sustained inflammatory response in the lung. Antibiotics are administered to CF patients in long-term treatment with the hope of maintaining quality of life, weight and lung function, as well as to decrease the number of exacerbations and hospital admission [7, 8].

Today there are few formulations, mostly solutions, approved for inhalation in CF patients and there is a continuous research in the development of new inhaled antibiotic therapeutic systems for management of chronic CF lung disease. New formulations and delivery devices are needed to improve efficiency, portability and possibly increase the dose locally available.

Besides chronic bacterial infections, chronic airway inflammation is uniformly observed in patients with CF [9, 10], as a consequence of over-expression of proinflammatory enzymes. Thus, the lung, dipped in an environment rich in oxygen as well as a defective antioxidant system, is susceptible to injury mediated by oxidative stress. Reactive oxygen species, ROS, such as super oxide anion ($O^{2\bullet-}$) and hydroxyl radical ($OH^{\bullet}$), and reactive nitrogen species, RNS, such as nitrogen dioxide and peroxynitrite, are unstable molecules with unpaired electrons, capable of initiating oxidation. In order to prevent tissue damage, lungs are endowed with several antioxidant defences, including glutathione, heme oxygenase, superoxide dismutase, vitamins C and E, beta-carotene, uric acid [11]. However, when the presence of ROS and RNS overcomes the physiologic antioxidant defences, an oxidative stress status, occurs. Thus, as an adjunct to optimal antibiotic therapy, antioxidant/anti-inflammatory therapy is warranted to avoid a decline in lung function and tissue damage.

1.1. Respiratory drug delivery

Inhalation drug therapy consists of drug administration directly to the lung in form of micronized droplets or solid microparticles, highly recommended especially in pathologies affecting the lung (i.e. asthma, cystic fibrosis, chronic obstructive pulmonary disease). The administration of the active compound directly in the airways can be of great advantage: after inhalation, the site where the drug is deposited is less aggressive in terms of pH and enzymatic attach; additionally, the hepatic first-passage effect is bypassed. Both aspects influence the dose administered, which can be decreased compared to oral route. Moreover, the permeability of pulmonary epithelium is higher than the intestinal mucosa, due to a reduced resistance to substance transport. Finally, the drug dissolution, critical for many compounds, is less relevant in the case of solids, since the active compound is a very fine powder that impacts with a high surface area. In addition to biopharmaceutical aspects, inhalation bioavailability requires the deposition of the dose in the lung i.e., the active compound must be formulated in a respirable form. Development of formulations for inhalation is particularly challenging since the preparation of a respirable formulation and the selection of an adequate device for the administration are both required. Formulation and device constitute the dosage forms and affect the bioavailability of the inhaled drug. Concerning the formulation, dry powder inhalers (DPI) are preferred to solutions/suspensions due to drug stability, high concentration at the site of action and lack of propellant. The biggest issue encountered when formulating a dry powder for inhalation is its size which has to be small enough to guarantee the aerosolization and the deposition at the appropriate site of the respiratory tract. A failure in deposition may result in a failure of efficacy. Given that any discussion about the right size of particles for inhalation is meaningless without the consideration of their geometry and density, the concept of aerodynamic diameter has been introduced. The aerodynamic diameter (Dae) is a spherical equivalent diameter and derives from the equivalence between the inhaled particle and a sphere of unit density (ρ_0] undergoing sedimentation at the same rate (Eq. 1).

$$Dae = \text{Dv} \sqrt{\frac{\rho}{\chi \rho_0}} \qquad (1)$$

where Dv is the volume-equivalent diameter, ρ is the particle density and χ is the shape factor.

Hence, the aerodynamic behaviour depends on particle geometry, density and volume diameter: a small spherical particle with a high density will behave aerodynamically as a bigger particle, being poorly transported in the lower airways. The Dae can be improved reducing the volume diameter and the density or increasing the shape factor of the particles, by means of different processes, i.e. dry or wet milling, spray-drying, spray-freeze drying, and supercritical fluid technology. Among these, spray drying is a commonly used technique for the preparation of dry powders for inhalation.

1.2. Spray drying

Spray drying is a one-step process able to convert liquid feeds (i.e., solutions, suspensions and emulsions) in a dry powder. Firstly, the liquid is broken into droplets by means of a nozzle atomizer (atomization step); then, droplets come in contact with a heated gas in the drying chamber and the drying step starts; finally, the dried particles are separated from the heated gas by means of a cyclone (separation step) and collected into a glass container. The optimization of the aerodynamic properties of the powders produced *via* spray drying can be achieved modulating process parameters, solvent composition, solute concentration, liquid feed rate, inlet temperature, gas pressure and aspiration.

1.3. The challenge of excipients for dry powder inhalers

The primary function of the lung is respiration. To fulfil this purpose, the lung has a large surface area and a thin membranes. Many compounds have been tested to overcome drug delivery outcomes related to the small particle size requested for deposition. For example, in the spray drying process the powder properties can be modulated adding excipients able to affect the evaporation of spray droplets during the drying and consequently the particle shape. The safety of an inhalation drug product has to be taken into account: the structural and functional integrity of respiratory epithelium must be respected. This hardly limits the choice of excipients available for the formulation to few compounds, like sugars (lactose, mannitol and glucose) and hydrophobic additive (magnesium stearate, DSPC). As a matter of fact, natural amino acids (AAs) possess good safety profiles and, recently, showed to enhance flow aid properties when co-spray-dried with active compounds. As a support to AAs pulmonary safety, a formulation of Aztreonam and lysine (Cayston®, powder for instant solution and inhalation) has been recently approved by FDA for CF patients.

2. Aerosolized antioxidant and anti-inflammatory agents in Cystic Fibrosis

Oxidative stress has been identified as an early complication in the airways of infants and young children affected by CF [12, 13]. Recent clinical data suggest that oxidative damage of pulmonary proteins during chronic infection may contribute to the decline of lung function in CF patients [14]. The massive infiltration of neutrophils in lungs of CF patients leads to the generation of oxygen-derived reactive oxygen species (ROS) and, in particular, H_2O_2 that contributes to irreversible lung damage and, ultimately, to patient death. Activated neutrophils migrate to the airways and release large amounts of ROS. On the other hand in CF epithelial cells, antioxidant defense systems appear to be defective in their ability to control the amount of ROS produced [15]. Therefore over-abundance of ROS and their products may cause tissue injury-events and modify intracellular signalling pathways leading to cell apoptosis and enhanced inflammatory processes. In addition to its Cl- channel function, CFTR has been proposed to carry antioxidant-reduced glutathione. A recent study demonstrated that oxidative stress can suppress CFTR expression and function while increasing the cellular GSH content. Chronic lung inflammation with episodes of acute exacerbations initiates several physiological and metabolic changes with harmful effects including weight loss and metabolic breakdown. Antioxidants (glutathione, vitamins, beta-carotene, selenium and flavonoids) as dietary support or pharmacological treatment can be a promising approach. Great attention has been focused on flavonoids [16, 17], polyphenolic compounds with antioxidant, anti-inflammatory and antibacteric activity, hugely present in fruits and vegetables. Among natural flavonoids, naringin (N, Fig. 1) extracted from grapefruits has shown anti-inflammatory, antioxidant and anticarcinogenic effects [18].

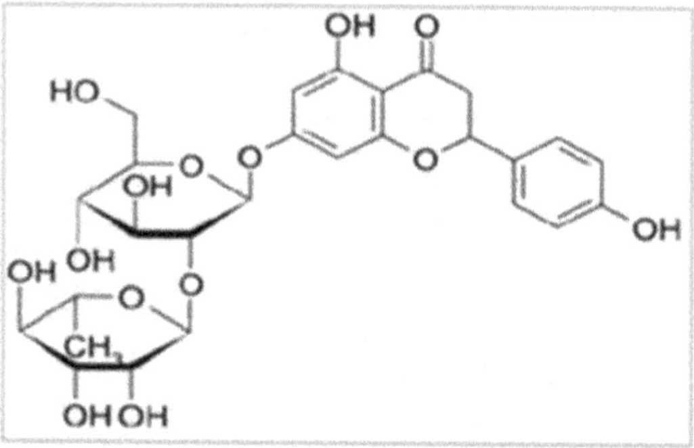

Figure 1. Naringin 4,5,7-trihydroxyflavanone 7-rhamnoglucosyde

In addition, recent studies have reported that flavonoids may act as CFTR direct activators, stimulating transepithelial chloride transport [19-21]. Although flavonoids are inhibitors of tyrosine kinases and phosphatases, their effects on CFTR are probably independent of these activities, resulting from direct binding to an NBD of phosphorylated CFTR [22].

With the aim to discover more effective activators of G551D-CFTR [19], some investigators have begun to examine the relationship between the chemical structure of flavonoids and their effects on CFTR Cl channels. This study served to identify the pharmacophore portion of the skeletons molecular basis for interaction with the NBD. The well-documented antioxidant effect of flavonoids is unfortunately more evident *in vitro* than *in vivo*, due to the high concentration needed, the susceptibility to oxidation and instability to the gastric pH in which they undergo hydrolysis and enzymatic degradation. Moreover, flavonoids show a very slight solubility in water, which leads to a very low dissolution rate, an irregular absorption of the drug from oral solid dosage forms in the gastrointestinal tract and a limited bioavailability. Despite a number of publications focused on the antioxidant effect of flavonoids, rather no attention has been addressed yet to their formulation in order to increase bioavailability. Recently, oral hydrophilic swellable matrices for a controlled release of some flavonoids [23, 24] and gastroresistant microparticles aiming at overcoming the acid environment have been formulated [25, 26]. An alternative strategy may be the direct aerosol delivery to the lung, which has the advantage to achieve higher locally available concentration of the antioxidant in the airways.

2.1. Naringin dry powders production and characterization

Naringin is a very slightly soluble molecule: its lipophilia can affect the dissolution of the drug when in contact with the liquids lining the lung. The micronization by means of spray drying process and addition of opportune additives able to improve powder wettability seem to be a valid strategy for the formulation of an efficacious dry powder inhaler. Micronized particles were produced by completely dissolving the active naringin (N) alone (#NET3) or with 5% w/w of leucine (#NET3-leu5) as dispersibility enhancer in 7/3 water/ethanol solutions [27, 28]. Spray drying conditions were: inlet temperature 110°C, drying air flow 500L/min, aspirator 100%, feed rate 5ml/min, nozzle 0.5mm. Aerodynamic properties were determined by means of both single stage glass impinger (SSGI) and Andersen cascade impactor (ACI). The device used for the DPI deposition tests was the Turbospin (kindly donated by PH&T SpA) in which the dose to be aerosolized was pre-metered in a size 2 gelatine capsule. Results demonstrated that the presence of leucine in the feed solution influenced particle size distribution, as well as powder density and morphology. Firstly, NET3-leu5 showed a d_{50} sensibly lower than NET3, evidencing a positive effect of leucine on particle diameter.

Code #	Leu content (% w/w)	Spray yield (%)	d_{50} (μm) and span	FPF (%)
NET3	0	59.4 ± 0.3	5.2 [1.6]	44.5 ± 1.5
NET3-leu5	5	60.7 ± 2.5	3.3 [1.7]	51.3 ± 1.6

FPF, fine particle fraction

Table 1. Composition, spray drying yield, particle size distribution and fine particle fraction after SSGI of Naringin powders.

Moreover, as showed by thermograms of NET3-leu5, DSC analyses indicated that spray-dried powders containing the AA were amorphous materials. Spray drying process caused the loss of crystalline habitus of both N and leu raw material as evidenced by the absence of the endotherms corresponding to N crystal melting point (247°C, Fig. 2b) and leu crystal melting point (275°C, Fig. 2a).

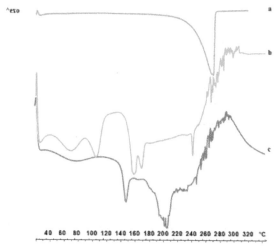

Figure 2. Differential scanning calorimetry thermograms of Naringin raw material (a), Leucine raw material (b) and NET3-leu5 (c).

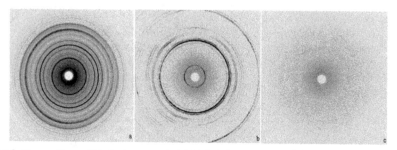

Figure 3. X-ray patterns of Naringin raw material (a), Leucine raw material (b) and NET3-leu5(c).

DSC results were confirmed by X-ray assessments, showing no crystalline state in NET3-leu5 powder. In figure 3 X-ray patterns of N (Fig. 3a) and leu (Fig. 3b) as raw materials were reported in comparison with X-ray patterns of NET3-leu5 (Fig. 3c). The loss in crystallinity is an important issue for drugs, such as N, very slightly soluble in water, bringing to an increase of solid solubility.

Microscopy observation revealed that particle morphology was affected by leucine content in the liquid feed: samples containing only N appeared as small particles, spherical in shape or very slightly corrugated and their SEM micrographs showed widespread aggregation (Fig. 4a).

On the contrary, micrographs of samples produced with 5% leu displayed well separated particles with corrugated, raisin-like surfaces (Fig. 4b), beneficial for particles intended for inhalation.

In fact, previous reports suggested that improvement of the respirable fraction may be obtained not only by lowering the size or the density of a powder, but also reducing interparticulate cohesion [29, 30]. Corrugated particles might also be more appropriate for dissolution in the lung fluid due to a larger area.

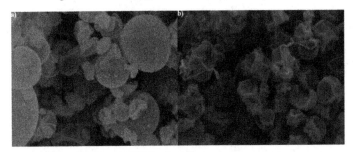

Figure 4. SEM picture of (a) NET3 and NET3-leu5

Regarding the *in vitro* deposition test by means of SSGI, the AA affected the aerodynamic properties of spray-dried powders as reported in table 1. NET3-leu5 showed an improvement of FPF due to both a reduction in the capsule and device retention and an increase in powder dispersibility. The latter is likely to be related to the absence of aggregates and high degree of particle corrugation, as observed by SEM analyses. These data were confirmed by ACI experiments (Fig. 5).

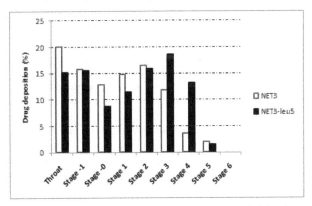

Figure 5. ACI deposition patterns of NET3 (white bars) and NET3-leu5 (black bars).

The powder containing the dispersibility agent (NET3-leu5) showed a lower deposition in the throat compared to NET3, with a resulting higher quantity of drug recovered from the deeper stages and an improving of the fine particle fraction.

These results are in agreement with previous report on the ability of surface corrugation to decrease interparticulate cohesion by reducing Van der Waals forces between particles and, consequently, increase powder respirability.

In conclusion, the use of leucine as excipient was useful to reduce adhesion between particles and improve powder dispersion, when delivered from dry powder inhalers. Therefore, a careful formulation plays a key role in the aerosol performance of N dry powders: NET3-leu5 showed optimezed bulk and aerodynamic behaviour.

Moreover, the spray drying process, reducing particle size while improving particle superficial area exposed to fluids, caused a greater (up to 30 fold higher, Fig. 6) immediate solubility of micronized powders (NET3 and NET3-leu5] when in contact with water at 37°C, compared to unprocessed commercial batch (rawN). Leucine addition to powder formulation (NET3-leu5) further increased N solubility which started declining very quikly, reaching a nearly constant value after 30 minutes, due to recrystallization of the amorphous material.

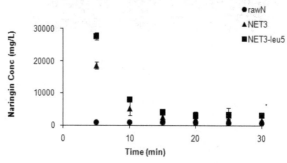

Figure 6. Aqueous solubility at 37°C of rawN (commercial batch, circles), NET3 (spray-dried batch without excipient, triangles) and NET3-leu5 (spray-dried batch with 5% leu, squares).

2.2. *In vitro* biological activities of N dry powders in bronchial epithelial cells

The developed dry powders have to be tested for verifying the ability to control airways inflammation. Two immortalized cell lines were selected as in vitro models: one, called CuFi1 (CF cells), was derived from human airway epithelial (HAE) cells of CFTR ΔF508/ΔF508 mutant genotype, the other, called NuLi1 (normal lung), was derived from a non-CF subject and used as control. These cell lines exhibited transepithelial resistance, maintained the ion channel physiology expected for the genotypes and retained NF-κB responses to inflammatory stimuli [31, 32] Cytotoxicity and effects on NF-κB pathway and on IL-6 and IL-8 release were examined.

2.2.1. *Effect of N and its formulations on cell viability*

Cytotoxicity (MTT assay) and cell viability (BrUd) evaluations (from 15 to 150μm) showed that neither rawN nor NET3 and NET3-leu5 are cytotoxic or cytostatic in both CF and non-

CF bronchial cells. After a 24 h treatment, rawN did not significantly affect cell viability, as determined by MTT assay in the concentration ranging from 15 to 150 μM (data not shown), but it caused a dose-dependent reduction of cell growth of different extent in NuLi1 and CuFi1 cells, from 60 to 150 μM (Fig. 7a). Interestingly, spray-dried powders containing leucine induced a dose-dependent and significant cell growth inhibition only in normal bronchial NuLi1 cells (Fig. 7c), while it determined a 14% increase of cell proliferation in CuFi1 cells at the highest dose (150 μM). To evaluate the contribution of the AA to the increased cell proliferation induced by NET3-leu5 in CuFi1, Leu spray-dried alone was also tested. The AA did not show any significant effect in NuLi1 cells while it was able to increase CuFi1 cell proliferation at all the concentrations tested (Fig. 7d).

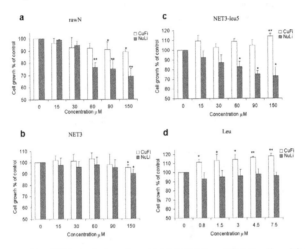

Figure 7. Naringin and its DPI formulations do not inhibit CuFi1 and NuLi1 cell proliferation at concentrations lower than 60 μM. Cells were treated for 24 h with: (a) raw Naringin (rawN), (b) spray-dried Naringin (NET3), (c) N co-sprayed with 5% leucine (NET3-leu5) (from 0.8 to 7.5 μM). Cell growth was determined using a colorimetric bromodeoxyuridine (BrdU) cell proliferation ELISA kit. The histograms report the percentage of growing cells in comparison with untreated cells (control, 100% proliferation). All data are shown as mean ± SD of three independent experiments each done in duplicate (*P < 0.05 and **P < 0.01 vs control).

This finding suggests that the technological improvement of immediate drug solubility and powder flowability, as well as the presence of the AA, may increase the drug uptake and improve the CF cell altered metabolism, reducing the toxicity observed for unprocessed rawN (Fig. 7a). In accordance, increased and altered basal protein catabolism has been reported in CF patients by many reports [33-35].

2.2.2. Effect of N and its formulations on NF-κB pathway

To study the anti-inflammatory effects of N in CuFi1 cells, we investigated the main molecular targets of NF-κB pathway in CuFi1 in comparison to normal bronchial NuLi1 cells. The NF-κB pathway is well known to play a crucial role in inflammatory process (36). In resting cells, the transcription factor NF-κB exists as homo- or heterodimer, maintained inactive in the cytosol by a family of inhibitor proteins named IκBs (IκBα, β, ε). In response to a wide range of stimuli such as cytokines and bacterial or viral products, IκB proteins are phosphorylated by IκB kinases (IKKα and β), ubiquitinated and degraded by the 26S proteasome. As a consequence, NF-κB dimers can localize into the nucleus and positively regulate the transcription of proinflammatory genes (37). This pathway is overactivated also in absence of any infection (38-40) in CF cells. In our experiments, CuFi1 cells exhibit higher expression levels of IKKβ and phosphoIKBα proteins compared to their normal counterpart NuLi1 cells (data from Western Blot analysis not shown). The effects of rawN, NET3 and NET3-leu5 at sub-toxic concentrations (30 μM) were evaluated at 2, 6 and 24 h on IKKβ and IκBα kinases, measuring both the expression levels and the phosphorylation status of the main molecular targets of the NF-κB pathway (i.e. IKKα, IKKβ and IκBα). Results are reported in figure 8.

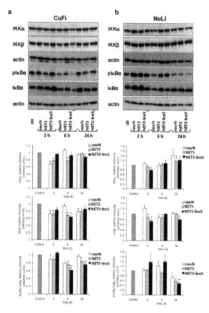

Figure 8. Naringin and its DPI formulations inhibit the key enzymes of the NF-κB pathway in CF bronchial epithelial cells. CuFi1 (a) and NuLi1 (b) cells were treated with raw Naringin (rawN), spray-dried Naringin (NET3) and N co-sprayed with 5% leucine (NET3-leu 5) at 30 μM concentration for the indicated time points. Cell lysates were analyzed by Western blot with antibodies against IKKα, IKKβ and pIκBα. Same filters were stripped and re-probed with total IκBα and anti-actin used as loading control. More representative results are shown (upper panels). Immunoreactive bands were quantified using Quantity One program. Densitometric analyses (mean ± SD) of three independent experiments are reported as relative intensity of IKKα, IKKβ or pIκBα/IκBα on actin and expressed as arbitrary units vs control (lower panels). (*P < 0.05 and **P < 0.01 vs control).

As regards to IKKα, NET3 and NET3-leu5 caused a reduction of IKKα but rawN did not in CuFi1 cells, while all powders did not cause any significant effect in normal airways epithelial cells (Fig. 8b). As IKKβ, its expression was generally reduced in CuFi1 cells: the highest decrease was observed at 6 h in NET3-leu5-treated cells (Fig. 8b). Interestingly, the observed reduction of expression levels of both the enzymatic subunits of the IKK complex in CuFi led to a significant and prolonged decrease of IκBα phoshorylation. In fact, this effect started early (2 h) and was retained all over the treatment time (24 h) in CF bronchial epithelial cells (Fig. 8a). On the contrary, in normal bronchial epithelial cells only a delayed (24 h) decrease of IκBα phosphorylation was observed as a consequence of the reduction of IKKβ subunit only expression level. Leucine spray-dried alone did not give any significant result in all Western Blot analyses (data not shown).

Previous evidence indicates that IKKβ plays a more crucial role for NF-κB activation in response to pro-inflammatory cytokines and microbial products [40], even though both the catalytic subunits of the IKK complex are able to regulate NF-κB activation and have a complementary role in the control of inflammation [41]. N formulations are effective in inhibiting both IKK subunits expression, and therefore caused a prolonged reduction of IκBα phosphorylation in CuFi1 cells.

2.2.3. Effect of N and its formulation on Interleukin-8 (IL-8) and interleukin-6 (IL-6) release

The direct effect of NET3-leu5 on the main cytokines involved in inflammatory response, interleukin 8 (IL-8) and interleukin 6 (IL-6) was also investigated. To this aim, CuFi1 cells were treated with NET3-Leu5 at 30 and 60 μM in the presence and absence of LPS-stimulation from *Pseudomonas aeruginosa*. Results (Fig. 9) showed that NET3-leu5 inhibited both cytokine production in unstimulated as well as in LPS-stimulated CuFi1 cells and the production of IL-8 more than IL-6.

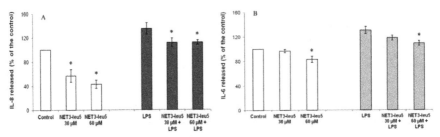

Figure 9. Effect of Naringin co-sprayed with 5% leucine (NET3-leu5) on basal and LPS-induced secretion of IL-8 (**A**) and IL-6 (**B**) in Cystic Fibrosis bronchial epithelial (CuFi1) cells. Data are presented as mean percentage of released cytokines in the control supernatants (untreated and unstimulated) ± SD of two independent experiments each done in duplicate. (*P < 0.05 vs control supernatants).

These data indicate that the inhibition of NFkB pathway by NET3-leu5 results in a reduction of the release of pro-inflammatory cytokines. NET3-leu5 seems involved in controlling the pro-inflammatory status of CF cells in the presence as well as in the absence of bacterial stimulation. However, LPS-stimulated cytokine secretion is dependent on Toll-like receptor-4 (TLR-4] signaling which expression is reduced in the CF airway epithelial cells, promoting the bacterial colonization and chronic infection in CF lung (42).

3. Aerosolized antibiotics in cystic fibrosis

Pulmonary infections are the major cause of morbidity and mortality in cystic fibrosis (CF), with Pseudomonas aeruginosa (Pa) acting as the princISOl pathogen. The viscous mucus lining the lung of CF patients impairs the mucociliary function, facilitating recurrent and chronic respiratory infections caused mainly by Pa but also by Haemophilus influenzae, Bulkolderia cepacia [7, 8]. Treatment of lung disease by antibiotics is an accepted standard in CF cure aiming at reducing decline in lung function and number of hospitalizations [43]. Aminoglycosides, such as gentamicin sulfate (G) (Fig. 10), are indicated in the management of acute exacerbations of CF as well as in the control of chronic infection and eradication of Pa infections. Various clinical studies on gentamicin inhalation treatment in cystic fibrosis patients chronically infected with Pseudomonas aeruginosa have shown that antibiotic solutions for aerosol treatment produce both subjective and objective improvement. Interestingly, among aminoglycosides, G has shown the ability to partially restore the expression of the functional protein CFTR (cystic fibrosis transmembrane conductance regulator) in CF mouse models bearing class I nonsense mutations [44-47]. In particular, Du and coll. [45] demonstrated that G was able to induce the expression of a higher CFTR level compared to tobramycin. Aminoglycoside antibiotics can suppress premature termination codons by allowing an amino acid to be incorporated in place of the stop codon, thus permitting translation to continue to the normal end of the transcript. Regarding the use of aminoglycosides in the treatment of airways infections and class I CFTR mutations, the main problem is their reduced penetration in the endobronchial space after intravenous (IV) administration, combined with their high systemic toxicity. Since aminoglycosides peak sputum concentrations are only 12 to 20% of the peak serum concentrations [48] to achieve adequate drug concentrations at the site of action, it is necessary to use large IV doses, which may produce serum levels associated with renal and oto-toxicity.

These problems can be overcome by the use of aerosolized aminoglycosides, which can deliver high dose of drug directly to the lungs, while minimizing systemic exposure. Therefore, the first aim of the research was to develop micronized gentamicin powders, easy to handle and stable for long time; the second goal was to obtain a dry powder suitable for pulmonary administration.

3.1. Design and development of a new dry powder inhaler of gentamicin

Differently from Naringin, Gentamicin is a very soluble drug: as its high hydrophilia guarantees a rapid drug solubility and diffusion in the fluids lining the lung, as it may cause high hygroscopicity and instability, preventing the formulation of a stable and respirable dry powder. As it is well known, hygroscopicity modulates the moisture content of the

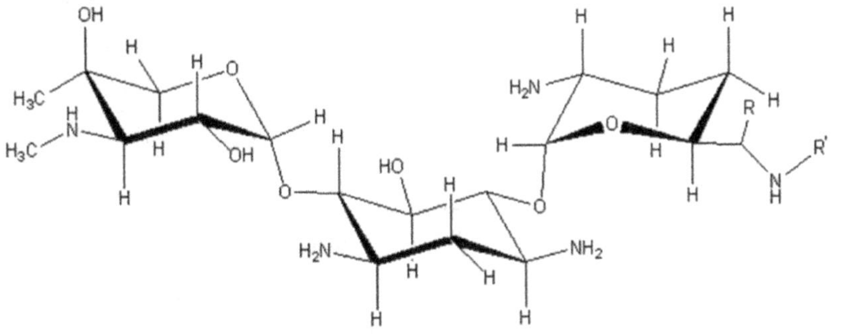

H_2SO_4

	R	R'
Gent.C1	CH$_3$	CH₃
Gent.C2	CH₃	H
Gent.C1a	H	H

Figure 10. Gentamicin sulfate structure.

particles in the final dosage form prior to aerosol generation and it is correlated to chemical or physical instability of the product. For aerosols formulation, the agglomeration leads to an inability to generate particles of respirable size. Moreover, as aerosol particles enter the lungs, they experience a high-humidity environment (99.5% relative humidity at 37°C): inhaled particles may be subject to hygroscopic growth, increasing their dimensions and affecting lung deposition. In this case, excipients able to modify the hygroscopic properties of a drug need to be considered. A dry powder formulation was obtained by co-spray-drying Gentamicin and leucine from 7/3 hydro-alcoholic solutions, using an organic solvent less polar than ethanol, the isopropanol. Microparticles were designed while studying the effect of leu, feed composition and process parameters on particle formation, physicochemical properties and aerosol performance. In addition, the effect of the engineered particles on cell viability and cell proliferation of CuFi1 cells was investigated.

3.1.1. Manufacturing and characterization of G/leu co-spray-dried powders

Due to its high polarity, G raw material was deliquescent, becoming liquid after 1 hour of exposure to room conditions. In order to reduce hygroscopicity and to increase powder dispersibility, G was subject to spray drying process alone or with leu as flowability enhancer using water or water-isopropanol (ISO) mixtures.

Preliminarly, the solubilities of the drug and excipient in the feed systems were determined; G freely soluble in water exhibited the lowest solubility in water/ISO 7/3 (v/v) system, the poor solubility of leu is even lower in water-co-solvent systems (Table 2).

Liquid feed composition	G (mg/ml)	Leu (mg/ml)
Water	Freely soluble	24.2±1.0
Water/ISO 8/2 (v/v)	351.8±25.1	11.2±0.5
Water/ISO 7/3 (v/v)	135.9±24.6	9.5±0.2

Table 2. Gentamicin and L-leucine solubility in liquid feeds used for spray drying at pH 7.0±0.1.

As reported in Table 3, addition of the organic co-solvent into the water feed was extremely helpful in terms of process yield suggesting a reduction in powder cohesiveness and, therefore, a potential enhancement of the aerosolisation properties (49). Differently, leu addition did not have a linear effect on spray drying yield (Table 3).

	Code #	Leu content (%w/w)	Process yield (%)	d_{50} (µm) and span
20% v/v ISO	GISO2	0	78.0 ±3.8	4.74 [2.10]
	GISO2-leu5	5	73.9 ±0.5	6.19 [1.88]
	GISO2-leu10	10	65.0 ±5.5	4.07 [1.81]
	GISO2-leu15	15	84.6 ±3.3	3.72 [1.58]
	GISO2-leu5	20	77.5 ±0.6	4.82 [1.73]
30% v/vISO	GISO3	0	85.5 ±0.7	4.24 [1.97]
	GISO3-leu5	5	86.6 ±1.2	3.77 [1.36]
	GISO3-leu10	10	85.9 ±0.9	3.69 [1.51]
	GISO3-leu15	15	82.0 ±2.1	3.90 [1.62]
	GISO3-leu20	20	80.8 ±1.3	4.11 [1.90]

Table 3. Physical characteristics of spray dried particles: liquid fees composition, process yield, particle size and bulk density.

Optimized process parameters led to micronized powders with d_{50} (ranging from 3.7 µm to 4.8 µm) similar for all batches produced (Table 3), with no evident effect of solvent and leu content on the particles diameter.

Organic co-solvent had a massive effect on hygroscopicity too (Fig. 11). In particular, by adding 30% v/v of ISO into the aqueous feed, humidity uptake by G powders was reduced from 10.5% (water) to 4.8% (water/ISO) after exposure at room conditions. In the presence of 10% w/w leu, G lost its water avidity [0.9% weight gained after 80 min). These effects may be explained by the addition of the lower-soluble component (leu) into the liquid feeds, able to reach the critical concentration for shell formation as the droplet evaporation progresses during spray-drying process [50]. Such enrichment in leu at the particle surface seems to slow down water uptake of hygroscopic drug such as G, in agreement with previous observations [51] and, potentially, increase powder flowability.

Leu effect on spray-dried powders appears clearly, after microscopy studies, as an evident increase in particle corrugation. Morphology studies showed an increase in particle corrugation as an effect of leu presence in spray-dried powders. As an example, SEM pictures of particles dried from 8:2 water/ISO ratio solutions were reported in figure 12.

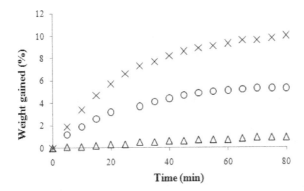

Figure 11. Weight gained after 80 min of exposure at room conditions by G raw material (cross), G spray-dried from 7:3 w water-ISO (circles) v/v systems, and G/10%leu spray-dried from water-ISO 7:3 v/v mixture (triangles).

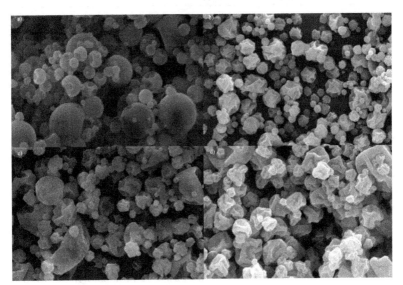

Figure 12. SEM pictures of powders dried from water/ISO 8:2 v/v systems containing: a) G; b) GISO2-leu5; c) GISO2-leu10; d) GISO2-leu5.

As well known, the morphology of spray-dried particles is strongly influenced by the solubility of the components and their initial saturation in the liquid feeds. G, freely soluble in water, led to the formation of spherical particles when spray dried alone (Fig. 12a, G). According to previous observations [52], during the co-spray drying process, the saturation of the lower-soluble component (leu) may increase faster than that of hydrophilic one (G), due to the preferential evaporation of alcohol and the associated change in the solvent/co-solvent ratio. This led to the formation of a primary solid shell which collapsed, hence corrugated microparticles were formed. As the relative amount of the less soluble component increased, particle corrugation was more and more evident; particles from almost spherical became raisins like (Fig. 12b, GISO2-leu5) or irregularly wrinkled (Fig.12d, GISO2-leu5). Such surface modification has been shown to be beneficial for particles intended for inhalation [29]: a corrugated surface improves powder dispersibility by minimizing contact areas and reducing interparticulate cohesion and, therefore, corrugated particles disperse better than spherical ones.

3.1.2. Aerodynamic behavior of G/leu powders

As aerodynamic properties, batches dried from water were hygroscopic, cohesive powders, difficult to insert into and come out from the capsule and with unsatisfying aerodynamic properties (data not shown). In particular, neat G dried from water was a cohesive and sticky material, unable to be aerosolized.

	Code #	Leu content (%w/w)	Charged Dose (mg)	ED (%)	FPF (%)	FPD (mg)
20% v/v ISO	GISO2	0	60	95.8±1.9	14.5±7.8	8.7±4.7
	GISO2-leu5	5	80	98.0±0.2	21.9±5.1	16.6±3.9
	GISO2-leu10	10	120	99.4±0.1	32.6±5.6	35.2±6.0
	GISO2-leu15	15	120	99.6±0.2	46.8±0.5	47.7±0.5
	GISO2-leu5	20	120	99.3±0.3	50.9±1.0	48.8± 0.9
30% v/vISO	GISO3	0	60	90.9±7.9	13.4±8.5	7.5±4.9
	GISO3-leu5	5	70	97.2±0.5	22.3±3.0	14.8±2.0
	GISO3-leu10	10	110	99.4±1.1	28.8±5.0	28.4± 5.0
	GISO3-leu15	15	120	99.1±0.3	49.4±0.8	50.4±0.8
	GISO3-leu20	20	120	99.2±0.0	50.2±1.0	48.2±0.9

ED, emitted dose; FPF, fine particle fraction; FPD, fine particle dose

Table 4. Aerodynamic properties of spray-dried powders after single stage glass impinger deposition experiments; device TURBOSPIN, charged with capsules type 2 (mean ± SD of three experiments).

G spray drying from hydroalcoholic solvent (GISO2 and GISO3) reduced powder cohesivity and enabled the aerosolization process; however, the resulting aerodynamic properties were still not satisfying (FPF less than 15%; Table 4). The inclusion of leu substantially increased emitted doses (ED up to 99.6% for #GISO2-leu15) and fine particle fractions (FPF up to 49.4% for #GISO3-leu15). Taking into account the relative reduction in drug content, further increase in the excipient/drug ratio up to 20/80 w/w did not improve DPI performance. The organic co-solvent led to the best

FPF and FPD values. As example, GISO3-leu15 formulations, containing 15% w/w of leu and obtained from 30% v/v of ISO/water feed, emitted 50.4 mg of fine G after one actuation of the Turbospin device. These results are in agreement with previous studies [29, 30, 53] evidencing the enhancement of powder aerosol performance as particle surface corrugation goes up to a certain degree; further corrugation enhancement did not improve aerodynamic properties. The plot in figure 13 allows to appreciate a dramatic increase in both particle corrugation (SEM micrographs) and FPF as the leu content increased.

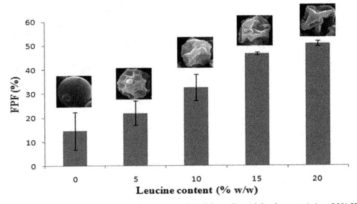

Figure 13. FPF and SEM images of G powders spray-dried from liquid feeds containing 20% ISO and increasing amount of leu.

MMAD, FPF and FPD values obtained by Andersen cascade impactor deposition studies (Table 5) confirmed the observed trend. Capsules charged with 120 mg of powder emitted almost the whole dose from the device after the pump actuation, as indicated by ED ≥ 99%. Among all formulations, GISO3-leu15 (G/15%leu from 30% v/v of ISO/water feed) showed very satisfying aerodynamic properties as proved by MMAD of 3.45 µm, FPF 58.1% and FPD of 56.4 mg (Table 5).

	Code #	ED (%)	MMAD (µm)	FPD (mg)	FPF (%)
20% v/v ISO	GISO2-leu15	99.7±0.3	4.0±0.1	49.3±1.7	46.0±2.7
	GISO2-leu5	99.6±0.4	4.2±0.1	39.3±0.3	42.5±0.2
30% v/v ISO	GISO3-leu15	99.2±0.3	3.4±0.2	56.4±1.1	58.1±3.6
	GISO3-leu20	99.2±0.2	3.3±0.1	54.7±2.2	58.0 ± 0.5

Table 5. Aerodynamic properties of G spray-dried powders containing 15 or 20% w/w leu after Andersen cascade impactor deposition experiments (mean ± SD)

3.1.3. Effect of G/leu powders on viability of cf airways epithelium

In order to establish whether the particle engineering has any cytotoxic or cytostatic effect on bronchial epithelial cells [31, 32], CuFi1 cells were treated for 24 h with increasing concentrations (from 0.0002 to 2 μM expressed as G content) of GISO3 or GISO-Leu15 powders in comparison to raw G. Results indicated that neither raw G nor its formulations generally inhibited cells viability as determined by MTT assay (Fig. 14 B). Only Raw G at concentrations higher than 0.02 μM showed a slight but significant decrease in cell survival. An interesting observation is that an increase in leu content up to 15%, as in GISO3-leu15 , faintly but not significantly decreased CuFi1 viability at concentration ranging from 0.02 to 0.2 μM (P<0.05) (Fig. 13 B) whereas at 2.0 μM did not. As previously oserved in formulations for inhalation containing leucine [27], this effect seems to be related to leu ability to improve cell proliferation and metabolism of bronchial epithelial CF cells.

Furthermore ELISA BrdU immunoassay confirmed that raw G slightly reduced CF cell growth only at the highest concentration [2 μM, P<0.01] (Fig. 14 A).

Therefore, G/leu systems had no cytotoxic or cytostatic effect on CF epithelial lung cells (CuFi1 model), at concentrations up to 2 μM.

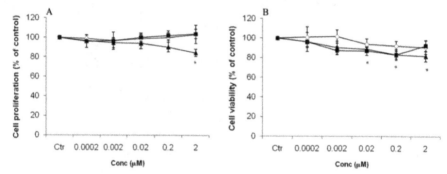

Figure 14. Effect of Gentamicin and its DPI formulations on CuFi1 cell proliferation and viability. Cells were treated for 24 h with: raw Gentamicin (rawG, ▲), spray-dried Gentamicin (GISO3 ◊) and G co-sprayed with 15%w/w leucine (GISO3-leu15 ■) at concentrations from 0.0002 μM to 2 μM. Cell growth (A) was determined using a colorimetric bromodeoxyuridine (BrdU) cell proliferation ELISA kit. Cell viability (B) was determined by MTT assay. All data are shown as mean ± SD of three independent experiments, each done in duplicate (*P<0.05 and **P<0.01 vs control).

An proper engineering process, use of hydro-alcoholic feeds and the AA addition, allow the preparation of micronized powders able to be aerosolized. The addition of small amount of the AA led to the production of dry formulations with excellent emitted dose and good aerodynamic properties after actuation of the Turbospin device. Finally, the engineered particles showed no cytotoxic or cytostatic effect on bronchial epithelial cells bearing a CFTR F508/F508 mutant genotype.

4. Conclusions

The engineering process by spray drying and the use of water-co-solvent systems as liquid feed allowed micronized powders to be produced with high yield, starting from Naringin or Gentamicin sulfate, drugs with different physicochemical properties. The addition of a small amount of a safe excipient, as leucine, led to powders with excellent emission doses, counteracting both G high hygroscopicity and N cohesiveness and low solubility. In particular, N DPI containing 5% leu (NET3-leu5) and G DPI containing 15% leu (GISO3-leu15) were able to deliver almost the total dose of drug loaded in the capsules, with about 60% of FPF. Finally, N and G engineered powders showed no cytotoxic or cytostatic effect on bronchial epithelial cells bearing a CFTR F508/F508 mutant genotype. As to efficacy, NET3-leu5 powder, containing natural polyphenol and AA, were able to negatively modulate NF-κB pathways in absence of stimulation in bronchial epithelia and to reduce the overexpressed IL-8 and IL-6 production both in basically and in LPS-stimulated conditions. These findings, together with the well-known G antibiotic activity support the use of G-leu and N-leu DPIs in the treatment of infections and intrinsic inflammation of CF lungs.

Author details

Paola Russo, Antonietta Santoro, Lucia Prota, Mariateresa Stigliani and Rita P. Aquino*

Department of Pharmaceutical and Biomedical Sciences, University of Salerno, Fisciano, Italy

5. References

[1] Cheng SH, Gregory RJ, Marshall J, Paul S, Souza DW, White GA, et al. Defective intracellular transport and processing of CFTR is the molecular basis of most cystic fibrosis. Cell. 1990;63(4):827-34. Epub 1990/11/16.

[2] Collins FS, Riordan JR, Tsui LC. The cystic fibrosis gene: isolation and significance. Hosp Pract (Off Ed). 1990;25(10):47-57. Epub 1990/10/15.

[3] Schwiebert EM, Egan ME, Hwang TH, Fulmer SB, Allen SS, Cutting GR, et al. CFTR regulates outwardly rectifying chloride channels through an autocrine mechanism involving ATP. Cell. 1995;81(7):1063-73. Epub 1995/06/30.

[4] Vankeerberghen A, Cuppens H, Cassiman JJ. The cystic fibrosis transmembrane conductance regulator: an intriguing protein with pleiotropic functions. J Cyst Fibros. 2002;1(1):13-29. Epub 2004/10/07.

[5] Mehta A. CFTR: more than just a chloride channel. Pediatr Pulmonol. 2005;39(4):292-8. Epub 2004/12/02.

[6] Quinton PM. Cystic fibrosis: impaired bicarbonate secretion and mucoviscidosis. Lancet. 2008;372(9636):415-7. Epub 2008/08/05.

[7] Mukhopadhyay S, Singh M, Cater JI, Ogston S, Franklin M, Olver RE. Nebulised antipseudomonal antibiotic therapy in cystic fibrosis: a meta-analysis of benefits and risks. Thorax. 1996;51(4):364-8. Epub 1996/04/01.

[8] Ramsey BW, Pepe MS, Quan JM, Otto KL, Montgomery AB, Williams-Warren J, et al. Intermittent administration of inhaled tobramycin in patients with cystic fibrosis. Cystic Fibrosis Inhaled Tobramycin Study Group. N Engl J Med. 1999;340(1):23-30. Epub 1999/01/08.

---

* Corresponding Author

[9] Doring G, Hoiby N. Early intervention and prevention of lung disease in cystic fibrosis: a European consensus. J Cyst Fibros. 2004;3(2):67-91. Epub 2004/10/07.

[10] Konstan MW, Hilliard KA, Norvell TM, Berger M. Bronchoalveolar lavage findings in cystic fibrosis patients with stable, clinically mild lung disease suggest ongoing infection and inflammation. Am J Respir Crit Care Med. 1994;150(2):448-54. Epub 1994/08/01.

[11] Rahman I, Biswas SK, Kode A. Oxidant and antioxidant balance in the airways and airway diseases. Eur J Pharmacol. 2006;533(1-3):222-39. Epub 2006/02/28.

[12] Brown RK, McBurney A, Lunec J, Kelly FJ. Oxidative damage to DNA in patients with cystic fibrosis. Free Radic Biol Med. 1995;18(4):801-6. Epub 1995/04/01.

[13] Cantin AM, White TB, Cross CE, Forman HJ, Sokol RJ, Borowitz D. Antioxidants in cystic fibrosis. Conclusions from the CF antioxidant workshop, Bethesda, Maryland, November 11-12, 2003. Free Radic Biol Med. 2007;42(1):15-31. Epub 2006/12/13.

[14] Starosta V, Griese M. Oxidative damage to surfactant protein D in pulmonary diseases. Free Radic Res. 2006;40(4):419-25. Epub 2006/03/07.

[15] Boncoeur E, Criq VS, Bonvin E, Roque T, Henrion-Caude A, Gruenert DC, et al. Oxidative stress induces extracellular signal-regulated kinase 1/2 mitogen-activated protein kinase in cystic fibrosis lung epithelial cells: Potential mechanism for excessive IL-8 expression. Int J Biochem Cell Biol. 2008;40(3):432-46. Epub 2007/10/16.

[16] Kumar P, Khanna M, Srivastava V, Tyagi YK, Raj HG, Ravi K. Effect of quercetin supplementation on lung antioxidants after experimental influenza virus infection. Exp Lung Res. 2005;31(5):449-59. Epub 2005/07/16.

[17] Kumar P, Sharma S, Khanna M, Raj HG. Effect of Quercetin on lipid peroxidation and changes in lung morphology in experimental influenza virus infection. Int J Exp Pathol. 2003;84(3):127-33. Epub 2003/09/17.

[18] Limasset B, le Doucen C, Dore JC, Ojasoo T, Damon M, Crastes de Paulet A. Effects of flavonoids on the release of reactive oxygen species by stimulated human neutrophils. Multivariate analysis of structure-activity relationships (SAR). Biochem Pharmacol. 1993;46(7):1257-71. Epub 1993/10/05.

[19] Springsteel MF, Galietta LJ, Ma T, By K, Berger GO, Yang H, et al. Benzoflavone activators of the cystic fibrosis transmembrane conductance regulator: towards a pharmacophore model for the nucleotide-binding domain. Bioorg Med Chem. 2003;11(18):4113-20. Epub 2003/08/21.

[20] Pyle LC, Fulton JC, Sloane PA, Backer K, Mazur M, Prasain J, et al. Activation of the cystic fibrosis transmembrane conductance regulator by the flavonoid quercetin: potential use as a biomarker of DeltaF508 cystic fibrosis transmembrane conductance regulator rescue. Am J Respir Cell Mol Biol. 2010;43(5):607-16. Epub 2010/01/01.

[21] Virgin F, Zhang S, Schuster D, Azbell C, Fortenberry J, Sorscher EJ, et al. The bioflavonoid compound, sinupret, stimulates transepithelial chloride transport in vitro and in vivo. Laryngoscope. 2010;120(5):1051-6. Epub 2010/04/28.

[22] Kunzelmann K, Schreiber R, Boucherot A. Mechanisms of the inhibition of epithelial Na(+) channels by CFTR and purinergic stimulation. Kidney Int. 2001;60(2):455-61. Epub 2001/07/28.

[23] Lauro MR, Torre ML, Maggi L, De Simone F, Conte U, Aquino RP. Fast- and slow-release tablets for oral administration of flavonoids: rutin and quercetin. Drug Dev Ind Pharm. 2002;28(4):371-9. Epub 2002/06/12.

[24] Lauro MR, Torre ML, De Simone F, Conte U, Aquino RP. Tablet formulation for the fast and sustained-release of flavonoids: naringin and naringenin. STP Pharma Sciences. 2001;11:265-9.

[25] Lauro MR, De Simone F, Sansone F, Iannelli P, Aquino RP. Preparations and release characteristics of Naringin and Naringenin gastro-resistant microparticles by spray-drying. J Drug Del Sci Tech. 2007;17:119-24.

[26] Lauro MR, Maggi L, Conte U, De Simone F, Aquino RP. Rutin and Quercetin gastro-resistant microparticles obtained by spray-drying technique. J Drug Del Sci Tech. 2005;15:363-9.

[27] Prota L, Santoro A, Bifulco M, Aquino RP, Mencherini T, Russo P. Leucine enhances aerosol performance of naringin dry powder and its activity on cystic fibrosis airway epithelial cells. International journal of pharmaceutics. 2011;412(1-2):8-19. Epub 2011/04/05.

[28] Sansone F, Aquino RP, Del Gaudio P, Colombo P, Russo P. Physical characteristics and aerosol performance of naringin dry powders for pulmonary delivery prepared by spray-drying. European journal of pharmaceutics and biopharmaceutics : official journal of Arbeitsgemeinschaft fur Pharmazeutische Verfahrenstechnik eV. 2009;72(1):206-13. Epub 2008/11/11.

[29] Chew NY, Chan HK. Use of solid corrugated particles to enhance powder aerosol performance. Pharm Res. 2001;18(11):1570-7. Epub 2002/01/05.

[30] Chew NY, Tang P, Chan HK, Raper JA. How much particle surface corrugation is sufficient to improve aerosol performance of powders? Pharm Res. 2005;22(1):148-52. Epub 2005/03/18.

[31] Dechecchi MC, Nicolis E, Norez C, Bezzerri V, Borgatti M, Mancini I, et al. Anti-inflammatory effect of miglustat in bronchial epithelial cells. J Cyst Fibros. 2008;7(6):555-65. Epub 2008/09/26.

[32] Zabner J, Karp P, Seiler M, Phillips SL, Mitchell CJ, Saavedra M, et al. Development of cystic fibrosis and noncystic fibrosis airway cell lines. Am J Physiol Lung Cell Mol Physiol. 2003;284(5):L844-54. Epub 2003/04/05.

[33] Holt TL, Ward LC, Francis PJ, Isles A, Cooksley WG, Shepherd RW. Whole body protein turnover in malnourished cystic fibrosis patients and its relationship to pulmonary disease. Am J Clin Nutr. 1985;41(5):1061-6. Epub 1985/05/01.

[34] Levy LD, Durie PR, Pencharz PB, Corey ML. Effects of long-term nutritional rehabilitation on body composition and clinical status in malnourished children and adolescents with cystic fibrosis. J Pediatr. 1985;107(2):225-30. Epub 1985/08/01.

[35] Switzer M, Rice J, Rice M, Hardin DS. Insulin-like growth factor-I levels predict weight, height and protein catabolism in children and adolescents with cystic fibrosis. J Pediatr Endocrinol Metab. 2009;22(5):417-24. Epub 2009/07/22.

[36] Yamamoto Y, Gaynor RB. Role of the NF-kappaB pathway in the pathogenesis of human disease states. Curr Mol Med. 2001;1(3):287-96. Epub 2002/03/20.

[37] Hayden MS, Ghosh S. Signaling to NF-kappaB. Genes Dev. 2004;18(18):2195-224. Epub 2004/09/17.

[38] Lyczak JB, Cannon CL, Pier GB. Lung infections associated with cystic fibrosis. Clin Microbiol Rev. 2002;15(2):194-222. Epub 2002/04/05.

[39] Rottner M, Kunzelmann C, Mergey M, Freyssinet JM, Martinez MC. Exaggerated apoptosis and NF-kappaB activation in pancreatic and tracheal cystic fibrosis cells. FASEB J. 2007;21(11):2939-48. Epub 2007/04/20.

[40] Verhaeghe C, Remouchamps C, Hennuy B, Vanderplasschen A, Chariot A, Tabruyn SP, et al. Role of IKK and ERK pathways in intrinsic inflammation of cystic fibrosis airways. Biochem Pharmacol. 2007;73(12):1982-94. Epub 2007/05/01.

[41] Descargues P, Sil AK, Karin M. IKKalpha, a critical regulator of epidermal differentiation and a suppressor of skin cancer. EMBO J. 2008;27(20):2639-47. Epub 2008/09/27.

[42] John G, Yildirim AO, Rubin BK, Gruenert DC, Henke MO. TLR-4-mediated innate immunity is reduced in cystic fibrosis airway cells. Am J Respir Cell Mol Biol. 2010;42(4):424-31. Epub 2009/06/09.

[43] Prayle A, Smyth AR. Aminoglycoside use in cystic fibrosis: therapeutic strategies and toxicity. Curr Opin Pulm Med. 2010;16(6):604-10. Epub 2010/09/04.

[44] Clancy JP, Bebok Z, Ruiz F, King C, Jones J, Walker L, et al. Evidence that systemic gentamicin suppresses premature stop mutations in patients with cystic fibrosis. Am J Respir Crit Care Med. 2001;163(7):1683-92. Epub 2001/06/13.

[45] Du M, Jones JR, Lanier J, Keeling KM, Lindsey JR, Tousson A, et al. Aminoglycoside suppression of a premature stop mutation in a Cftr-/- mouse carrying a human CFTR-G542X transgene. J Mol Med (Berl). 2002;80(9):595-604. Epub 2002/09/13.

[46] Wilschanski M, Yahav Y, Yaacov Y, Blau H, Bentur L, Rivlin J, et al. Gentamicin-induced correction of CFTR function in patients with cystic fibrosis and CFTR stop mutations. N Engl J Med. 2003;349(15):1433-41. Epub 2003/10/10.

[47] Wilschanski M, Famini C, Blau H, Rivlin J, Augarten A, Avital A, et al. A pilot study of the effect of gentamicin on nasal potential difference measurements in cystic fibrosis patients carrying stop mutations. Am J Respir Crit Care Med. 2000;161(3 Pt 1):860-5. Epub 2000/03/11.

[48] Mendelman PM, Smith AL, Levy J, Weber A, Ramsey B, Davis RL. Aminoglycoside penetration, inactivation, and efficacy in cystic fibrosis sputum. Am Rev Respir Dis. 1985;132(4):761-5. Epub 1985/10/01.

[49] Li HY, Seville PC, Williamson IJ, Birchall JC. The use of amino acids to enhance the aerosolisation of spray-dried powders for pulmonary gene therapy. J Gene Med. 2005;7(3):343-53. Epub 2004/10/30.

[50] Vehring R. Pharmaceutical particle engineering via spray drying. Pharm Res. 2008;25(5):999-1022. Epub 2007/11/28.

[51] Shur J, Nevell TG, Ewen RJ, Price R, Smith A, Barbu E, et al. Cospray-dried unfractionated heparin with L-leucine as a dry powder inhaler mucolytic for cystic fibrosis therapy. J Pharm Sci. 2008;97(11):4857-68. Epub 2008/03/21.

[52] Lechuga-Ballesteros D, Charan C, Stults CL, Stevenson CL, Miller DP, Vehring R, et al. Trileucine improves aerosol performance and stability of spray-dried powders for inhalation. J Pharm Sci. 2008;97(1):287-302. Epub 2007/09/08.

[53] Weiler C, Egen M, Trunk M, Langguth P. Force control and powder dispersibility of spray dried particles for inhalation. J Pharm Sci.99(1):303-16. Epub 2009/06/18.

Chapter 2

The Role of Carrier in Dry Powder Inhaler

Hamed Hamishehkar, Yahya Rahimpour and Yousef Javadzadeh

Additional information is available at the end of the chapter

1. Introduction

Increasing prevalence of pulmonary diseases with high mortality and morbidity such as chronic obstructive pulmonary disease (COPD), asthma, cystic fibrosis, infectious diseases, tuberculosis and lung cancer, makes pulmonary drug delivery as a non-invasive and attractive approach for the local drug administration and treatment of these pathologies (Marianecci et al., 2011). In this case, lower dosages than by the oral route can be used with comparable effectiveness which will reduce unwanted side effects (Timsina et al., 1994).The lung also provides a non-invasive route of delivery for the systemic circulation, due to its unique characteristics such as large surface area, thin epithelial barrier and high blood flow. Lack of first pass metabolism and less enzymatic activity make pulmonary delivery as an ideal administration route for extensively degraded drugs following oral delivery and for macromolecules, such as proteins and peptides, respectively(Hamishehkar et al., 2010; Rytting et al., 2008; Sakagami, 2006). Following approving the first inhaled therapeutic macromolecule for systemic delivery, human insulin (Exubera™) by the Food and Drug Administration (FDA) and the European Agency for the Evaluation of Medicinal Products in 2006, the scientific community look for other candidates that would benefit from pulmonary delivery for systemic action (Patton et al., 2004; Furness, 2005). In contrast to injection therapy, inhalation therapy is not associated with pain and this should increase patient comfort and compliance, causing improved treatment outcome (Laube, 2005). Drug deposition in the lung is mainly controlled by its aerodynamic diameter (Wolff et al., 1993). Particles larger than 5 μm are mostly trapped by oropharyngeal deposition and incapable of reaching the lungs while smaller than 1 μm are mostly exhaled without deposition (Sakagami, 2006). Particles with aerodynamic diameters between 1 and 5 μm are expected to efficiently deposit in the lung periphery (Heyder et al., 1986). The effective inhalation performance of dry-powder products is dependent on the drug formulation and the inhaler device. Dry powder formulations are usually prepared by mixing the micronized drug particles with larger carrier particles. The aerosolization efficiency of a powder is highly dependent on the carrier characteristics, such as particle size distribution, shape and surface properties. The main objective in the inhalation field is to achieve reproducible, high pulmonary deposition. This could be achieved by successful carrier selection and careful process optimization (Pilcer et al., 2012). Therefore, the purpose of this chapter is to review the used carriers in inhalable formulations, their production and the impact of the physicochemical properties of carriers on carrier-drug dispersion is discussed in detail. This chapter offers a perspective on current reported studies to modify carrier for its better performance. Several methodologies have been discussed.

2. Dry powder inhalers

Pressurized metered-dose inhaler (MDI), nebulizer and dry powder inhaler (DPI) are main delivery systems in pulmonary delivery (Timsina et al., 1994). Among these, DPI appears to be the most promising for future use (Todo et al., 2001).They are propellant-free, portable, easy to operate and low-cost devices with improved stability of the formulation as a result of the dry state(Carpenter et al., 1997; Prime et al., 1997).Spinhaler®, the first dry powder inhaler, came into the market in 1970 and since then a new are started in the subject of pulmonary drug delivery. Dry powder inhalers and dry powder inhalation technology became the second most frequently used inhalation devices for pulmonary drug administration after Montreal Protocol in 1987 in limitation of using CFC in products. Dry powder inhalers have even become the first choice of inhalation devices in European countries (Marriott et al., 2012).They are a widely accepted inhaled delivery dosage form where they are currently used by an estimated 40% of patients to treat asthma and chronic obstructive pulmonary disease (Atkins, 2005). Using the DPI system, respiratory delivery of potent drugs such as insulin (Edwards et al., 1997), antibiotics (Geller et al., 2007; Hickey et al., 2006), drugs for neurological disorders like Parkinson's disease(Stoessl, 2008), antituberculosis (Anon, 2008), antihypertensive nifedipine(Plumley et al., 2009), anticoagulant heparin (Rawat et al., 2008),drugs for sexual dysfunction (Cheatham et al., 2006), opioids and fentanyl for cancer pain (Farr et al., 2006; Kleinstreuer et al., 2008; Fleischer et al., 2005) and delivery of atropine sulphate nanoparticle as an antidote for organophosphorus poisoning with better bioavailability (Ali et al., 2009) have been studied. DPI formulations of measles vaccine (LiCalsi et al., 2001), mucosal vaccination for influenza virus (Edwards et al., 2005), have all been studied with considerable achievement. DPIs have to overcome various physical difficulties for effective drug delivery either local or systemic purposes (Prime et al., 1997). First, small size of inhalable particles subjected them to forces of agglomeration and cohesion, resulting in poor flow and non-uniform dispersion (Crowder et al., 2002).

3. The role of carrier on DPI performance

DPI is generally formulated as a powder mixture of coarse carrier particles and micronized drug particles with aerodynamic particle diameters of 1–5 μm (Iida et al., 2003). Carrier particles are used to improve drug particle flowability, thus improving dosing accuracy and minimizing the dose variability observed with drug formulations alone while making them easier to handle during manufacturing operations (Timsina et al., 1994; Schiavone et al., 2004). With the use of carrier particles, drug particles are emitted from capsules and devices more readily, hence, the inhalation efficiency increases (Iida et al., 2001). Moreover, usually no more than a few milligrammes of a drug needs to be delivered (e.g., between 20 µg and 500 µg of corticosteroids for asthma therapy), and thus carrier provides bulk, which improves the handling, dispensing, and metering of the drug (Pilcer et al., 2012). The presence of the carrier material is the taste/sensation on inhaling, which can assure the patient that a dose has been taken (Prime et al., 1997).Consequently, the carrier forms an important component of the formulation and any change in the physico-chemical properties of the carrier particles has the potential to alter the drug deposition profile (Zeng et al., 2000). Therefore, the design of the carrier particle is important for the development of dry powder inhalations (Hamishehkar et al., 2010). Carrier particles should have several characteristics such as physico-chemical stability, biocompatibility and biodegradability, compatible with the drug substance and must be inert, available and economical. During insufflation, the drug particles are detached from the surface of the carrier particles by the energy of the inspired air flow that overcomes the adhesion forces between drug and carrier. The larger carrier particles impact in the upper airways, while the small drug particles go through the lower parts of lungs (Pilcer et al., 2012). Unsatisfactory detachment of drug from the carrier due to strong inter-particulate forces may be one of the main reasons of inefficient drug delivery encountered with most DPIs (Zeng et al., 2000; Zhou et al., 2011). Therefore, in the best case, the adjusted balance between adhesive and cohesive forces provides enough adhesion between drug and carrier to produce a stable formulation (homogeneous mixture with no powder segregation and proper content uniformity) yet allows for easy separation during inhalation. Consequently, it has been stated that the efficiency of a DPI formulation is extremely dependent on the carrier characteristics and the selection of carrier is a crucial determinant of the overall DPI performance (Pilcer et al., 2012). Obviously, the effect of the carrier material on DPI formulation should be carefully evaluated. The range of materials which can be proposed to be as carriers in inhaled products are restricted for toxicological reasons. Lactose and other sugars have been studied and used, therefore modifications to these materials may allow further formulation optimization (Prime et al., 1997).

4. Inhaler testing equipments

Cascade impactors operate on the base of inertial impaction. Each stage of the impactor contains a single or series of nozzles or jets through which the sample laden air is drawn directing any airborne particles towards the surface of the collection plate for that particular stage. Whether a particular particle impacts on that stage is dependent on its aerodynamic diameter. Particles having sufficient inertia will impact on that particular stage collection plate whilst smaller particles with insufficient inertia will remain entrained in the air stream and pass to the next stage where the process is repeated. The stages are normally assembled in a stack in order of decreasing particle size. As the jets get smaller, the air velocity increases and finer particles are collected. Any remaining particles are collected on an after filter (or by a –Micro-Orifice Collector). The term 'Impactor' is generally used for an instrument where the particles 'impact' on a dry impaction plate or cup. If the collection surface is liquid, as in the case of the Multi-Stage Liquid Impinger (MSLI), then the term 'impinger' is used. The general principles of inertial impaction apply to both 'impactors' and 'impingers'. The US and European Pharmacopoeia list no less than five different cascade impactors/impingers suitable for the aerodynamic assessment of fine particles. However, only the Andersen Cascade Impactor (ACI), the Next Generation Impactor (NGI) and the Multi-Stage Liquid Impinger (MSLI) appear in both pharmacopoeia. In research applications, in vitro/in vivo correlation and bioequivalence may be important and so detailed particle size data may be required. In routine quality control, where the concern is batch-to-batch variation a coarser test may be acceptable. The Glass Twin Impinger, for example has been retained as Apparatus A in the European Pharmacopoeia, because of its value as a simple and inexpensive quality control tool. In general however, it is accepted that an Impactor/impinger should have a minimum of five stages and preferably more, if it is to provide detailed particle size distribution data. The aerodynamic particle size distribution of the drug leaving an inhaler device can define the manner in which an aerosol deposits in the respiratory tract during inhalation. This characteristic of the aerosol is often used in judging inhaler performance and is particularly relevant in the development of inhalation formulations during research, production, quality assurance and equivalency testing. The results of characterizations using cascade impaction techniques are additionally used for the determination of fine particle fraction or fine particle dose which may be correlated to the dose or fraction of the drug that penetrates to the lung during inhalation by a patient. Dry Powder Inhaler (DPI) testing could require added options for preventing stage overloading and necessary to achieve the specified pressure drop through the device. Upper stage mass overloading can be prevented with the addition of a high capacity preseparator or pre-collector. The feature traps non-inhalable aerosols. To achieve the proper pressure drop of 4 kPa (40.8 cm water) in the inhaler, a higher vacuum flow rate at 60 or 90 L/minute may be needed.Impactors/impingers are specifically designed to meet the highest criteria laid down in the various Pharmacopoeia (e.g. United States Pharmacopeia Chapter <601>; European Pharmacopoeia Chapter 29.9.18 for characterizing aerosol clouds emitted by inhalers). By analyzing the drug deposited on the individual stages and the final filter, the Fine Particle Fraction (FPF), the Fine Particle Dose (FPD), the Mass Median Aerodynamic Diameter (MMAD) and Geometric Standard Deviation (GSD) can all be calculated (The Copley Scientific Limited, 2010).

5. Expressions used to define drug lung deposition

The American and European pharmacopoeias have explained methods based on inertial impaction to assess the in vitro inhalation performance of formulations by determination of the fine particles (Pilcer et al., 2012).

5.1. Fine Particle Dose (FPD) and fine particle fraction (FPF)

The aerodynamic evaluation methods of fine particles permit the determination of the fine-particle dose (FPD), which corresponds to the mass of drug particles that have an aerodynamic diameter less than 5 μm. Such particles can theoretically be deposited in the deep lung after inhalation. The fine-particle fraction (FPF), which is the percentage of the

FPD usually related to either the nominal dose (total drug mass contained in the device) or the recovered drug (sum of the drug collected in the device and in the different parts of the impingers or impactors after inhalation) (Pilcer et al., 2012).

5.2. Emitted dose

The emitted dose expresses the drug mass exiting the device after inhalation. In some cases, FPF can be calculated from emitted dose instead of total or recovered dose of drug from impingers or impactors. The ability of the powder to be fluidised by the airflow through an inhaler is usually indicated by the emission dose, whilst the FPD and FPF measure the capability of the formulation to be fluidised and deagglomerated in time to release the drug from the carrier to be deposited in the appropriate level of the impactors and impingers (Pilcer et al., 2012).

5.3. Dispersibility

The dispersibility is calculated as the ratio of FPD to emitted dose (Zeng et al., 2000).

5.4. Mass median aerodynamic diameter (MMAD)

Mass median diameter of an aerosol means the particle diameter that has 50% of the aerosol mass residing above and 50% of its mass below it. The concept of aerodynamic diameter is central to any aerosol measurements and respiratory drug delivery. The aerodynamic diameter relates the particle to the diameter of a sphere of unit density that has the same settling velocity as the particle of interest regardless of its shape or density. The mass–mean aerodynamic diameter (MMAD) is read from the cumulative distribution curve at the 50% point (Labiris et al., 2003).The theoretical mass–mean aerodynamic diameter (d_{aero}) was determined from the geometric particle size and tap density using the following relationship:

$$d_{aero} = d_{geo} \left[\frac{(\rho / \rho_{ref})^{0.5}}{\gamma} \right]$$

Where d_{geo}=geometric diameter, γ=shape factor (for a spherical particle, $\gamma=1$), ϱ=particle bulk density and ϱ_{ref}=water mass density (1 g/cm^3). Tapped density measurements underestimate particle bulk densities since the volume of particles measured includes the interstitial space between the particles. The true particle density, and the aerodynamic diameter of a given powder, is expected to be slightly larger than reported (El-Gendy et al., 2009).

5.5. Geometric standard deviation (GSD)

The degree of dispersity is an important consideration for both quality and efficacy of pharmaceutical aerosols (Chew et al., 2002). The nature of the aerosol distribution must be established accurately if its implications for deposition and efficacy are to be understood

(Telko et al., 2005). The degree of dispersion in a lognormally distributed aerosol is characterized by the geometric standard deviation (GSD). A larger GSD implies a longer large particle size tail in the distribution(Musante et al., 2002). GSD for a well-functioning stage should ideally be less than 1.2 (the GSD for an ideal size fractionators would be 1.0 and indicates a monodisperse aerosol) (Marple et al., 2003). GSD is a measure of the variability of the particle diameters within the aerosol and is calculated from the ratio of the particle diameter at the 84.1% point on the cumulative distribution curve to the MMAD. For a log-normal distribution, the GSD is the same for the number, surface area or mass distributions (Labiris et al., 2003). The GSD was determined as

$$GSD = \sqrt{\frac{sizes\ X}{sizes\ Y}}$$

where sizes X and Y are particle sizes for which the line crosses the 84% and 16% mark, respectively (Emami et al., 2009).Mostly, particle size distributions are log-normal, for which type of distributions the geometric mean diameter (GMD) and GSD are frequently used as the characteristic parameters. Aerosols from dry powder inhalers are not log-normal however, because they are nearly always a mixture of primary and secondary particles. Agglomerates in the aerosol are the reason for a tail-off at the side of the larger diameters. Therefore, the mass median diameter is a better parameter, although the size fraction for which mass median diameter is calculated should be defined also. For inhalation drugs, the mass median aerodynamic diameter (MMAD) is the most frequently used parameter(Bosquillon et al., 2001).

6. Carrier qualifications for application in DPIs

6.1. Carrier size

Different and controversy reports have been published about the suitable carrier size for inhalation purposes. Some previous studies have reported improvements in the amount of respirable drug delivered from a DPI by way of reducing the particle size of the carrier (Steckel et al., 1997; Gilani et al., 2004; Louey et al., 2003). For example, increased respirable fraction of salbutamol sulphate (Kassem et al., 1989; Zeng et al., 2000), terbutaline (Kassem et al., 1989), disodium chromoglycate(Braun et al., 1996) and budesonide (Steckel et al., 1997) were concluded with decreased carrier size. It was proposed that smaller agglomerates meet more forceful shear in the turbulent airstreams causing more effective deagglomeration (Islama et al., 2012). However, the use of too small a carrier will result in poor flow properties of the powder, which is one of the primary reasons for incorporating a coarse carrier within the formulation (Zeng et al., 2001).On the other hand, it was reported that larger carrier particles, normally exhibit larger surface discontinuities than fine crystals (De Boer et al., 2003). This may have the advantage of providing shelter to drug particles from the press-on forces during mixing, as the drug particles tend to assemble in these discontinuities during mixing (Iida et al., 2003; De Boer et al., 2005). Therefore, a high carrier particle size does not necessarily have a negative effect on the drug deposition profiles after inhalation (Hamishehkar et al., 2010). In a study, formulations of respirable recombinant human granulocyte-colony stimulating factor with larger carriers (90–125 µm) showed a higher drug dispersion than the same formulation with 38–75 µm carriers, and it is interpreted that this is due to the lower inter-particle forces among the larger sized particles (French et al., 1996). Similar results was shown for enhanced inhalation performance of terbutaline sulphate from a formulation containing coarse lactose (53–105 µm) than the same drug containing fine lactose carriers with size less than 53 µm (Byron et al., 1990). Recently, an increase in carrier size resulted better aerosolisation behavior of insulin loaded PLGA microparticles mixed with mannitol carrier. The authors conclude that the use of larger particles of mannitol carrier with a lower carrier/microcapsule ratio leads to higher dispersion of the drug due to increase flowability (Hamishehkar et al., 2010).

6.2. Carrier shape

Although the influence of carrier particle shape on the drug dispersibility from the DPI formulation is not well recognized but it is known that the attractive forces between drug and carrier particles can be shape dependent (Mullins et al., 1992; Crowder et al., 2001). In fact most commonly used particles for DPI formulations have irregular shapes. In vitro inhalation studies have indicated that elongated (Larhrib et al., 2003; Zeng et al., 2000), needle-like (Ikegami et al., 2002), porous and wrinkled particles (Chew et al., 2005)have improved lung deposition properties of various formulations. Increasing the elongation ratio of the lactose carrier particles also appeared to increase the FPF of salbutamol sulphate (Zeng et al., 2000).Recently, it was reported pollen-shaped hydroxyapatite carrier increased dispersibility of budesonide particles due to reduction in particle interactions (Hassan et al., 2010; 2010). Definitely surface shape effects agglomeration strength but it was also discussed that the aerodynamic diameter of the agglomerates can be changed by shape factor. Because of their larger shape factor, elongated particles have a smaller aerodynamic diameter than spherical particles and thus agglomerations of active drug particles and elongated carriers remain aerosolized for a longer time, and greater distance along the inhalation path, then deagglomeration is enhanced (Islama et al., 2012). The figure 1 shows the presence of loose agglomerates in freeze dried mannitol samples adapted from reference (Hamishehkar et al., 2010), applied mannitol particles in different shapes for formulation of DPI form of insulin-loaded biodegradable polymeric microparticles. Spray dried and freeze dried mannitol, both showed smooth surfaces while formulation composed of freeze dried mannitol showed higher FPF and emitted dose than spray dried mannitol. This was interesting when it was found that spray dried mannitol had lower true density than freeze dried mannitol, possible resulting in better emitted dose and consequently improved FPF. This aerosolization behavior of freeze dried mannitol can be attributed to its needle shape particle morphology. Spatial hindering effect of rod shape particles can lead their easier aerosolization, and hence higher emission and higher FPF. The results of FPF and emitted dose for different formulations can partially be explained by elongation ratio and shape factors reported in this article. Freeze dried mannitol had higher elongation ratio and lower shape factor than spray dried mannitol which indicates more irregular shape. In vitro inhalation studies have indicated that elongated, fibrous particles improve lung deposition properties (Chan et al., 1989; Fults et al., 1997).

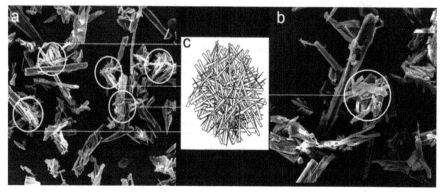

Figure 1. Scanning electron micrographs of freeze-dried mannitol (FDM) (a, b) and schematic image of formed loose agglomerates of needle shape FDM particles (c) adapted from reference (Hamishehkar et al., 2010)

6.3. Carrier surface

The in vitro inhalation properties of DPI are reported to be related to the surface properties of the carrier particles (Zeng et al., 2000; Heng et al., 2000; Iida et al., 2001; 2003). Surface morphology has been demonstrated to directly influence the contact area between drug particle and carrier, leading to variations in interparticulate adhesion. Several studies have reported that variations in contact area, as a result of differing surface structure, could potentially compromise the aerosolization performance of the drug particles (Zeng et al., 2000; Flament et al., 2004; Young et al., 2002). Some surface modifications of carrier particles have been reported to improve inhalation performance of DPI (Kawashima et al., 1998; Chan et al., 2003). Previous investigations reported that the carrier surface morphology directly affected the aerosolization efficiency from a DPI (Podczeck, 1998; Larhrib et al., 1999). In general terms, a decrease in roughness is believed to improve aerosolization efficiency of a drug-carrier blend (Ganderton et al., 1992; Kawashima et al., 1998; Zeng et al., 2001). However, it was shown that coarse carrier particles which normally exhibit large surface discontinuities may provide shelter to drug particles from the press-on forces during mixing, as the drug particles tend to assemble in these discontinuities during mixing (Iida et al., 2003). Therefore, high carrier rugosity drug-to-carrier interaction (Kawashima et al., 1998; Podczeck, 1998; Zeng et al., 2000). These interaction forces have to be strong enough to guarantee good mixture stability during handling and proper drug deaggregation does not necessarily have a negative effect on the drug detachment from carrier crystals during inhalation, providing that inertial detachment forces are applied. Chan et al. also reported that a positive linear trend was established between the roughness of the lactose surface and the FPF and dispersibility of the drug (Chan et al., 2003). Therefore, an important balance between the surface morphologies of both the drug and carrier can exist (Young et al., 2002). It was shown by Heng et al. that an optimum lactose surface roughness (Ra) was required for an increased fine particle fraction of salbutamol sulphate (Heng et al., 2000). All these studies demonstrated that the different surface roughness of the carrier led to different adhesion forces between the drug and carrier, which was reflected in the in vitro deposition results. The carrier surface plays an important role in, but weak enough to enable the separation forces during inhalation to detach a substantial fraction of the drug dose from the carrier crystals. This requires that the size distributions of the interaction forces (during mixing) and separation forces (during inhalation) are balanced properly (De Boer et al., 2003).The assumed role of carrier surface on the separation of microcapsules aggregation during preparation of DPI formulations and detachment of microcapsules after aerosolization from the surface of carriers is shown schematically in Figure 2 which is adapted from reference (Hamishehkar et al., 2010).This figure shows the dry powder inhalation formulations containing the blend of microcapsules and carriers. It can be seen that there are not enough active sites on the surface of spray dried mannitol and freeze dried mannitol for microcapsules to be deposited on, so carriers cannot disaggregate microcapsules. In the case of sieved sorbitol, microcapsules immersed on the surface of carrier and did not detach easily from its surface after aerosolization. Therefore in spite of better emission of microcapsules from the formulation containing sieved sorbitol, the FPF of the drug decreased. In this article, sieved mannitol showed higher FPF for insulin-loaded PLGA microparticles due to its appropriate surface roughness characteristics.

6.4. Fine carrier particles

The addition of fine particles to DPI formulations was shown to improve the inhalation efficiency of drugs (Zeng et al., 1998; Lucas et al., 1998). Islam et al. confirmed that the presence of fine lactose associated with large carriers or added as an excipient, played a key role in the drug dispersion process in this study (Islam et al., 2004). Similar observations were made by Louey et al. using salbutamol sulphate with various lactose carriers (Louey et al., 2003). The addition of ternary components like magnesium stearate and leucine (French et al., 1996; Islam et al., 2004; Staniforth, 1996) has also enhanced drug dispersion by decreasing the cohesive forces between drug particles. The addition of 10% fine carriers (lactose, glucose, mannitol and sorbitol) in the interactive mixtures of salmeterol xinafoate and coarse carriers demonstrated the same conclusion that fines enhance the detachment of the drug from the large carriers (Adi et al., 2007). On the other hand, the opposite results have been concluded about the role of fines from few studies. It was reported that the concentration of added fine lactose has to be carefully controlled such that a desired dispersibility of the drug can be achieved without substantially affecting powder flow properties (Zeng et al., 1998). The presence of "fines" tend to inhibit flow because fines can fit into the voids between larger particles and encourage packing and consequent powder densification, and fines are inherently poor flowing (Augsburger, 1974) due to various surface forces (Hickey et al., 2007) and high cohesive energy. It was recently reported that the presence of fines caused a decrease in FPF (Steckel et al., 2004; Hamishehkar et al., 2010). Also the use of micronized fine carrier may introduce extra amorphous content to the powder because a large portion of micronized lactose is in the amorphous form, which is thermodynamically unstable and will convert to the more stable crystalline form on exposure to moisture (Saleki-Gerhardt et al., 1994). Such a transformation is likely to change the performance characteristics of the bulk powder, such as flowability and drug dispersion (Ward et al., 1994).

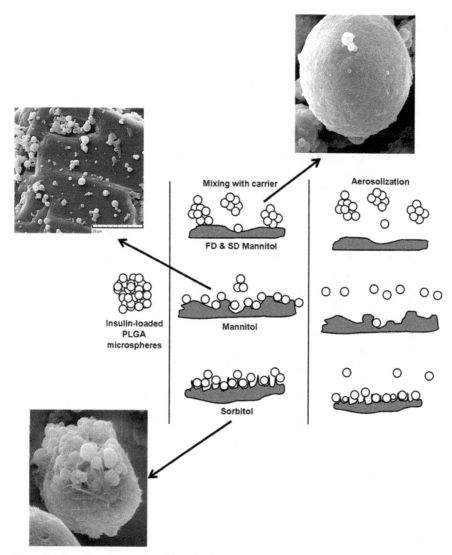

Figure 2. Schematic representation of the role of carrier surface asperities on the drug entrapment and its fluidization capabilities adapted from reference (Hamishehkar et al., 2010).

6.5. Carrier crystallinity

The amorphous part shows a higher surface adhesion energy compared to crystalline surfaces (Young et al., 2004). As a result of increase in adhesion energy, poor deaggregation of drug particles is observed (Podczeck et al., 1997). Therefore it can be hypothesized that, the presence of amorphous material may cause problems, for example, due to the fusion of particles, resulting in poor dispersion (Young et al., 2004; Ward et al., 1995; Podczeck et al., 1997). In addition, the amorphous regions can present difficulties such as decreased chemical stability (Pikal et al., 1978). Partially amorphous or unstable polymorphic forms and changes therein (Harjunen et al., 2002) make the interparticulate contact quite unpredictable and the powder formulation rather unstable (De Boer et al., 2003). It was reported that the maximum fine particle dose of terbutalinesulphate is obtained with the crystallized form of mannitol comparing to different polymorphs of mannitol (Saint-Lorant et al., 2007). Furthermore, previous reports have suggested increased amorphous content in DPI systems resulted in decreased aerosolization performance (Young et al., 2004; Ward et al., 1995).

7. Lactose as the most frequently used carrier in DPIs

Lactose, 4-(b-D-galactosido-)-D-glucose, can be obtained in either two basic isomeric forms, α and β-lactose, or as an amorphous form (Zeng et al., 2000). Historically, lactose monohydrate was an obvious choice for use as a carrier excipient. Lactose accompanying with glucose and mannitol is allowed as carriers in DPIs by the US Food and Drug Administration department (Labiris et al., 2003).Lactose is the most common and frequently used carrier in DPIs formulations and nowadays various inhalation grades of lactose with different physico-chemical properties are available on the market. The advantages of lactose are its well-investigated toxicity profile, physical and chemical stability, compatibility with the drug substance, its broad availability and relatively low price (Steckel et al., 2004; Pilcer et al., 2010).α-lactose monohydrate is the most common lactose grade used in the inhalation field.Almost all DPI formulations on the market are based on a-lactose monohydrate as a carrier. Therefore, wealth of literatures refers to the optimization of lactose carrier particles for better inhalation performance. More than 250 articles have been published in the past 40 years regarding the role of lactose in adhesive mixtures used in DPIs. However, in spite of these extensive investigations, the relationship between physico-chemical properties of the lactose in adhesive mixtures and the performance of the DPIs remains largely indistinct (Marriott et al., 2012).

8. Lactose engineering for application in DPIs

8.1. Surface modification

Iida et al. prepared lactose carrier particles for dry powder inhalations by its surface modification with aqueous ethanol solution and evaluated the inhalation efficiency of salbutamol sulfate from its mixture with modified lactose. The degree of adhesion between drug particles and carrier particles and the separation characteristics of drug particles from carrier particles in air flow were assessed by the ultracentrifuge separation and the air jet sieve methods, respectively. It was shown that the average adhesion force between the surface-treated lactose carrier and drug particles was considerably lower than that of powder mixed with the un-treated lactose carrier, indicating better drug separation from carrier and consequently an improvement of in vitro inhalation properties. The authors claimed that surface-smoothing of lactose by aqueous ethanol solution resulted a well balanced drug-carrier adhesion force so that the drug particles could be emitted together with the carrier particles and efficiently separated in airflow after emission(Iida et al., 2003). Fine lactose particles were immobilized on the lactose surface by spray coating with liquid suspensions consisting of micronized lactose dispersed in isopropyl alcohol and/or water mixtures to modify surface of lactose. The produced lactose was used as a carrier in the formulation of inhalable salbutamol sulfate powder. It was found that the roughness of the lactose surface established by immobilization of fine lactose increased the FPF and dispersibility of the drug. The authors claimed that unlike crevices and valleys, these microscopic undulations did not accommodate the drug particles and instead enhanced the detachment of drug from the lactose surface and improved the drug inhalation efficiency (Chan et al., 2003). Spray dried amorphous, spray dried crystallized and fluidized bed granulated lactose were prepared and used as carrier for inhalation of pranlukast hydrate. Fluidized bed granulated lactose emitted drug particles effectively from the inhalation device, whereas most part of drug captured in the upper stage of twin impinger, resulting in lower inhalation efficiency, due to strong adhesion of drug to the carrier lactose. The spray dried amorphous lactose, smoothed sphere particle, did not so improve the inhalation efficiency as expected, because of fairly strong adhesion between drug and lactose particles. But the spray dried crystallized lactose having lots of microscopical projection on its surface increased the respirable particle percent of the emitted particles. The conclusion was that the surface roughness should be optimized to gain improved inhalation efficiency of particles (Kawashima et al., 1998). In the other study, a Wurster fluidized bed was used for surface-coating of lactose particles with lactose aqueous solution containing hydroxypropyl methyl cellulose. The authors could be able to increase the inhalation performance of salbutamol sulfate 2.5 times more than commercial lactose (Pharmatose® 200M) and reported that surface coating of carrier particles may be an effective technique for improving the inhalation performance of DPI (Iida et al., 2005).Lactose carrier particles were layered with vegetable magnesium stearate by physical mixing and their effect of on the dry powder inhalation properties of salbutamol sulfate was investigated. The in vitro inhalation performance of drug was enhanced compared with the powder mixed with unlayered lactose carrier. It was stated that using this surface layering system would thus be valuable for increasing the inhalation properties of dry powder inhalation (Iida et al., 2004). For example, increasing the surface smoothness of lactose carrier particles was shown to improve the potentially respirable fraction of albuterol sulfate from the Rotahaler®(Littringer et al., 2012).

8.2. Shape modification

Lactose crystallization from Carbopol gel in different conditions (named Carbo lactose) produced a more regular shape lactose with smoother surface as compared with the control lactose. The Carbo lactose caused a higher and reproducible salbutamol sulphate emission and FPF after aerosolisation via a Rotahaler® tested in multi-stage impinge. It was concluded that engineered crystal growth under controlled conditions can enhance the potential inhalable fraction of drug from dry powder inhalers (Zeng et al., 2001).More recently, the use of more elongated crystals of lactose was also found to produce a higher inhalation efficiency of albuterol sulfate(Zeng et al., 2000).However, the improvement in drug dispersion that can be achieved by increasing the elongation ratio of the carrier particles is limited (Zeng et al., 2001).

8.3. Composite lactose

Lactose carrier particles were prepared by fusing sub units of lactose (either2, 6 or 10 μm prepared by spray drying) in saturated lactose slurry, sieve fractioned to obtain a 63–90 μm carriers and used for inhalation of salbutamol sulfate. The surface morphology and physico-chemical properties of the composite carriers were considerably different from regular α-lactose monohydrate.In all cases the composite carriers resulted in improved drug aerosol performance. It was suggested that composite based carriers are a potential route to control drug–carrier adhesion forces and variability thus allowing more precise control of formulation performance (Young et al., 2009).

8.4. Engineered lactose-mannitol mixture

Mannitol and lactose were co-crystallised to prepare crystals with more desirable characteristics than either lactose or mannitol alone appropriate for application as carriers in the formulations of salbutamol sulfate DPIs. In vitro deposition evaluation showed that crystallized carriers resulted more efficient delivery of salbutamol sulphate compared to formulations containing commercial grade carriers. It was concluded that simultaneous crystallization of lactose-mannitol can be a new approach to enhance inhalation performance of DPI formulations (Kaialy et al., 2012).

9. Mannitol

Because of clinical considerations lactose or other sugars cannot be used for drug delivery to diabetic patients. Moreover, for some drugs, e.g., formoterol, or for specific applications, e.g., peptide or protein drugs, lactose monohydrate may not be the carrier of choice due to its reducing sugar function that may interact with functional groups of the drug or the protein (Patton et al., 1992)In addition, lactose monohydrate is produced from bovine or with bovine-driven additives so that the transmissible spongiform encephalopathy (TSE) is still an issue for this compound (European Commission-Health & Consumer Protection Directorate, 2002)Lactose intolerance is a problem that necessitates the patient to use lactose-free formulations (Glasnapp, 1998).It is therefore logical to look for substitute carriers that still possess the positive aspects but overcome the above mentioned drawbacks of lactose monohydrate (Hamishehkar et al., 2010). Mannitol, a hexahydric alcohol, has been mainly used as a pharmaceutical excipient. Its potential use as a carrier for aerosol delivery has been reported (Tee et al., 2000; Steckel et al., 2004). Mannitol does not have a reducing sugar function, is less hygroscopic than lactose (Saint-Lorant et al., 2007)and gives a suitable sweet after-taste which has a benefit to patients confirming them that a dose has been properly administered (Kaialy et al., 2010).Mannitol proved to be the most promising candidate for this application than the more hygroscopic sugar alcohols such as sorbitol, xylitol and maltitol. D-mannitol is currently marketed in some countries as a pulmonary diagnostic dry powder inhalation aerosol (Aridol™) and as a therapeutic dry powder inhalation aerosol for the treatment of cystic fibrosis and chronic bronchitis (Bronchitol™) which are recently approved by US food and drug administration office and a European regulatory committee, respectively(Mansour et al., 2010).Spherical mannitol particles used in Aridol™ were produced by spray drying (Tang et al., 2009).A DPI formulation for inhalation of ciprofloxacin hydrochloride (an antibacterial fluoroquinolone) was prepared by its co-spray drying with different percentages of mannitol. The combination formulation containing 50% (w/w) mannitol showed the best inhaltion performance, good stability and lowest particle cohesion (as measured by colloid probe microscopy). It was proposed that the combination of co-spray-dried mannitol and ciprofloxacin from a DPI is an attractive approach to promote mucous clearance in the respiratory tract while simultaneously treating local chronic infection, such as chronic obstructive pulmonary disease and cystic fibrosis (Adi et al., 2010). Spray drying method was used to prepare several types of mannitol differ in shape and surface roughness. In this study besides the introducing the spray drying method as a proper technique for preparation of mannitol as a carrier for inhlation purposes, it was concluded that the highest fine particle fraction was achieved with carrier particles of spherical shape and a rough surface (Littringer et al., 2012).Despite the above mentioned study, in another study it was shown that the use of elongated mannitol as the carrier particle produced improved DPI performance. It was also indicated that mannitol particles crystallized from either acetone or ethanol (α-mannitol) showed the best aerosolisation performance while poorest aerosolisation performance was obtained from grounded mannitol (β-mannitol) (Kaialya et al., 2011).The same research group in another study again reported the better inhalation performance of salbutamol sulfate from elongated mannitol. In this study mannitol was crystallized from different binary mixtures of acetone/water and its carrier role in DPI formulations of salbutamol sulfate was investigated (Kaialy et al., 2010).Mannitol particles, produced by spray drying, have been used commercially (Aridol™) in bronchial provocation test (mannitol particle itself as an active ingredient not as a carrier). In a study, a confined liquid impinging jets (CLIJs) followed by jet milling was applied and introduced as an alternative method for spray drying. Although the inhalation performance of mannitol particles prepared by CLIJ method was not higher than those prepared from spray drying method (FPF 30% for particles prepared by CLIJ method compared to FPF 47% of those prepared by spray dying method) but CLIJ method offers several advantages. A main advantage of using the CLIJ method is that it can be scaled up with an acceptable yield as the precipitate can be largely collected and recovered on a filter, compared with spray drying which has a low collection efficiency for fine particles below 2 μm (Tang et al., 2009).Lactose, mannitol and glucose were used as the carriers in the formulations of inhalation powders of budesonide and salbutamol sulphate. The highest respirable fraction of drugs were achieved when mannitol was used as the carrier (Harjunen et al., 2003).

10. Sorbitol

Reducing sugars such as lactose may have an impact on the stability of proteins and peptides (Li et al., 1996; Dubost et al., 1996). Actuality, the use of lactose with protein powders may cause a reaction with lysine residues present in the protein, generating lactosylated protein molecules (Cryan, 2005).In this case, polyols such as sorbitol can play a crucial role in the formulation of respirable protein powder. Sorbitol can also serve as stability enhancers during processing. It was reported that the stability of interferon β to jet milling, required to produce a respirable powder, was found to be dependent on the presence of sorbitol in the formulation (Platz et al., 1991; Platz et al., 1994).Sorbitol showed a comparable inhalation outcome for salbutamol sulfate with lactose and mannitol but failed to produce efficient dispersion of drug (FPF less than10%) (Tee et al., 2000).

11. Erythritol

Erythritol, a meso-compound of 1,2,3,4-butanetetrol, is a natural occurring sugar alcohol existing in various fruits and fermented foods, as well as in body fluids of humans and animals. Industrially, it is prepared by glucose fermentation (Lopes Jesus et al., 2010). Erythritol has been administered as a suitable excipient in pharmaceutical formulations due to its thermal stability, very low hygroscopicity (Cohen et al., 1993) sweetness taste, low toxicity (Munro et al., 1998) and high compatibility with drugs (Endo et al., 2005; Gonnissen et al., 2007).Due to above desirable characteristics, erythritol was recently entered in the European Pharmacopoiea (Traini et al., 2006). Endo et al. used erythritol as carrier in the DPI formulation of glucagon, a key regulatory element of glycogen metabolism which is known to be effective in the clinical treatment of hypoglycemia and the maintenance of normal circulating glucose levels in patients with total pancreatectomy. This hormone has been restricted to parenteral administration. The in vitro and in vivo studies were indicated the suitability of erythritol for application in DPI formulation. Moreover, it was claimed that this dry powder inhalation of glucagon can be administered to the clinical treatment of hypoglycemia, and the maintenance of normal circulating glucose levels in patients with total pancreatectomy (Endo et al., 2005). In a comparative study, erythritol andlactose monohydrate were used as carriers in the DPI formulation of salbutamol sulfate. Drug-carrier adhesion was measured using atomic force microscope colloid probe technique and showed a higher adhesion force for erythritol than lactose. Consequently lower inhalation performance of salbutamol sulfate was resulted from DPI formulations containing erythritol than lactose. However, it was concluded that even though erythritol may show a reduced DPI functionality, with this drug, it may offer some potential advantages in terms of its reproducible chemical structure and stability (Traini et al., 2006).

12. Trehalose

Trehalose dihydrate is a disaccharide sugar and crystalline hydrate like lactose. However, trehalose dihydrate is a non-reducing sugar and lactose monohydrate is a reducing sugar. As a reducing sugar, it participates in solid-state chemical degradation by the Maillard reaction with certain types of small molecular weight drugs (such as formoterol and budesonide) and polypeptide/protein-type drugs. Therefore, some attempts have been carried out on the application of trehalose in the formulation of DPIs. In a study, trehalose was used as a carrier for DPI formulation of albuterol sulfate, ipratropium bromide monohydrate, disodium cromoglycate, and fluticasone propionate (Mansour et al., 2010).The highest inhalation performance was reported for the blend of albuterol and ipratropium with trehalose dihydrate in comparison with lactose monohydrate and mannitol (Cline et al., 2002).

13. Other carriers

Recently, the feasibility of using pollen-shape hydroxyapatite particles as carrier in DPI formulation of budesonide is investigated. The hydroxyapatite carriers showed better flowability and capability of higher drug attachment than commonly used lactose carrier with similar size range. Consequently, DPI formulations with hydroxyapatite carriers gave higher drug emission and respirable fraction than traditional lactose carriers (Hassan et al., 2010). Many different non-lactose carriers have been investigated, such as cyclodextrins, dextrose, glucose monohydrate, maltitol, maltose, raffinosepentahydrate and xylitol.Anhydrous glucose is already used in the marketed product Bronchodual® (Boehringer) (Pilcer et al., 2010).Sucrose, trehalose and raffinose are non-reducing sugars and as such have the advantage that they will not undergo the Maillard browning reaction with proteins (Ógáin et al., 2011). But in contrast to lactose monohydrate which was found to only take up moisture on its surface, and showing only a small reduction in its FPF after storage at 75% RH (Young et al., 2007; Zeng etal., 2007), a main difficulty with these sugars, especially with the more hygroscopic substances – sorbitol, maltitol and xylitol – has attributed to their sensitivity to humidity. In fact, the capillary forces, arisen from the dynamic condensation of water molecules onto particle surfaces, seem to be less prominent with mannitol and lactose as carriers, probably because of their less hygroscopic characteristics than the other carbohydrates (Zeng et al., 2007; Young et al., 2007). However, it was proposed that the difficulties arising from their hygroscopicity can be overcome by adding an ultrafine hydrophobic excipient to the powder blend (Steckel et al., 2004).Comparing the different forms of mannitol, lactose and maltitol mixed with terbutaline sulfate resulted in higher FPF with crystallized mannitol for terbutaline sulfate (Saint-Lorant et al., 2007).Hooton et al, used beta cyclodextrin, lactose, raffinose, trehalose and xylitol for the formulation of salbutamol sulfate DPI and applied the cohesive-adhesive balance technique for analyzing quantitative AFM measurements to interpret inhalation behavior of drug. The rank order of the FPF of the salbutamol sulfate based carrier DPI formulations was beta cyclodextrin> lactose >raffinose>trehalose> xylitol which had a linear correlation with cohesive-adhesive ratios of the AFM force measurements (Hooton et al., 2006).

14. Large porous particles

A new type of aerosol formulation is the large porous hollow particles. These particles have the mean diameters >5 μm and mass densities <0.1g/cm^3 (Edwards et al., 1997). Although these particles have large geometric diameters because of their low density, they exhibit aerodynamic diameters comparable to smaller particles having higher densities (Koushik et al., 2004). They may be ideal for pulmonary drug delivery because of their low density and large surface area which causes excellent dispersibility (Labiris et al., 2003). Furthermore, their large geometric size may reduce clearance by macrophage action, thereby improving the bioavailability of inhaled pharmaceuticals (Musante et al., 2002).To show the ability of large porous aerosols to increase systemic bioavailability as well as to provide sustained-release capability in the lungs, Edwards et al. encapsulated insulin into a biodegradable polymers and indicated the better inhalation performance and controlled-release capability of these particles in the lung (Edwards et al., 1997).Ungaro et al. confirmed the same observations with delivery of insulin into rat lung by preparation of PLGA large porous particle with the aid of cyclodextrins (Ungaro et al., 2009).These particles can be prepared using polymeric or nonpolymeric excipients, by solvent evaporation and spray-drying techniques (Edwards et al., 1998). Pulmospheres™ is an example which is made of phosphatidylcholine, the primary component of human lung surfactant (Labiris et al., 2003). In two interesting studies, highly porous large biodegradable polymeric particles were fabricated using ammonium bicarbonate as an effervescent porogen (Ungaro et al., 2010; Yang et al., 2009).

15. Conclusion

The number of diseases that are being considered candidates for the aerosol therapy has increased considerably. Until recently, asthma and chronic obstructive pulmonary diseases were only the apparent examples of diseases that could be treated via drug delivery to lungs. But now other pulmonary diseases such as cystic fibrosis, lung cancer and pulmonary infectious diseases and also systemic disorders such as diabetes, cancer, neurobiological disorders are considered to be managed by pulmonary drug delivery. Interest in DPIs has increased in the last decade due to its numerous advantages over other pulmonary drug delivery dosage forms. Currently, the inhalation performance of DPIs are being improved by changing formulation strategy, drug and carrier particle engineering. Regarding formulation development, micronised drug particles are cohesive with poor flow properties. Addition of large carrier particles into powders to enhance their flow characteristics has been an appropriate approach. The main goal in the inhalation field is to obtain reproducible, high pulmonary deposition which can be highly effected by physico-chemical characteristics of carrier. This could be achieved by successful carrier selection and careful process optimization. Technologies for engineering carrier particle shape, density, and size will continue to develop to enhance the effectiveness of pulmonary drug formulations. This approach may enable more drugs to be delivered through this route for local treatment of lung diseases or systemic therapy.

Author details

Hamed Hamishehkar
Pharmaceutical Technology Laboratory, Drug Applied Research Center,
Tabriz University of Medical Sciences, Tabriz, Iran

Yahya Rahimpour
Student Research Committee and Faculty of Pharmacy,
Tabriz University of Medical Sciences, Tabriz, Iran

Yousef Javadzadeh *
Biotechnology Research Center andFaculty of Pharmacy,
Tabriz University of Medical Sciences, Tabriz, Iran

16. References

Adi, H.; Larson, I. & Stewart, P.J., (2007). Adhesion and redistribution of salmeterol xinafoate particles in sugar-based mixtures for inhalation. *Int J Pharm*, Vol. 337, No. 1-2, pp. 229-238, ISSN: 0378-5173.

Adi, H.; Young, P.M.; Chan, H.-K.; Agus, H. & Traini, D., (2010). Co-spray-dried mannitol-ciprofloxacin dry powder inhaler formulation for cystic fibrosis and chronic obstructive pulmonary disease. *Eur J Pharm Sci*, Vol. 40, pp. 239-247, ISSN: 0928-0987.

Ali, R.; Jain, G.K.; Iqbal, Z.; Talegaonkar, S.; Pandit, P.; Sule, S.; Malhotra, G.; Khar, R.K.; Bhatnagar, A. & Ahmad, F.J., (2009). Development and clinical trial of nano-atropine sulfate dry powder inhaler as a novel organophosphorous poisoning antidote. *Nanomed-Nanotechnol*, Vol. 5, No. 1, pp. 55-63, ISSN: 1549-9634.

Anon, (2008). Method of and apparatus for effecting delivery of fine powders. *IP Com J*, Vol. 8, No. 1B, pp. 13,

Atkins, P.J., (2005). Dry powder inhalers: an overview. *Resp Care*, Vol. 50, No. 10, pp. 1304-1312, ISSN: 0020-1324.

Augsburger, L.L., (1974). Powdered dosage forms. *Sprowls' American Pharmacy: An Introduction to Pharmaceutical Techniques and Dosage Forms 7th ed Philadelphia: JB Lippincott Company*, pp. 301-343,

Bosquillon, C.; Lombry, C.; Preat, V. & Vanbever, R., (2001). Influence of formulation excipients and physical characteristics of inhalation dry powders on their aerosolization performance. *J Control Release*, Vol. 70, No. 3, pp. 329-339, ISSN: 0168-3659.

Braun, M.A.; Oschmann, R. & Schmidt, P.C., (1996). Influence of excipients and storage humidity on the deposition of disodium cromoglycate (DSCG) in the twin impinger. *Int J Pharm*, Vol. 135, No. 1, pp. 53-62, ISSN: 0378-5173.

Byron, P.R. & Jashnani, R., (1990). Efficiency of aerosolization from dry powder blends of terbutaline sulphate and lactose NF with different particle size distributions. *Pharm Res*, Vol. 7, pp. S81, ISSN: 0724-8741.

Carpenter, J.F.; Pikal, M.J.; Chang, B.S. & Randolph, T.W., (1997). Rational design of stable lyophilized protein formulations: some practical advice. *Pharm Res*, Vol. 14, pp. 969-975, ISSN: 0724-8741.

Chan, H.K. & Gonda, I., (1989). Aerodynamic properties of elongated particles of cromoglycic acid. *J Aerosol Sci*, Vol. 20, No. 2, pp. 157-168, ISSN: 0021-8502.

---

* Corresponding Author

Chan, L.W.; Lim, L.T. & Heng, P.W.S., (2003). Immobilization of fine particles on lactose carrier by precision coating and its effect on the performance of dry powder formulations. *J Pharm Sci*, Vol. 92, No. 5, pp. 975-984, ISSN: 1520-6017.

Cheatham, W.W.; Leone-Bay, A.; Grant, M.; Fog, P.B. & Diamond, D.C., (2006). Pulmonary delivery of inhibitors of phosphodiesterase type 5. Application: WO. USA: Mannkind Corporation; p. 23 .

Chew, N.Y. & Chan, H.K., (2002). Effect of powder polydispersity on aerosol generation. *J Pharm Pharm Sci* Vol. 5, pp. 162-168, ISSN: 1482-1826.

Chew, N.Y.K.; Tang, P.; Chan, H.K. & Raper, J.A., (2005). How much particle surface corrugation is sufficient to improve aerosol performance of powders? *Pharm Res*, Vol. 22, No. 1, pp. 148-152, ISSN: 0724-8741.

Cline, D. & Dalby, R., (2002). Predicting the quality of powders for inhalation from surface energy and area. *Pharm Res*, Vol. 19, No. 9, pp. 1274-1277, ISSN: 0724-8741.

Cohen, S.; Marcus, Y.; Migron, Y.; Dikstein, S. & Shafran, A., (1993). Water sorption, binding and solubility of polyols. *J Chem Soc, Faraday Trans*, Vol. 89, pp. 3271-3275,

Crowder, T.M.; Louey, M.D.; Sethuraman, V.V.; Smyth, H.D.C. & Hickey, A.J., (2001). An odyssey in inhaler formulation and design. *Pharm Technol*, Vol. 25, No. 7, pp. 99-113, ISSN: 0147-8087.

Crowder, T.M.; Rosati, J.A.; Schroeter, J.D.; Hickey, A.J. & Martonen, T.B., (2002). Fundamental effects of particle morphology on lung delivery: Predictions of Stokes' law and the particular relevance to dry powder inhaler formulation and development. *Pharm Res*, Vol. 19, No. 3, pp. 239-245, ISSN: 0724-8741.

Cryan, S.A., (2005). Carrier-based strategies for targeting protein and peptide drugs to the lungs. *The AAPS journal*, Vol. 7, No. 1, pp. 20-41,

De Boer, A.H.; Dickhoff, B.H.J.; Hagedoorn, P.; Gjaltema, D.; Goede, J.; Lambregts, D. & Frijlink, H.W., (2005). A critical evaluation of the relevant parameters for drug redispersion from adhesive mixtures during inhalation. *Int J Pharm*, Vol. 294, No. 1, pp. 173-184, ISSN: 0378-5173.

De Boer, A.H.; Hagedoorn, P.; Gjaltema, D.; Goede, J. & Frijlink, H.W., (2003). Air classifier technology (ACT) in dry powder inhalation. Part 1. Application of a Force Distribution Concept (FDC) to explain the performance of a basic classifier on adhesive mixtures. *Int J Pharm*, Vol. 260, pp. 187-200, ISSN: 0378-5173.

De Boer, A.H.; Hagedoorn, P.; Gjaltema, D.; Goede, J.; Kussendrager, K.D. & Frijlink, H.W., (2003). Air classifier technology (ACT) in dry powder inhalation Part 2. The effect of lactose carrier surface properties on the drug-to-carrier interaction in adhesive mixtures for inhalation. *Int J Pharm*, Vol. 260, No. 2, pp. 201-216, ISSN: 0378-5173.

Dubost, D.C.; M.J., K.; Zimmerman, J.A.; Bogusky, M.J.; Coddington, A.B. & Pitzenberger, S.M., (1996). Characterization of a solid state reaction product from a lyophilized formulation of a cyclic heptapeptide: a novel example of an excipient-induced oxidation. *Pharm Res*, Vol. 13, pp. 1811-1814, ISSN: 0724-8741.

Edwards, D.A.; Chen, D.; Wang, J. & Ben-Jebria, A., (1998). Controlled-release inhalation aerosols. In Respiratory drug delivery, 6th edn, eds Dalby RN, Byron PR, Farr SJ. Buffalo Grove, IL: Interpharm Press Inc., 187–192.

Edwards, D.A.; Hanes, J.; Caponetti, G.; Hrkach, J.; Ben-Jebria, A. & Eskew, M.L., (1997). Large porous particles for pulmonary drug delivery. *Science*, Vol. 276, pp. 1868-1871, ISSN: 0036-8075.

Edwards, D.A.; Sung, J.; Pulliam, B.; Wehrenberg-Klee, E.; Schwartz, E.; Dreyfuss, P. & al., e., (2005). Pulmonary delivery of malarial vaccine in the form of particulates.Application:WO: USA: President and Fellows of Harvard College; p. 25

El-Gendy, N. & Berkland, C., (2009). Combination chemotherapeutic dry powder aerosols via controlled nanoparticle agglomeration. *Pharm Res*, Vol. 26, No. 7, pp. 1752-1763, ISSN: 0724-8741.

Emami, J.; Hamishehkar, H.; Najafabadi, A.R.; Gilani, K.; Minaiyan, M.; Mahdavi, H.; Mirzadeh, H.; Fakhari, A. & Nokhodchi, A., (2009). Particle size design of PLGA microspheres for potential pulmonary drug delivery using response surface methodology. *J Microencapsul*, Vol. 26, No. 1, pp. 1-8, ISSN: 1464-5246.

Endo, K.; Amikawa, S.; Matsumoto, A.; Sahashi, N. & Onoue, S., (2005). Erythritol-based dry powder of glucagon for pulmonary administration. *Int J Pharm*, Vol. 290, pp. 63-71, ISSN: 0378-5173.

European Commission-Health & Consumer Protection Directorate, (2002). Provisional statement on the safety of calf-derived rennet for the manufacture of pharmaceutical grade lactose.

Farr, S.J. & Otulana, B.A., (2006). Pulmonary delivery of opioids as pain therapeutics. *Adv Drug Deliv Rev*, Vol. 58, No. 9, pp. 1076-1088, ISSN: 0169-409X.

Flament, M.P.; Leterme, P. & Gayot, A., (2004). The influence of carrier roughness on adhesion, content uniformity and the in vitro deposition of terbutaline sulphate from dry powder inhalers. *Int J Pharm*, Vol. 275, No. 1, pp. 201-209, ISSN: 0378-5173.

Fleischer, W.; Reimer, K. & Leyendecker, P. Opioids for the treatment of the chronic obstructive pulmonary disease. Euro-Celtique S.A2005.

French, D.L.; Edwards, D.A. & Niven, R.W., (1996). The influence of formulation on emission, deaggregation and deposition of dry powders for inhalation. *J Aerosol Sci*, Vol. 27, No. 5, pp. 769-783, ISSN: 0021-8502.

Fults, K.A.; Miller, I.F. & Hickey, A.J., (1997). Effect of particle morphology on emitted dose of fatty acid-treated disodium cromoglycate powder aerosols. *Pharm Dev Technol*, Vol. 2, No. 1, pp. 67-79, ISSN: 1083-7450.

Furness, G., (2005). Is systemic pulmonary delivery really in a make-or-break position? . *Pharm Dev Technol*, Vol. 5 No. pp. 24-27, ISSN: 1083-7450.

Ganderton, D. & Kassem, N.M., (1992). Dry powder inhalers. *Adv Pharm Sci*, Vol. 6, No. pp. 165-191,

Geller, D.E.; M.W., K.; Smith, J.; Noonberg, S.B. & Conrad, C., (2007). Novel tobramycin inhalation powder in cystic fibrosis subjects: pharmacokinetics and safety. *Pediatr Pulm* Vol. 42, pp. 307-313, ISSN: 8755-6863.

Gilani, K.; Najafabadi, A.R.; Darabi, M.; Barghi, M. & Rafiee-Tehrani, M., (2004). Influence of formulation variables and inhalation device on the deposition profiles of cromolyn sodium dry powder aerosols. *DARU J Pharm Sci*, Vol. 12, No. 3, ISSN: 1560-8115.

Gonnissen, Y.; Remon, J.P. & Vervaet, C., (2007). Development of directly compressible powders via co-spray drying *Eur J Pharm Biopharm*, Vol. 67, pp. 220-226, ISSN: 0939-6411.

Hamishehkar, H.; Emami, J.; Najafabadi, A.R.; Gilani, K.; Minaiyan, M.; Hassanzadeh, K.; Mahdavi, H.; Koohsoltani, M. & Nokhodchi, A., (2010). Pharmacokinetics and pharmacodynamics of controlled release insulin loaded PLGA microcapsules using dry powder inhaler in diabetic rats. *Biopharm Drug Dispos*, Vol. 31, No. 2-3, pp. 189-201, ISSN: 1099-081X

Hamishehkar, H.; Emami, J.; Najafabadi, A.R.; Gilani, K.; Minaiyan, M.; Mahdavi, H. & Nokhodchi, A. Do fines always improve dry powder inhalation performance? Lactose as a carrier for inhalation products congress; 2010; Parma-Italy2010.

Hamishehkar, H.; Emami, J.; Najafabadi, A.R.; Gilani, K.; Minaiyan, M.; Mahdavi, H. & Nokhodchi, A., (2010). Effect of carrier morphology and surface characteristics on the development of respirable PLGA microcapsules for sustained-release pulmonary delivery of insulin. *Int J Pharm*, Vol. 389, No. 1-2, pp. 74-85, ISSN: 1873-3476

Hamishehkar, H.; Emami, J.; Najafabadi, A.R.; Gilani, K.; Minaiyan, M.; Mahdavi, H. & Nokhodchi, A., (2010). Influence of carrier particle size, carrier ratio and addition of fine ternary particles on the dry powder inhalation performance of insulin-loaded PLGA microcapsules. *Powder Technol*, Vol. 201 pp. 289-295, ISSN: 0032-5910.

Harjunen, P.; Lankinen, T.; Salonen, H.; Lehto, V.P. & Järvinen, K., (2003). Effects of carriers and storage of formulation on the lung deposition of a hydrophobic and hydrophilic drug from a DPI. *Int J Pharm*, Vol. 263, No. 1, pp. 151-163, ISSN: 0378-5173.

Harjunen, P.; Lehto, V.P.; Martimo, K.; Suihko, E.; Lankinen, T.; Paronen, P. & Järvinen, K., (2002). Lactose modifications enhance its drug performance in the novel multiple dose Taifun® DPI. *Eur J Pharm Sci*, Vol. 16, No. 4-5, pp. 313-321, ISSN: 0928-0987.

Hassan, M.S. & Lau, R., (2010). Feasibility study of pollen-shape drug carriers in dry powder inhalation. *J Pharm Sci*, Vol. 99, pp. 1309-1321, ISSN: 1520-6017.

Hassan, M.S. & Lau, R., (2010). Inhalation performance of pollen-shape carrier in dry powder formulation with different drug mixing ratios: comparison with lactose carrier. *Int J Pharm*, Vol. 386, pp. 6-14, ISSN: 0378-5173.

Heng, P.W.S.; Chan, L.W. & Lim, L.T., (2000). Quantification of the surface morphologies of lactose carriers and their effect on the in vitro deposition of salbutamol sulphate. *Chem Pharm Bull*, Vol. 48, pp. 393-398, ISSN: 0009-2363.

Heyder, J.; Gebhart, J.; Rudolf, G.; Schiller, C.F. & Stahlhofen, W., (1986). "Deposition of particles in the human respiratory tract in the size range 0.005 - 5 μm". *J Aerosol Sci*, Vol. 17, No. 5, pp. 811-825, ISSN: 0021-8502.

Hickey, A.J.; Lu, D.; Ashley, E.D. & Stout, J., (2006). Inhaled azithromycin therapy *J Aerosol Med*, Vol. 19, pp. 54-60,

Hickey, A.J.; Mansour, H.M.; Telko, M.J.; Xu, Z.; Smyth, H.D.C.; Mulder, T.; Mclean, R.; Langridge, J. & Papadopoulos, D., (2007). Physical characterization of component particles included in dry powder inhalers. II. Dynamic characteristics. *J Pharm Sci*, Vol. 96, pp. 1302-1319, ISSN: 1520-6017.

Hooton, J.C.; Jones, M.D. & Price, R., (2006). Predicting the behavior of novel sugar carriers for dry powder inhaler formulations via the use of a cohesive–adhesive force balance approach. *J Pharm Sci*, Vol. 95, No. 6, pp. 1288-1297, ISSN: 1520-6017.

Iida, K.; Hayakawa, Y.; Okamoto, H.; Danjo, K. & Leuenberger, H., (2001). Evaluation of flow properties of dry powder inhalation of salbutamol sulfate with lactose carrier. *Chem Pharm Bull*, Vol. 49, No. 10, pp. 1326-1330, ISSN: 0009-2363.

Iida, K.; Hayakawa, Y.; Okamoto, H.; Danjo, K. & Leuenberger, H., (2003). Preparation of dry powder inhalation by surface treatment of lactose carrier particles. *Chem Pharm Bull*, Vol. 51, No. 1, pp. 1-5, ISSN: 0009-2363.

Iida, K.; Hayakawa, Y.; Okamoto, H.; Danjo, K. & Luenberger, H., (2003). Effect of surface covering of lactose carrier particles on dry powder inhalation properties of salbutamol sulfate. *Chem Pharm Bull*, Vol. 51, No. 12, pp. 1455-1457., ISSN: 0009-2363.

Iida, K.; Hayakawa, Y.; Okamoto, H.; Danjo, K. & Luenbergerb, H., (2004). Effect of surface layering time of lactose carrier particles on dry powder inhalation properties of salbutamol sulfate. *Chem Pharm Bull*, Vol. 52 No. 3, pp. 350-353, ISSN: 0009-2363.

Iida, K.; Todo, H.; Okamoto, H.; Danjo, K. & Leuenberger, H., (2005). Preparation of dry powder inhalation with lactose carrier particles surface-coated using a Wurster fluidized bed. *Chem Pharm Bull*, Vol. 53, No. 4, pp. 431-434, ISSN: 0009-2363.

Ikegami, K.; Kawashima, Y.; Takeuchi, H.; Yamamoto, H.; Isshiki, N.; Momose, D. & Ouchi, K., (2002). Improved inhalation behavior of steroid KSR-592 in vitro with Jethaler® by polymorphic transformation to needle-like crystals (β-form). *Pharm Res*, Vol. 19, No. 10, pp. 1439-1445, ISSN: 0724-8741.

Islam, N.; Stewart, P.; Larson, I. & Hartley, P., (2004). Lactose surface modification by decantation: are drug-fine lactose ratios the key to better dispersion of salmeterol xinafoate from lactose-interactive mixtures? *Pharm Res*, Vol. 21, No. 3, pp. 492-499, ISSN: 0724-8741.

Islama, N. & Clearyb, M.J., (2012). Developing an efficient and reliable dry powder inhaler for pulmonary drug delivery – A review for multidisciplinary researchers. *Med Eng Phs*, Vol. 34, pp. 409-427, ISSN: 1350-4533.

Kaialy, W.; Larhrib, H.; Martin, G.P. & Nokhodchi, A., (2012). The effect of engineered mannitol-lactose mixture on dry powder inhaler performance. *Pharm Res*, pp. 1-18, ISSN: 0724-8741.

Kaialy, W.; Martin, G.P.; Ticehurst, M.D.; Momin, M.N. & Nokhodchi, A., (2010). The enhanced aerosol performance of salbutamol from dry powders containing engineered mannitol as excipient. *Int J Pharm*, Vol. 392, No. 1, pp. 178-188, ISSN: 0378-5173.

Kaialy, W.; Alhalaweh, A.; Velaga, S.P. & Nokhodchi, A., (2011). Effect of carrier particle shape on dry powder inhaler performance. *Int J Pharm*, Vol. 421, pp. 12-23, ISSN: 0378-5173.

Kassem, N.M.; Ho, K.K.l. & Ganderton, D., (1989). The effect of air flow and carrier size on the characteristics of an inspirable cloud. *J Pharm Pharmacol*, ISSN: 0022-3573.

Kawashima, Y.; Serigano, T.; Hino, T.; Yamamoto, H. & Takeuchi, H., (1998). Effect of surface morphology of carrier lactose on dry powder inhalation property of pranlukast hydrate. *Int J Pharm*, Vol. 172, No. 1, pp. 179-188, ISSN: 0378-5173.

Kleinstreuer, C.; Zhang, Z. & Donohue, J.F., (2008). Targeted drug-aerosol delivery in the human respiratory system. *Annu Rev Biomed Eng*, Vol. 10, pp. 195-220, ISSN: 1523-9829.

Koushik, K. & Kompella, U.B., (2004). Preparation of large porous deslorelin–PLGA microparticles with reduced residual solvent and cellular uptake using a supercritical carbon dioxide process. *Pharm Res*, Vol. 21, No. 3, pp. 524-535, ISSN: 0724-8741.

Labiris, N.R. & Dolovich, M.B., (2003). Pulmonary drug delivery. Part I: Physiological factors affecting therapeutic effectiveness of aerosolized medications. *Br J Clin Pharmacol*, Vol. 56, pp. 588-599, ISSN: 1365-2125.

Labiris, N.R. & Dolovich, M.B., (2003). Pulmonary drug delivery. Part II: the role of inhalant delivery devices and drug formulations in therapeutic effectiveness of aerosolized medications. *Br J Clin Pharmacol*, Vol. 56, No. 6, pp. 600-612, ISSN: 1365-2125.

Larhrib, H.; Martin, G.P.; Marriott, C. & Prime, D., (2003). The influence of carrier and drug morphology on drug delivery from dry powder formulations. *Int J Pharm*, Vol. 257, No. 1, pp. 283-296, ISSN: 0378-5173.

Larhrib, H.; Zeng, X.M.; Martin, G.P.; Marriott, C. & Pritchard, J., (1999). The use of different grades of lactose as a carrier for aerosolised salbutamol sulphate. *Int J Pharm*, Vol. 191, No. 1, pp. 1-14, ISSN: 0378-5173.

Laube, B.L., (2005). The expanding role of aerosols in systemic drug delivery, gene therapy, and vaccination. *Resp Care*, Vol. 50, No. 9, pp. 1161-1176, ISSN: 0020-1324.

Li, S.; Patapoff, T.W.; Overcashier, D.; Hsu, C.; Nguyen, T.H. & Borchardt, R.T., (1996). Effects of reducing sugars on the chemical stability of human relaxin in the lyophilized state. *J Pharm Sci*, Vol. 85, pp. 873-877, ISSN: 1520-6017.

LiCalsi, C.; Maniaci, M.J.; Christensen, T.; Phillips, E.; Ward, G.H. & Witham, C., (2001). A powder formulation of measles vaccine for aerosol delivery. *Vaccine*, Vol. 19, No. 17, pp. 2629-2636, ISSN: 0264-410X.

Littringer, E.; Mescher, A.; Schroettner, H.; Achelis, L.; Walzel, P. & Urbanetz, N., (2012). Spray dried mannitol carrier particles with tailored surface properties–The influence of carrier surface roughness and shape. *Eur J Pharm Biopharm*, ISSN: 0939-6411.

Littringer, E.M.; Mescher, A.; Schroettner, H.; Achelis, L.; Walzel, P. & Urbanetz, N.A., (2012). Spray dried mannitol carrier particles with tailored surface properties –The influence of carrier surface roughness and shape. *Eur J Pharm Biopharm* *http://dxdoiorg/101016/jejpb201205001*, ISSN: 0939-6411.

Lopes Jesus, A.J.; Nunes, S.C.C.; Ramos Silva, M.; Matos Beja, A. & Redinha, J., (2010). Erythritol: Crystal growth from the melt. *Int J Pharm*, Vol. 388, No. 1-2, pp. 129-135, ISSN: 0378-5173.

Louey, M.D.; Razia, S. & Stewart, P.J., (2003). Influence of physico-chemical carrier properties on the in vitro aerosol deposition from interactive mixtures. *Int J Pharm*, Vol. 252, No. 1, pp. 87-98, ISSN: 0378-5173.

Lucas, P.; Anderson, K. & Staniforth, J.N., (1998). Protein deposition from dry powder inhalers: fine particle multiplets as performance modifiers. *Pharm Res*, Vol. 15, No. 4, pp. 562-569, ISSN: 0724-8741.

Mansour, H.M.; Xu, Z. & Hickey, A.J., (2010). Dry powder aerosols generated by standardized entrainment tubes from alternative sugar blends: 3.Trehalose dihydrate and D-mannitol carriers. *J Pharm Sci*, Vol. 99, No. 8, pp. 3430-3441, ISSN: 1520-6017.

Marianecci, C.; Di Marzio, L.; Rinaldi, F.; Carafa, M. & Alhaique, F., (2011). Pulmonary delivery: innovative approaches and perspectives. *Journal of Biomaterials and Nanobiotechnology*, Vol. 2, No. 5, pp. 567-575, ISSN: 2158-7027.

Marple, V.A.; Olson, B.A.; Santhanakrishnan, K.; Mitchell, J.P.; Murray, S.C. & Hudson-Curtis, B.L., (2003). Next generation pharmaceutical impactor. Part II: Calibration. . *J Aerosol Med*, Vol. 16, pp. 301-324,

Marriott, C. & Frijlink, H.W., (2012). Lactose as a carrier for inhalation products: breathing new life into an old carrier. *Adv Drug Deliv Rev*, Vol. 64, No. 3, pp. 217, ISSN: 0169-409X.

Mullins, M.E.; Michaels, L.P.; Menon, V.; Locke, B. & Ranade, M.B., (1992). Effect of geometry on particle adhesion. *Aerosol Sci Tech*, Vol. 17, No. 2, pp. 105-118, ISSN: 0278-6826.

Munro, I.C.; Bernt, W.O.; Borzelleca, J.F.; Flamm, G.; Lynch, B.S.; Kennepohl, E.; Bär, E.A. & Modderman, J., (1998). Erythritol: an interpretive summary of biochemical,metabolic, toxicological and clinical data. *Food Chem Toxicol* Vol. 36, pp. 1139-1174, ISSN: 0278-6915.

Musante, C.J.; Schroeter, J.D.; Rosati, J.A.; Crowder, T.M.; Hickey, A.J. & Martonen, T.B., (2002). Factors affecting the deposition of inhaled porous drug particles. *J Pharm Sci*, Vol. 91, No. 7, pp. 1590-1600, ISSN: 1520-6017.

Ógáin, O.N.; Li, J.; Tajber, L.; Corrigan, O.I. & Healy, A.M., (2011). Particle engineering of materials for oral inhalation by dry powder inhalers. I—Particles of sugar excipients (trehalose and raffinose) for protein delivery. *Int J Pharm*, Vol. 405, No. 1, pp. 23-35, ISSN: 0378-5173.

Patton, J.S. & Bossard, M.J., (2004). Drug delivery strategies for proteins and peptides from discovery and development to life cycle management. *Pharm Dev Technol*, Vol. 4, No. 8, pp. 73-77, ISSN: 1083-7450.

Patton, J.S. & Platz, R.M., (1992). Pulmonary delivery of peptides and proteins for systemic action. *Adv Drug Deliv Rev*, Vol. 8, pp. 179-228, ISSN: 0169-409X.

Pikal, M.J.; Lukes, A.L.; Lang, J.E. & Gaines, K., (1978). Quantitative crystallinity determinations for beta-lactamantibiotics by solution calorimetry: correlations with stability. *J Pharm Sci*, Vol. 67, pp. 767-772, ISSN: 1520-6017.

Pilcer, G. & Amighi, K., (2010). Formulation strategy and use of excipients in pulmonary drug delivery. *Int J Pharm*, Vol. 392, pp. 1-19, ISSN: 0378-5173.

Pilcer, G.; Wauthoz, N. & Amighi, K., (2012). Lactose characteristics and the generation of the aerosol. *Adv Drug Deliv Rev*, Vol. 64 pp. 233-256, ISSN: 0169-409X.

Platz, R.; Ip, A. & Whitham, C.L., (1994). Process for preparing micronized polypeptide drugs.US Patent 5,354,562., Vol., No.

Platz, R.; Utsumi, J.; Satoh, Y. & Naruse, N. Pharmaceutical aerosol formulation of solid polypeptide microparticles and method for the preparation thereof. World Patent 9,116,038. 1991.

Plumley, C.; Gorman, E.M.; El-Gendy, N.; Bybee, C.R.; Munson, E.J. & Berkland, C., (2009). Nifedipine nanoparticle agglomeration as a dry powder aerosol formulation strategy. *Int J Pharm*, Vol. 369, No. 1-2, pp. 136-143, ISSN: 0378-5173.

Podczeck, F., (1998). The relationship between physical properties of lactose monohydrate and the aerodynamic behaviour of adhered drug particles. *Int J Pharm*, Vol. 160, No. 1, pp. 119-130, ISSN: 0378-5173.

Podczeck, F.; Newton, J.M. & James, M.B., (1997). Variations in the adhesion force between a drug and carrier particles as a result of changes in the relative humidity of the air. *Int J Pharm*, Vol. 149, pp. 151-160, ISSN: 0378-5173.

Prime, D.; Atkins, P.J.; Slater, A. & Sumby, B., (1997). Review of dry powder inhalers. *Adv Drug Deliv Rev*, Vol. 26, No. 1, pp. 51-58, ISSN: 0169-409X.

Rawat, A.; Majumder, Q.H. & Ahsan, F., (2008). Inhalable large porous microspheres of low molecular weight heparin: in vitro and in vivo evaluation. *J Control Release*, Vol. 128, No. 3, pp. 224-232, ISSN: 0168-3659.

Rytting, E.; Nguyen, J.; Wang, X. & Kissel, T., (2008). Biodegradable polymeric nanocarriers for pulmonary drug delivery. *Expert Opin Drug Deliv*, Vol. 5, No. 6, pp. 629-639   ISSN: 1742-5247.

Saint-Lorant, G.; Leterme, P.; Gayot, A. & Flament, M.P., (2007). Influence of carrier on the performance of dry powder inhalers. *Int J Pharm*, Vol. 334, No. 1, pp. 85-91, ISSN: 0378-5173.

Sakagami, M., (2006). In vivo, in vitro and ex vivo models to assess pulmonary absorption and disposition of inhaled therapeutics for systemic delivery. *Adv Drug Deliv Rev*, Vol. 58, No. 9, pp. 1030-1060, ISSN: 0169-409X.

Saleki-Gerhardt, A.; Ahlneck, C. & Zografi, G., (1994). Assessment of disorder in crystalline solids. *Int J Pharm*, Vol. 101, pp. 237-247, ISSN: 0378-5173.

Schiavone, H.; Palakodaty, S.; Clark, A.; York, P. & Tzannis, S.T., (2004). Evaluation of SCF-engineered particle-based lactose blends in passive dry powder inhalers. *Int J Pharm*, Vol. 281, No. 1, pp. 55-66, ISSN: 0378-5173.

Staniforth, J.N., (1996). Improvement in dry powder inhaler performance: surface passivation effects. *Drug Delivery to the Lungs VII*.

Steckel, H. & Bolzen, N., (2004). Alternative sugars as potential carriers for dry powder inhalations. *Int J Pharm*, Vol. 270, No. 1, pp. 297-306, ISSN: 0378-5173.

Steckel, H.; Markefka, P.; TeWierik, H. & Kammelar, R., (2004). Functionality testing of inhalation grade lactose. *Eur J Pharm Biopharm*, Vol. 57, No. 3, pp. 495-505, ISSN: 0939-6411.

Steckel, H. & Muller, B.W., (1997). In vitro evaluation of dry powder inhalers II: influence of carrier particle size and concentration on in vitro deposition. *Int J Pharm*, Vol. 154, No. 1, pp. 31-37, ISSN: 0378-5173.

Stoessl, A.J., (2008). Potential therapeutic targets for Parkinson's disease. *Expert Opin Ther Tar* Vol. 12, pp. 425-436, ISSN: 1472-8222.

Tang, P.; Chan, H.-K.; Chiou, H.; Ogawa, K.; Jones, M.D.; Adi, H. & Buckton, G., (2009). Characterisation and aerosolisation of mannitol particles produced via confined liquid impinging jets. *Int J Pharm*, Vol. 367, pp. 51-57, ISSN: 0378-5173.

Tee, S.K.; Marriott, C.; Zeng, X.M. & Martin, G.P., (2000). The use of different sugars as fine and coarse carriers for aerosolised salbutamol sulphate. *Int J Pharm*, Vol. 208, pp. 111-123., ISSN: 0378-5173.

Telko, M.J. & Hickey, A.J., (2005). Dry powder inhaler formulation. *Resp Care*, Vol. 50, No. pp. 1209-1227, ISSN: 0020-1324.

The Copley Scientific Limited, (2010). Quality Solutions for Inhaler Testing, inhaler testing equipment brochure, edition 2010.

Timsina, M.P.; Martin, G.P.; Marriott, C.; Ganderton, D. & Yianneskis, M., (1994). Drug delivery to the respiratory tract using dry powder inhalers. *Int J Pharm*, Vol. 101, No. 1-2, pp. 1-13, ISSN: 0378-5173.

Todo, H.; Okamoto, H.; Iida, K. & Danjo, K., (2001). Effect of additives on insulin absorption from intratracheally administered dry powders in rats. *Int J Pharm*, Vol. 220, pp. 101-110, ISSN: 0378-5173.

Traini, D.; Young, P.M.; Jones, M.; Edge, S. & Price, R., (2006). Comparative study of erythritol and lactose monohydrate as carriers for inhalation: Atomic force microscopy and in vitro correlation. *Eur J Pharm Sci*, Vol. 27, No. 2, pp. 243-251, ISSN: 0928-0987.

Ungaro, F.; d'Emmanuele di Villa Bianca, R.; Giovino, C.; Miro, A.; Sorrentino, R.; Quaglia, F. & La Rotonda, M.I., (2009). Insulin-loaded PLGA/cyclodextrin large porous particles with improved aerosolization properties: in vivo deposition and hypoglycaemic activity after delivery to rat lungs. *J Control Release*, Vol. 135, No. 1, pp. 25-34, ISSN: 0168-3659.

Ungaro, F.; Giovino, C.; Coletta, C.; Sorrentino, R.; Miro, A. & Quaglia, F., (2010). Engineering gas-foamed large porous particles for efficient local delivery of macromolecules to the lung. *Eur J Pharm Sci*, Vol. 41, pp. 60-70, ISSN: 0928-0987.

Ward, G.H. & Schultz, R.K., (1994). Process-induced crystallinity changes of albuterol sulphate and its effect on powder physical stability. *Pharm Res*, Vol. 12, pp. 773-779, ISSN: 0724-8741.

Ward, G.H. & Schultz, R.K., (1995). Processed-induced crystallinity changes in albuterol sulphate and its effect on powder physical stability. *Pharm Res*, Vol. 12, pp. 773-779, ISSN: 0724-8741.

Wolff, R.K. & Dorato, M.A., (1993). Toxicologic testing of inhaled pharmaceutical aerosols. *Crit Rev Toxicol*, Vol. 23 pp.343-369,

Yang, Y.; Bajaj, N.; Xu, P.; Ohn, K.; Tsifansky, M.D. & Yeo, Y., (2009). Development of highly porous large PLGA microparticles for pulmonary drug delivery. *Biomaterials*, Vol. 30, pp. 1947-1953, ISSN: 0142-9612.

Young, P.; Cocconi, D.; Colombo, P.; Bettini, R.; Price, R.; Steele, D. & Tobyn, M., (2002). Characterization of a surface modified dry powder inhalation carrier prepared by "particle smoothing". *J Pharm Pharmacol*, Vol. 54, No. 10, pp. 1339-1344, ISSN: 2042-7158.

Young, P.M.; Cocconi, D.; Colombo, P.; Bettini, R.; Price, R.; Steele, D.F. & Tobyn, M.J., (2002). Characterization of a surface modified dry powder inhalation carrier prepared by "particle smoothing". *J Pharm Pharmacol*, Vol. 54, pp. 1339-1344, ISSN: 0022-3573.

Young, P.M.; Kwok, P.; Adi, H.; Chan, H.-K. & Traini, D., (2009). Lactose composite carriers for respiratory delivery. *Pharm Res*, Vol. 26, No. 4, pp. 802-810, ISSN: 0724-8741.

Young, P.M. & Price, R., (2004). The influence of humidity on the aerolisation of micronised and SEDS produced salbutamol sulphate. , . *Eur J Pharm Sci*, Vol. 22, pp. 235-240, ISSN: 0928-0987.

Young, P.M.; Sung, A.; Traini, D.; Kwok, P.; Chiou, H. & Chan, H.K., (2007). Influence of humidity on the electrostatic charge and aerosol performance of dry powder inhaler carrier based systems. *Pharm Res*, Vol. 24, No. 5, pp. 963-970, ISSN: 0724-8741.

Zeng, X.M.; MacRitchie, H.B.; Marriott, C. & Martin, G.P., (2007). Humidity-induced changes of the aerodynamic properties of dry powder aerosol formulations containing different carriers. *Int J Pharm*, Vol. 333, No. 1, pp. 45-55, ISSN: 0378-5173.

Zeng, X.M.; Martin, G.P.; Marriott, C. & Pritchard, J., (2000). The effects of carrier size and morphology on the dispersion of salbutamol sulphate after aerosolization at different flow rates. *J Pharm Pharmacol*, Vol. 52, No. 10, pp. 1211-1221, ISSN: 0022-3573.

Zeng, X.M.; Martin, G.P.; Marriott, C. & Pritchard, J., (2000). The influence of carrier morphology on drug delivery by dry powder inhalers. *Int J Pharm*, Vol. 200 pp. 93-106, ISSN: 0378-5173.

Zeng, X.M.; Martin, G.P.; Marriott, C. & Pritchard, J., (2001). Lactose as a carrier in dry powder formulations: the influence of surface characteristics on drug delivery. *J Pharm Sci*, Vol. 90, No. 9, pp. 1424-1434, ISSN: 1520-6017.

Zeng, X.M.; Martin, G.P.; Marriott, C. & Pritchard, J., (2001). The use of lactose recrystallised from carbopol gels as a carrier for aerosolised salbutamol sulphate. *Eur J Pharm Biopharm* Vol. 51, No. 1, pp. 55-62, ISSN: 0939-6411.

Zeng, X.M.; Martin, G.P.; Marriott , C. & Pritchrd, J., (2000). The Influence of crystallization conditions on the morphology of lactose intended for use as a carrier for dry powder aerosols. *J Pharm Pharmacol*, Vol. 52, pp. 633-643, ISSN: 0022-3573.

Zeng, X.M.; Martin, G.P.; Tee, S.K. & Marriott, C., (1998). The role of fine particle lactose on the dispersion and deaggregation of salbutamol sulphate in an air stream in vitro. *Int J Pharm*, Vol. 176, No. 1, pp. 99-110, ISSN: 0378-5173.

Zeng, X.M.; Pandhal, K.H. & Martin, G.P., (2000). The influence of lactose carrier on the content homogeneity and dispersibility of beclomethasone dipropionate from dry powder aerosols. *Int J Pharm*, Vol. 197, pp. 41-52, ISSN: 0378-5173.

Zhou, Q.T. & Morton, D.A.V., (2011). Drug-lactose binding aspects in adhesive mixtures: controlling performance in dry powder Inhaler formulations by altering lactose carrier surfaces. *Adv Drug Deliv Rev,*Vol.64 , pp. 275–284 ISSN: 0169-409X.

Chapter 3

Hot-Melt Extrusion (HME): From Process to Pharmaceutical Applications

Mohammed Maniruzzaman, Dennis Douroumis,
Joshua S. Boateng and Martin J. Snowden

Additional information is available at the end of the chapter

1. Introduction

Over the last three decades hot-melt extrusion (HME) has emerged as an influential processing technology in developing molecular dispersions of active pharmaceutical ingredients (APIs) into polymers matrices and has already been demonstrated to provide time controlled, modified, extended and targeted drug delivery resulting in improved bioavailability [1, 2, 3, 4]. HME has now provided opportunity for use of materials in order to mask the bitter taste of active substances. Since industrial application of the extrusion process back in the 1930's HME has received considerable attention from both the pharmaceutical industry and academia in a range of applications for pharmaceutical dosage forms, such as tablets, capsules, films and implants for drug delivery through oral, transdermal and transmucosal routes [5]. This makes HME an excellent alternative to other conventionally available techniques such as roll spinning and spray drying. In addition to being a proven manufacturing process, HME meets the goal of the US Food and Drug Administration's (FDA) process analytical technology (PAT) scheme for designing, analyzing as well as controlling the manufacturing process through quality control measurements during active extrusion process [6]. In this chapter we review the hot-melt extrusion technique, based on a holistic perspective of its various components, processing technologies as well as the materials and novel formulation design and developments to its varied applications in oral drug delivery systems.

2. Hot-melt extrusion (HME): Process technology

Joseph Brama first invented the extrusion process for the manufacturing of lead pipes at the end of the eighteenth century [7]. Since then, it has been used in the plastic, rubber and food manufacturing industries to produce items ranging from pipes to sheets and bags. With the advent of high throughput screening, currently more than half of all plastic products including bags, sheets, and pipes are manufactured my HME and therefore various polymers have been used to melt and form different shapes for a variety of industrial and domestic applications. The technology (HME) has proven to be a robust method of producing numerous drug delivery systems and therefore it has been found to be useful in the pharmaceutical industry as well [8]. Extrusion is the process of pumping raw materials at elevated controlled temperature and pressure through a heated barrel into a product of uniform shape and density [9]. Breitenbach first introduced the development of melt extrusion process in pharmaceutical manufacturing operations [10], however, Follonier and his co-workers first examined the hot melt technology to manufacture sustained release polymer based pellets of various freely soluble drugs [11]. HME involves the compaction and conversion of blends from a powder or a granular mix into a product of uniform shape [9]. During this process, polymers are melted and formed into products of different shapes and sizes such as plastic bags, sheets, and pipes by forcing polymeric components and active substances including any additives or plasticisers through an orifice or die under controlled temperature, pressure, feeding rate and screw speed [9, 12]. However, the theoretical approach to understanding the melt extrusion process could be summarized by classifying the whole procedure of HME compaction into the followings [13]:

1. Feeding of the extruder through a hopper
2. Mixing, grinding, reducing the particle size, venting and kneading
3. Flow through the die.
4. Extrusion from the die and further down-stream processing.

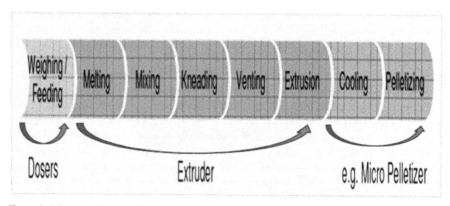

Figure 1. Schematic diagram of HME process [12].

The extruder generally consists of one or two rotating screws (either co-rotating or counter rotating) inside a stationary cylindrical barrel. The barrel is often manufactured in sections in order to shorten the residence time of molten materials. The sectioned parts of the barrel are then bolted or clamped together. An end-plate die is connected to the end of the barrel which is determined according to the shape of the extruded materials.

3. Equipment: Single screw and twin screw extruder

A single screw extruder consists of one rotating screw positioned inside a stationary barrel at the most fundamental level. In the more advanced twin-screw systems, extrusion of materials is performed by either a co-rotating or counter-rotating screw configuration [9]. Irrespective of type and complexity of the function and process, the extruder must be capable of rotating the screw at a selected predetermined speed while compensating for the torque and shear generated from both the material being extruded and the screws being used. However, regardless of the size and type of the screw inside the stationary barrel a typical extrusion set up consists of- a motor which acts as a drive unit, an extrusion barrel, a rotating screw and an extrusion die [13]. A central electronic control unit is connected to the extrusion unit in order to control the process parameters such as screw speed, temperature and therefore pressure [14]. This electronic control unit acts as a monitoring device as well. The typical length diameter ratios (L/D) of screws positioned inside the stationary barrel are another important characteristic to consider whether the extrusion equipment is a single screw or twin screw extruder. The L/D of the screw either in a single screw extruder or a twin screw extruder typically ranges from 20 to 40:1(mm). In case of the application of pilot plant extruders the diameters of the screws significantly ranges from 18-30 mm.   In pharmaceutical scale up, the production machines are much larger with diameters typically exceeding 50-60mm [15]. In addition, the dimensions of a screw change over the length of the barrel. In the most advanced processing equipment for extrusion, the screws could be separated by clamps or be extended in proportion to the length of the barrel itself. A basic single screw extruder consists of three discrete zones: feed zone, compression and a metering zone (Fig. 2). Under the compression zone which is basically know as processing zone could be accompanied by few other steps such as mixing, kneading, venting etc [13, 15].

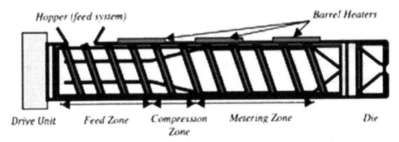

Figure 2. Schematic diagram of a single screw extruder [10].

The depth along with the pitch of the screw flights (both perpendicular and axial) differ within each zone, generating dissimilar pressures along the screw length (Fig. 3). Normally the pressure within the feed zone is very low in order to allow for consistent feeding from the hopper and gentle mixing of API, polymers and other excipients and therefore the screw flight depth and pitch are kept larger than that of other zones. At this stage of the process the pressure within the extruder is very low which subsequently gets increased in the compression zone. This results in a gradual increase in pressure along the length of the compression zone which effectively imparts a high degree of mixing and compression to the material by decreasing the screw pitch and/or the flight depth [9, 15]. Moreover the major aim of the compression zone is not only to homogenize but also compress the extrudate to ensure the molten material reaches the final section of the barrel (metering zone) in a form appropriate for processing. Finally the final section which is known as the metering zone stabilizes the effervescent flow of the matrix and ensures the extruded product has a uniform thickness, shape and size. A constant and steady uniform screw flight depth and pitch helps maintain continuous high pressure ensuring a uniform delivery rate of extrudates through the extrusion die and hence a uniform extruded product.

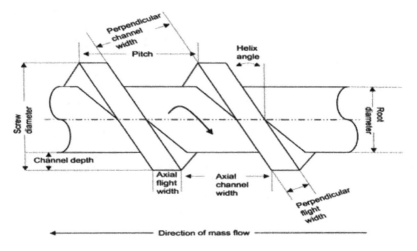

Figure 3. Screw geometry (extrusion) [9].

In addition to the above mentioned systems, downstream auxiliary equipment for cooling, cutting, collecting the finished product is also typically employed. Mass flow feeders to accurately meter materials into the feed hopper, pelletizers, spheronizer, roller/calendaring device in order to produce continuous films and process analytical technology such as near infra-red (NIR) and Raman, ultra sound, DSC systems are also options. Throughout the whole process, the temperature in all zones are normally controlled by electrical heating bands and monitored by thermocouples.

The single screw extrusion system is simple and offers lots of advantages but still does not acquire the mixing capability of a twin-screw machine and therefore is not the preferred approach for the production of most pharmaceutical formulations. Moreover, a twin-screw extruder offers much greater versatility (process manipulation and optimisation) in accommodating a wider range of pharmaceutical formulations making this set-up much more constructive. The rotation of the screws inside the extruder barrel may either be co-rotating (same direction) or counter-rotating (opposite direction), both directions being equivalent from a processing perspective. A greater degree of conveying and much shorter residence times are achievable with an intermeshing set-up. Furthermore, the use of reverse-conveying and forward-conveying elements, kneading blocks and other intricate designs as a means of improving or controlling the level of mixing required can help the configuration of the screws themselves to be varied [16].

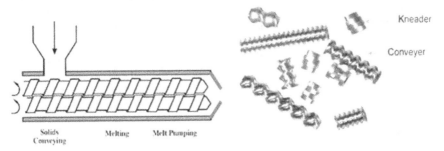

Figure 4. A twin screw extruder and screws [9].

4. Advantages of HME

HME offers several advantages over conventionally available pharmaceutical processing techniques including: (a) increased solubility and bioavailability of water insoluble compounds, (b) solvent free non ambient process, (c) economical process with reduced production time, fewer processing steps, and a continuous operation, (d) capabilities of sustained, modified and targeted release, (e) better content uniformity in extrudates, (f) no requirements on the compressibility of active ingredients, (g) uniform dispersion of fine particles, (h) good stability at changing pH and moisture levels and safe application in humans, (i) reduced number of unit operations and production of a wide range of performance dosage forms, and (j) a range of screw geometries [17, 18, 19, 20, 21].

However, HME has some disadvantages as well. The main drawbacks of HME include: thermal process (drug/polymer stability), limited polymers, high flow properties of polymers and excipients required and not suitable for relatively high heat sensitive molecules such as microbial species, proteins etc [20, 21].

5. Applications of HME

Extrusion technology is one of the most important fabrication processes in the plastic and rubber industries. Products made from melt extruded polymers range from pipes to hoses through to the insulated wires, cables, rubber sheeting and polystyrene tiles. Plastics that are commonly processed by HME technique include acrylics and cellulosics, polyethylene, poly propylene, polystyrene and vinyl plastics [9, 22]. In the food industry, extrusion has been utilized for pasta production with a widely used multitalented technique combines cooking and extrusion in a self-styled extrusion cooker [23]. In the animal feed industry and veterinary science, extrusion is commonly applied as a means of producing pelletized feeds, implants or injection moulding [24]. HME has successfully been applied in the formulation of fast dispersing PVP melt extrudates of poorly soluble active agents as solid molecular dispersions in the crop protection field [25].

HME technology has already achieved a strong place in the pharmaceutical industry and academia due to several advantages over traditional processing methods such as roll spinning, grinding [18]. In addition to being an efficient manufacturing process, HME enhances the quality and efficacy of manufactured products and therefore over the past few years HME has emerged as a novel technique in the pharmaceutical applications [15, 28]. The main use of HME is to disperse active pharmaceutical ingredients (APIs) in a matrix at the molecular level, thus forming solid solutions [26]. In the pharmaceutical industry, HME has been used for various applications, such as i) enhancing the dissolution rate and bioavailability of poorly soluble drug by forming a solid dispersion or solid solution, ii) controlling or modifying the release of the drug, iii) taste masking of bitter APIs, and iv) formulation of various thin films [27].

The bioavailability of an active ingredient is controlled by its aqueous solubility. Therefore increasing the solubility of water insoluble drugs is still a real challenge in the formulation development process [26]. Due to the advent of high throughput screening (HTS) in the drug discovery process, the resultant compounds are often high molecular weight and highly lipophilic and therefore exhibit poor solubility [29]. Scientists have already tried to address solubility issues by various pharmaceutical interventions. Among the many methods available to improve solubility and dissolution rate, preparation of solid dispersions and solid solutions has gained vast attention. For that reason HME has been successfully applied to prepare solid molecular dispersion of APIs into different hydrophilic polymer matrices [26, 29].

6. Formulation research and developments to dates

Despite the fact that initial research developments have focused on the effects of formulation and processing variables on the properties of the final dosage forms, [9, 30, 31, 34, 35] more recent investigations have focused on the use of HME as a novel manufacturing technology of solid molecular dispersions through to the development of mini-matrices, taste masked formulations and also sustained release formulations as well as paediatric formulations [26, 48]. Early work by De Brabander et al. (2000) described the preparation of matrix mini-tablets which was followed by further investigations into the properties of sustained release mini-matrices manufactured from ethyl cellulose, HPMC and ibuprofen [32, 33]. Extruded mini tablets showed minimised risk of dose dumping, reduced inter- and intra-subject variability. Very recently, Roblegg et al. (2011) reported the development of retarded release pellets using vegetable calcium stearate (CaSt) as a thermoplastic excipient processed through HME, where pellets with a drug loading of 20% paracetamol released only 11.54% of the drug after 8 hours due to the significant densification of the pellets. As expected, the drug release was influenced by the pellet size and the drug loading [36]. A microbicide intravaginal ring (IVRs) IVR was prepared and developed from polyether urethane (PU) elastomers for the sustained delivery of UC781 (a highly potent nonnucleoside reverse transcriptase inhibitor of HIV-1). PU IVRs containing UC781 were fabricated using a hot-melt extrusion process [37].

Moreover, a fourfold increase in the availability of propanolol in the systemic circulation was observed when the HME formulation was compared with a commercially available formulation (Inderal®). Over the last five years HME has been used largely to manufacture granules, pellets, immediate and modified release tablets, transmucosal/ transdermal films and implantable reservoir devices [3, 4, 9,35]. For instance, with respect to drug administration through the oral route, molecular solid dispersions of nifedipine [38], nimodipine [29] and itraconazole [39, 40,41] have been successfully produced using HME technology. Amorphous indomethacin dispersions have been manufactured using pharmaceutically acceptable hydrophilic polymers by using HME technology [26, 42,43].

Furthermore, HME research developments have driven targeted drug delivery systems including enteric matrix tablets and capsule systems over the last few years [44, 45]. Miller *et al.* (2007) have demonstrated the ability of HME to act as an efficient dispersive process for aggregated, fine engineering particles to improve dissolution rate properties by enhancing particles' wettability [46]. A very interesting investigation of Verreck and co-workers (2006) [47] determined the use of supercritical carbon dioxide (scCO2) as a temporary plasticiser during the manufacture of ethylcellulose through HME. A significant reduction in the processing temperature was achieved using scCO2 without any disadvantageous effects on the extrudate. Macroscopic morphology was significantly altered due to expansion of the scCO2 in the die. The use of scCO2 increased the surface area, porosity and hygroscopicity of the final dosage forms. More recently Douroumis and co-workers used HME technique to effectively enhance the solubility of ibuprofen, indomethacin and famotidine [26, 42].

The taste masking of bitter APIs is a major challenge especially for the development of orally disintegrating tablets (ODT). HME has been reported to be an effective technique to mask the bitter tastes of various APIs by the use of taste masking polymers that create solid dispersions to prevent bitter drugs from coming in contact with the patient's taste buds. Breitkruitz et al. (2008) successfully applied HME in taste masking of sodium benzoate for the formulation of paediatric drugs [48]. More recently Grycze *et al.* (2011) and Maniruzzaman *et al.* (2012) developed taste masked formulations of ibuprofen and paracetamol, respectively [26, 48]. Basically taste masking is achieved through intermolecular forces (e.g. hydrogen bonding) between the active substance and the polymer matrix by processing oppositely charged compounds through HME [49, 50]. The extrusion of solid lipids using twin–screw extruders was introduced for the preparation of immediate or sustained release taste masked matrices [51]. In this process, occasionally called "solvent – free cold extrusion" the lipids are extruded below their melting ranges. Consequently, the lipids are not melted during extrusion and build a coherent matrix with low porosity. In these few studies the effect of lipid composition and processing parameters such as the die diameter, the size of the extruded pellets, the screw speed and the powder feeding rates on the obtained drug release patterns were thoroughly investigated. Very recently, Breitkreutz *et al.* (2012) applied solid lipid extrusion at room temperature for the taste masked formulation development of the BCS Class II drug NXP 1210. In this study, the authors investigated powdered hard fat (Witocan® 42/44 mikrofein), glycerol distearate (Precirol® ato 5) and glycerol trimyristate (Dynasan® 114) as lipid binders. The lipid based formulations design in this study was feasible for taste-masked granules or pellets containing poorly soluble drugs [52].

6.1. Films by hot-melt extrusion

Only a handful of researchers have reported the use of hot-melt extrusion for the manufacture of films. Films can be defined as thin sheets containing one or more polymers with or without a plasticiser and may be used as a drug delivery system (device) or directly applied to facilitate a therapeutic effect as in wound dressings. Films are currently being produced mainly by solvent casting in which polymers (and excipients such as plasticisers) are dissolved in a suitable solvent until they form clear viscous solution (gel). While film preparation using the solvent–casting approach allows film uniformity, clarity, flexibility and adjustable thickness to accommodate drug loadings they are limited by decreased elongation or elasticity and increased film tensile strength when physical aging is applied [53]. Another, limitation associated with solvent cast films is the use of organic solvents for water insoluble polymers. The hazardous nature of most organic solvents and the residual solvents after drying affect the selection of the appropriate solvent [54–57] as well as complicated processing conditions and disposal of the associated waste, all of which create significant environmental concerns. As a result, alternative technologies are needed in the pharmaceutical industry to overcome some of challenges described above. The two commonly used approaches include spray coating and hot melt extrusion with the latter becoming increasingly popular due to the many advantages it provides. Firstly, no solvents are used and fewer processing steps are required. In fact one of the key advantages of HME is the fact that extrudates can be obtained in a single processing step making it very economical. As far as films are concerned, there is no requirement for compressing of the active ingredients together with the excipients. The melting of the polymer into the molten state, coupled with the thorough initial mixing allows a more uniform dispersion of fine particles. Further, molecular dispersion of the drug helps improve its bioavailability [58]. Hot melt extruded films are produced through a simple process involving blending of appropriate amounts relevant polymer, drug and plasticiser into a uniform powdered mixture prior to feeding through the hopper of the preheated extruder and transferred into the heated barrel by a rotating extruder screw. Homogeneous films are obtained with thickness generally expected to be in the range less than 1mm. Generally three main ingredients are required for successful formulation of hot melt films i.e. film forming polymer, active ingredient and plasticiser [59]. The latter is required to impart flexibility to the final film which ensures ease of handling and application to the site of action. Occasionally, other additives are added to affect other functionally important properties such as bioadhesive agent which ensures that the film adheres to the mucosal surface for a long enough time to allow drug absorption or action. Different polymers and drugs have been employed and reported in the literature for obtaining drug loaded hot-melt extruded films for various indications and are summarised in table 1.

Film	Main polymer(s)	Plasticiser/additive	Main active ingredient(s)	Author
1	Acrylic Eudragit	- Triacetin - Triethylcitrate	Lidocaine	[60]
2	Hydroxypropylcellulose Polyethylene oxide	N/A	Ketoconazole	[61]
3	Hydroxypropylcellulose Hydroxypropylmethylcellulose Polyethylene oxide	Polyethylene glycol 3350	Lidocaine	[62]
4	Hydroxypropylcellulose	Polyethylene glycol 400	Hydrocortisone	[65]
5	Hydroxypropylcellulose Polycarbophil	Polyethylene glycol 3350	Clotrimazole	[58]
6	Polyethylene oxide	N/A	Ketoprofen	[59]

Table 1. Different hot-melt extruded films comprising different polymeric materials, plasticisers and active ingredients for various indications.

Repka and co-workers have conducted extensive research on the use of HME for the manufacture of mucoadhesive buccal films. They successfully evaluated different matrix formers and additives for the processing of the blend prior to extrusion [61, 62, 63, 64]. In an early investigation, it was found that even though films containing exclusively HPC could not be obtained, the addition of plasticizers, such as triethyl citrate, PEG 2000/8000, or acetyltributyl citrate, allowed for the manufacture of thin, flexible, and stable HPC films [65]. It has also been found that increasing the molecular weight of HPC decreased the release of drugs from hot-melt extruded films which resulted in dissolution profiles exhibiting zero-order drug release. According to the models applied in the research, the drug release was solely determined by erosion of the buccal film [66, 67, 68].

Development of films by HME may present future opportunities to develop gastro-retentive films for prolonged drug delivery and multi-layer films to modulate drug release for oral and transdermal applications. The growing market in medical devices, including incorporating drugs such as biodegradable stents and drug-loaded catheters will undoubtedly require HME manufacturing processes. These are required to be commercialised and perhaps may lead to new areas of collaboration across pharmaceutical, medical device and biotechnology research.

7. HME in commercial products

HME related patents which have been issued for pharmaceutical systems have steadily increased since the early 1980's. So far, the USA and Germany hold approximately more than half (56%) of all issued patents for HME in the market [69]. Despite this increased interest, only a handful of commercialized HME pharmaceutical products are currently marketed. Several companies have been recognized to specialize in the use of HME as a drug delivery technology, such as PharmaForm and SOLIQS (Abbott). Recently, SOLIQS has developed a proprietary formulation which is known as Meltrex® and re-developed a protease-inhibitor combination product, Kaletra®. Kaletra is mainly used for the treatment of human immunodeficiency virus (HIV) infections. The formulated, melt extruded product was shown to have a significant enhancement in the bioavailability of active substances [70]. Furthermore, HME Kaletra® tablets were shown to have significant advantages for patient compliance (i.e. reduced dosing frequency and improved stability) compared to the previous soft-gel capsule formulation as recognized by the FDA decision to fast-track approval. Additionally, Nurofen (Meltlets® lemon) is available on the market as a fast dissolving tablet prepared by HME [42]. Ibuprofen has been used as active substance in the Meltlets® tablets where its bitter taste was successfully masked by similar technique to HME. Moreover, SOLIQS has also developed a fast-onset ibuprofen system and a sustained-release formulation of verapamil (Isoptin® SR-E) through a HME related technology called 'Calendaring' that was the first directly shaped HME product on the market.

8. Summary

HME has proven to be a robust method of producing numerous drug delivery systems and therefore it has been found to be useful in the pharmaceutical industry enlarging the scope to include a range of polymers and APIs that can be processed with or without plasticizers. It has also been documented that HME is a solvent-free, robust, quick and economy favoured manufacturing process for the production of a large variety of pharmaceutical dosage forms.

Author details

Mohammed Maniruzzaman *, Dennis Douroumis, Joshua S. Boateng and Martin J. Snowden
School of Science, University of Greenwich, Central Avenue, Chatham Maritime, Chatham, Kent, ME4 4TB, UK

9. References

[1] Maniruzzaman M, Boateng JS, Bonnefille M, Aranyos A, Mitchell JC, Douroumis D. Taste Masking of Paracetamol by Hot Melt Extrusion: an *in vitro* and *in vivo* evaluation. Euro J Pharm Biopharm 2012;80(2):433-42.

[2] Repka MA, Shah S, Lu J, Maddineni S, Morott J, Patwardhan K, Mohammed NN. Melt extrusion: process to product. Expert Opin Drug Deliv 2012; 9(1):105-25.

[3] Repka MA, Majumdar S, Kumar Battu S, Srirangam R, Upadhye SB. Applications of hot-melt extrusion for drug delivery. Expert Opin Drug Deliv 2008; 5(12):1357-76.

---

* Corresponding Author

[4] Repka MA, Battu SK, Upadhye SB, Thumma S, Crowley MM, Zhang F, Martin C, McGinity JW. Pharmaceutical applications of hot-melt extrusion: Part II. Drug Dev Ind Pharm 2007; (10):1043-57.

[5] Crowley MM, Thumma S, Updhye SB. Pharmaceutical applications of hot melt extrusion: part-1. Drug Dev Ind Pharm 2007; 33(9):909-26.

[6] Charlie M. Continuous mixing of solid dosage forms via Hot-Melt Extrusion. Pharm Tech 2008; 32(10):76-86.

[7] James S. Encyclopedia of Pharmaceutical Technology. 2004; 3rd Ed (3); P-20.

[8] Andrews GP and Jones DS. Formulation and Characterization of Hot Melt Extruded Dosage Forms: Challenges and Opportunities. Cheminform 2010; 41(43).

[9] Breitenbach J. Melt extrusion: from process to drug delivery technology. Eur J Pharm and Biopharm 2002 54:107–117.

[10] Andrews GP, David S, Osama AM, Daniel NM, Mark.S. Hot Melt Extrusion: An Emerging Drug Delivery Technology. Pharm Tech Europe 2009; 21 (1):24-27.

[11] Follonier N, Doelker E, Cole ET. Evaluation of hot-melt extrusion as a new technique for the production of polymerbased pellets for sustained release capsules containing high loadings of freely soluble drugs. Drug Dev Ind Pharm 1994; 20(8):1323-133.

[12] Gryczke A. Melt Extrusion with EUDRAGIT® Solubility Enhancement Modified Release. Degussa. RÖHM GmbH & Co. KG, Darmstadt. 2006-06-13.

[13] Chokshi R, Zia H. Hot-Melt Extrusion Technique: A Review. Iranian J of Pharm Res 2004; 3: 3-16.

[14] Whelan T, Dunning D (Eds.). The Dynisco Extrusion Processors Handbook 1st ed., London School of Polymer Technology 1988, Polytechnic of North London, London.

[15] Andrews GP, Margetson DN, Jones DS, McAllister SM, Diak OA. A basic Guide: Hot-melt Extrusion. UKICRS 2008; Vol.13.

[16] White JL. Twin Screw Extrusion: Technology and Principles Hanser/ Gardner Publications Inc. 1991; Cincinnati, Ohio. ISBN 1-56990-109-0.

[17] http://www.pharinfo.net/reviews/melt granulation techniques/reviews.

[18] McGnity JW, KOleng JJ. Preparation and Evaluation of Rapid Release Granules Using Novel Melt Extrusion Technique. AAPS.org.2004; 153-54.

[19] Jones DS. Engineering Drug Delivery Using Polymer Extrusion/Injection Moulding Technologies. School of Pharmacy, Queen's University, Belfast: 2008; 4-9, 18, 25, 27.

[20] Grunhagen HH, Muller O. Melt extrusion technology. Pharm. Manu. Int.1995 1, 167–170.

[21] Singhal S, Lohar VK, Arora V. Hot-melt extrusion technique. WebmedCentral Pharmaceutical Sciences 2011;2(1): 001459

[22] Mollan M. Historical overview, in: I. Ghebre-Sellassie, C. Martin (Eds.), Pharmaceutical Extrusion Technology, CRC Press 2003; pp. 1–18.

[23] Senouci A, Smith A, Richmond A. Extrusion cooking, Chem. Eng. 417 (1985) 30–33.

[24] Sebestyen E. Flour and animal feed milling 1974; 10;24–25.

[25] Wedlock DJ, Wijngaarden DV. Fast dispersing solid PVP-containing crop protection formulation and process therefore, US Patent 1992; 5,665,369.

[26] Maniruzzaman M, Rana M, Boateng JS, Douroumis D. Dissolution enhancement of indomethacin and famotidine processed by hot-melt extrusion. Drug developments and Ind Pharmacy 2012; In press.

[27] Morales JO, McConville JT. Manufacture and characterization of mucoadhesive buccal films. European Journal of Pharmaceutics and Biopharmaceutics 2011; 77;187–199.

[28] M. Repka, M. Munjal, M. ElSohly, S. Ross. Temperature stability and bioadhesive properties of D9-tetrahydrocannabinol incorporated hydroxypropylcellulose polymer matrix systems, Drug Development and Industrial Pharmacy 2006; 32: 21–32.

[29] Zheng X, Yang R, Tang X and Zheng L. Part I: Characterization of Solid Dispersions of Nimodipine Prepared by Hot-melt Extrusion. Drug Development and Industrial Pharmacy 2007; 33:791–802.

[30] M.A. Repka, S.K. Battu, S.B. Upadhye, S. Thumma, M.M. Crowley, F. Zhang, C. Martin, J.W. McGinity, Pharmaceutical applications of hot-melt extrusion: Part II, Drug Development and Industrial Pharmacy 2007; 33:1043–1057.

[31] Cilurzo F, Cupone I, Minghetti P, Selmin F, Montanari L. Fast dissolving films made of maltodextrins, European Journal of Pharmaceutics and Biopharmaceutics 2008; 70: 895-900.

[32] De Brabander C, Vervaet C, Fiermans L, Remon JP. Matrix mini-tablets based on starch/microcrystalline wax mixtures. Int J Pharm 2000; 199: 195-203.

[33] De Brabander C, Vervaet C, Remon JP. Development and evaluation of sustained release mini-matrices prepared via hot melt extrusion. J Cont Rel 2003; 89: 235–247.

[34] Zhang F, McGinity JW. Properties of sustained-release tablets prepared by hot-melt extrusion. Pharmaceut Dev Tech 1999; 4(2), 241–250.

[35] Crowley MM, Zhang F, Koleng JJ, McGinity JW. Stability of polyethylene oxide in matrix tablets prepared by hot-melt extrusion. Biomaterials 2002; 23: 4241-4248.

[36] Roblegg E, Jäger E, Hodzic A, Koscher G, Mohr S, Zimmer A, Khinast J. Development of sustained-release lipophilic calcium stearate pellets via hot melt extrusion. Eur Jl Pharms and Biopharms 2011; 79:635–645.

[37] Clark MR, Johnson TJ, McCabe RT, Clark JT, Tuitupou A, Elgendy H, Friend DR, Kiser PF. A hot-melt extruded intravaginal ring for the sustained delivery of the antiretroviral microbicide UC781.J Pharm Sci 2011. In Press

[38] Li L, AbuBaker O, Shao Z, (2006). Characterization of poly(ethylene oxide) as a drug carrier in hot-melt extrusion. Drug Dev Ind Pharm 2006; 32: 991–1002.

[39] Rambali B, Verreck G, Baert L, Massart DL. Itraconazole formulation studies of the melt-extrusion process with mixture design. Drug Dev Pharm 2003; 29(6): 641–652.

[40] Six K, Berghmans H, Leuner C, Dressman J, Van Werde K, Mullens J, Benoist L, Thimon M, Meublat L, Verreck G, Peeters J, Brewster M, Van den Mooter G. Characterization of solid dispersions of itraconazole and hydroxypropylmethylcellulose prepared by melt extrusion, Part II. Pharm Res 2003; 20(7): 1047–1054.

[41] Six K, Daems T, de Hoon J, Van Hecken A, Depre M, Bouche MP, Prinsen P, Verreck G, Peeters J, Brewster ME, Van den Mooter G. Clinical study of solid dispersions of itraconazole prepared by hot-stage extrusion. Eur J Pharm Sci 2005; 24(2–3): 179–186.

[42] Grycze A, Schminke GS, Maniruzzaman M, Beck J, Douroumis D. Development and evaluation of orally disintegrating tablets (ODTs) containing ibuprofen granules prepared by hot melt extrusion. Colloids Surf B Biointerface 2011; 86: pp. 275-84.

[43] Chokshi RJ, Shah NHS, Sandhu KH, Malick AW, Zia H. Stabilization of Low Glass Transition Temperature Indomethacin Formulations: Impact of Polymer-Type and Its Concentration. Journal of Pharmaceutical Sciences 2007, Published online in Wiley InterScience (www.interscience.wiley.com). DOI 10.1002 jps.21174

[44] Andrews GP, Jones DS, Abu Diak O, McCoy CP, Watts AB, McGinity JW (In press). The manufacture and characterization of hot melt extruded enteric tablets. Eur J Pharm Biopharm 2008; 69(1):264-73.

[45] Mehuys E, Remon JP, Vervaet C. Production of enteric capsules by means of hot-melt extrusion. Eur J Pharm Sci 2005; 24: 207-212.

[46] Miller DA, Jason TM, Yang W, Robert OW, McGinity JW. Hot-Melt Extrusion for Enhanced Delivery of Drug Particles. J Pharm Sci 2007, 96(2): 361-376.

[47] Verreck G, Decorte A, Heymans K, Adriaensen J, Liu D, Tomasko D, Arien A, Peeters J, Van den Mooter G, Brewster ME. Hot stage extrusion of p-amino salicylic acid with EC using CO2 as a temporary plasticizer. Int J Pharm 2006; 327: 45-50.

[48] Breitkreutz J, El-Saleh F, Kiera C, Kleinebudde P, Wiedey W. Pediatric drug formulations of sodium benzoate: II. Coated granules with a lipophilic binder. Eur. J. Pharm. Biopham 2003; 56, pp. 255-60.

[49] Douroumis D. Practical approaches of taste masking technologies in oral solid forms. Expert Opin. Drug Deliv 2007; 4 , pp. 417–426.

[50] Douroumis D. Orally disintegrating dosage forms and taste-masking technologies. Expert Opin Drug Deliv 2010; 8, pp. 665-75.

[51] Breitkreutz J, El Saleh F, Kiera C, Kleinebudde P, Wiedey W. Pediatric drug formulations of sodium benzoate II. Coated granules with a lipophilic binder. Eur. J. Pharm. Biopharm. 2003, 56: 255–260.

[52] Vaassena J, Bartscherb K, Breitkreutza J. Taste masked lipid pellets with enhanced release of hydrophobic active Ingredient. Int. J. Pharm 2012, 429:99– 103.

[53] Gutierrez-Rocca JC, McGinity JW. Influence of aging on the physical-mechanical properties of acrylic resin films cast from aqueous dispersions and organic solutions. Drug Development and Industrial Pharmacy 1993, 19:315–332.

[54] Steuernagel CR. Latex emulsions for controlled drug delivery. In McGinity JW. (Ed.), Aqueous polymeric coatings for pharmaceutical dosage forms (Vol. 79, pp. 582). New York: Marcel Dekker Inc.1997

[55] Barnhart S, Thin film oral dosage forms, in: Rathbone MJ, Hadgraft J, Roberts MS, Lane ME (Eds.), Modified-release Drug Delivery Technology, Informa Healthcare, 2008:209–216.

[56] International Conference on Harmonization, ICH topic Q3C(R3) Impurities: Residual Solvents, 2009.
<http://www.emea.europa.eu/pdfs/human/ich/028395en.pdf>.

[57] Morales JO, McConvill JT. Manufacture and characterization of mucoadhesive buccal films. Eur J Pharm Biopharm.2011, 77:187-99.

[58] Repka MA, McGinity JW, Zhang F, Koleng JJ. Encyclopedia of pharmaceutical technology, in: J. Boylan (ed.), Marcel Dekker, NewYork, 2002.

[59] Venkat S. Tumuluri, Mark S. Kemper, Ian R. Lewis, Suneela Prodduturi,[c] Soumyajit Majumdar, Bonnie A. Avery, and Michael A. Repka Off-line and On-line Measurements of Drug-loaded Hot-Melt Extruded Films Using Raman Spectroscopy.

[60] Mididoddi PK, Repka MA. Characterization of hot-melt extruded drug delivery systems for onychomycosis. Eur J Pharm Biopharm. 2007, 66:95–105.

[61] Prodduturi S, Manek R, Kolling W, Stodghill S, Repka M. Solid-state stability and characterization of hot-melt extruded poly(ethylene oxide) films, Journal of Pharmaceutical Sciences 2005; 94:2232–2245.

[62] Repka M, Gutta K, Prodduturi S, Munjal M, Stodghill S. Characterization of cellulosic hot-melt extruded films containing lidocaine, European Journal of Pharmaceutics and Biopharmaceutics 2005; 59:189–196.

[63] Repka M, McGinity J. Bioadhesive properties of hydroxypropylcellulose topical films produced by hot-melt extrusion, Journal of Controlled Release 2001; 70:341–351.

[64] Thumma S, Majumdar S, ElSohly M, Gul W, Repka M. Preformulation studies of a prodrug of D9-tetrahydrocannabinol, AAPS Pharmaceutical Science and Technology 2008a; 9:982–990.

[65] Repka M, Gerding T, Repka S, McGinity J. Influence of plasticizers and drugs on the physical–mechanical properties of hydroxypropylcellulose films prepared by hot melt extrusion, Drug Development and Industrial Pharmacy 1999; 25:625–633.

[66] Prodduturi S, Manek R, Kolling W, Stodghill S, Repka M. Water vapour sorption of hot-melt extruded hydroxypropyl cellulose films: effect on physico-mechanical properties, release characteristics, and stability, Journal of Pharmaceutical Sciences 2004; 93: 3047–3056.

[67] Kopcha M, Tojo KJ, Lordi NG. Evaluation of methodology for assessing release characteristics of thermosoftening vehicles, Journal of Pharmacy and Pharmacology 1990; 42: 745–751.

[68] Thumma S, ElSohly M, Zhang S, Gul W, Repka M. Influence of plasticizers on the stability and release of a prodrug of [Delta]9-tetrahydrocannabinol incorporated in poly (ethylene oxide) matrices, European Journal of Pharmaceutics and Biopharmaceutics 2008b; 70 :605–614.

[69] Crowley MM., Zhang F, Repka MA, Thumma S, Upadhye SB, Battu SK, McGinity J, Martin C. Pharmaceutical Applications of Hot- Melt Extrusion: Part I. Drug Development and Industrial Pharmacy 2007; 33: 909-926.

[70] Klein CE, Chiu Y, Awni W, Zhu T, Heuser RS, Doan T, Breitenbach J, Morris JB, Brun SC, Hanna GJ. The tablet formulation of lopinavir/ritonavir provides similar bioavailability to the soft-gelatin capsule formulation with less pharmacokinetic variability and diminished food effect. J Acquir Immune Defic Syndr 2007; 44: 401-410.

Nanocarriers in Drug Delivery

Chapter 4

Nanotechnology in Drug Delivery

Martins Ochubiojo Emeje, Ifeoma Chinwude Obidike,
Ekaete Ibanga Akpabio and Sabinus Ifianyi Ofoefule

Additional information is available at the end of the chapter

1. Introduction

Nanoscience has been variously defined at different fora, books, journals and the web, yet one thing is common; it involves the study of the control of matter on an atomic and molecular scale. This molecular level investigation is at a range usually below 100 nm. In simple terms, a nanometer is one billionth of a meter and the properties of materials at this atomic or subatomic level differ significantly from properties of the same materials at larger sizes. Although, the initial properties of nanomaterials studied were for its physical, mechanical, electrical, magnetic, chemical and biological applications, recently, attention has been geared towards its pharmaceutical application, especially in the area of drug delivery.

This is because of the challenges with use of large size materials in drug delivery, some of which include poor bioavailability, in vivo stability, solubility, intestinal absorption, sustained and targeted delivery to site of action, therapeutic effectiveness, generalized side effects, and plasma fluctuations of drugs. Of recent, several researches in nanodrug delivery have been designed to overcome these challenges through the development and fabrication of nanostructures. It has been reported that, nanostructures have the ability to protect drugs from the degradation in the gastrointestinal tract, the technology can allow target delivery of drugs to various areas of the body. The technology enables the delivery of drugs that are poorly water soluble and can provide means of bypassing the liver, thereby preventing the first pass metabolism Nanotechnology increases oral bioavailability of drugs due to their specialized uptake mechanisms such as absorptive endocytosis and are able to remain in the blood circulation for a long time, releasing the incorporated drug in a controlled fashion, leading to less plasma fluctuations and minimized side-effects. Nanoscale size nanostructures are able to penetrate tissues and are easily taken up by cells, allowing for efficient delivery of drugs to target sites of action. Uptake of nanostructures has been reported to be 15–250 times greater than that of microparticles in the 1–10 um range. Nanotechnology improves performance and acceptability of dosage forms by increasing their effectiveness, safety, patient adherence, as well as ultimately reducing health care costs. It may also enhance the performance of drugs that are unable to pass clinical trial phases. Nanotechnology definitely promises to serve as drug delivery carrier of choice for the more challenging conventional drugs used for the treatment and management of chronic diseases such as cancer, asthma, hypertension, HIV and diabetes.

2. Nanotechnology-based drug delivery systems

2.1. Smart drug delivery systems

Ideally, nanoparticulate drug delivery system should selectively accumulate in the required organ or tissue and at the same time, penetrate target cells to deliver the bioactive agent. It has been suggested (1, 2) that, organ or tissue accumulation could be achieved by the passive or antibody-mediated active targeting (3, 4), while the intracellular delivery could be mediated by certain ligands (5, 6) or by cell-penetrating peptides (7, 8). Thus, a drug delivery system (DDS) should be multifunctional and possess the ability to switch on and switch off certain functions when necessary. Another important requirement is that different properties of the multifunctional DDS are coordinated in an optimal fashion. Thus, for example, if the system is to be constructed that can provide the combination of the longevity allowing for the target accumulation and specific cell surface binding allowing, two requirements must be met; the half-life of the carrier in the circulation should be long enough and second, the internalization of the DDS by the target cells should proceed fast enough not to allow for the carrier degradation and drug loss in the interstitial space. Intracellular transport of bioactive molecules is one of the key problems in drug delivery. Nanoparticulate DDS, such as liposomes and micelles, are frequently used to increase the efficacy of drug and DNA delivery and targeting (9, 10). So far, very few successful attempts have been made to deliver various drug carriers directly into the cell cytoplasm, bypassing the endocytic pathway, to protect drugs and DNA from the lysosomal degradation, thus enhancing drug efficiency and DNA incorporation into the cell genome (11-14). Within the multifunctional DDS, it has been postulated that, the development of a DDS built in such a way that during the first phase of delivery, a nonspecific cell-penetrating function is shielded by the organ/tissue-specific delivery will be possible. Upon accumulating in the target, protecting polymer or antibody attached to the surface of the DDS via the stimuli-sensitive bond should detach under the action of local pathological conditions such as abnormal pH or temperature and expose the previously hidden second function allowing for the subsequent delivery of the carrier and its cargo inside cells. While such DDS should be stable in the blood for a long time to allow for an efficient target accumulation, it has to lose the protective coat inside the target almost instantly to allow for fast internalization thereby minimizing the washing away of the released drug or DNA. Intracellular trafficking, distribution, and fate of the carrier and its cargo can be additionally controlled by its charge and composition, which can drive it to the nuclear compartment or toward other cell organelles.

It has been reported within the past few years, that certain proteins and peptides (such as TAT peptide) can enter cell cytoplasm directly and even target cell nuclei (15, 16). Certain proteins and peptides have also been used for the intracellular delivery of small drug molecules, large molecules (enzymes, DNA), and nanoparticulates (quantum dots, iron oxide nanoparticles, liposomes) (13, 17-22). The mechanism of this phenomenon is currently a subject of investigation, although important progress has been made, as some reports show that electrostatic interactions and hydrogen bonding lay behind certain proteins and peptides-mediated direct transduction of small molecules (23, 24), while the energy-dependent macropinocytosis is responsible for certain proteins and peptides-mediated intracellular delivery of large molecules and nanoparticulates with their subsequent enhanced release from endosomes into the cell cytoplasm (25 – 28).

One of the most outstanding achievements in the drug delivery field was the development of smart drug delivery systems (SDDSs), also called stimuli-sensitive delivery systems. The concept is based on rapid transitions of a physicochemical property of polymer systems upon a stimulus. This stimulus includes physical (temperature, mechanical stress, ultrasound, electricity, light), chemical (pH, ionic strength), or biological (enzymes, biomolecules) signals and such stimuli can either be internal, resulting from changes in the physiological condition of a living subject, or "external" signals, artificially induced to provoke desired events. SDDS provides a programmable and predictable drug release profile in response to various stimulation sources. Fig 1 below shows a typical smart drug delivery system;

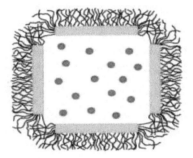

Figure 1. Smart drug delivery system -- Gold nanocage covered with polymer

Depending on the desired applications, one may design different drug delivery systems for enhanced therapeutic efficiency with low systemic toxicity and side effects. SDDS has several advantages compared to conventional drug delivery systems. The conventional controlled release systems are based on the predetermined drug release rate irrespective of the environmental condition at the time of application. On the other hand, SDDS is based on the release-on-demand strategy, allowing a drug carrier to liberate a therapeutic drug only when it is required in response to a specific stimulation. The best example of SDDS has been self-regulated insulin delivery systems that can respond to changes in the environmental glucose level (29, 30). One of the most widely used SDDSs has been polymeric micelles. Many polymeric micelles consisting of hydrophobic and hydrophilic polymer blocks have been developed. They have been found to dissolve water-insoluble drugs, such as doxorubicin or paclitaxel, at high concentrations. When administered to the body, drug release from polymeric micelles usually depends on simple diffusion, degradation of the micelle blocks, or disruption of the micelles by body components.

The release kinetics of the loaded drug can be modulated by varying the degradation rate of hydrophobic polymer blocks, but because the degradation rate is usually very slow, the loaded drug is released by diffusion from polymeric micelles. This slow release by passive diffusion may not be desirable, as the polymeric micelles reaching the target site need to release their contents fast. To solve this problem, smart polymeric micelles have been designed to liberate the loaded therapeutic agent at the targeted site fast. For example, Lee et al, (31) reported that Poly (ethylene glycol)-b-polyhistidine (PEG-b-PHis) forms micelles only over the pKb of the polyhistidine block (pH 6.5–7.0). It is interesting to know that, the pKb can be adjusted by varying the molecular weight of polyhistidine. Since solid tumors have a slightly acidic environment, a small reduction in pH to less than 7 at the tumor site triggers dissociation of the polymeric micelle to release its contents. In a separate study, Lee et al (32) reported that, PEG-b- polyhistidine micelles containing doxorubicin effectively killed multi-drug resistant MCF-7 cells at pH 6.8. Similarly, Hruby et al, (33) reported that, SDDS can achieve a highly localized drug accumulation at target sites even though it is administered parenterally. It is therefore postulated that, SDDS with enhanced targeting property is highly promising in increasing the efficiency and efficacy of therapy while at the same time minimizing side effects.

2.2. Polymer–drug conjugates

Polymer–drug conjugates are a class of polymer therapeutics that consists of a water-soluble polymer that is chemically conjugated to a drug through a biodegradable linker. The idea started in 1975 when Ringsdorf proposed the use of polymer–drug conjugates to deliver hydrophobic small molecules (34). The reasoning was that, small molecule drugs, especially hydrophobic compounds, have a low aqueous solubility and a broad tissue distribution profile such that, administration of the free drug may result in serious side effects. Therefore, conjugation of these compounds to hydrophilic, biocompatible polymers would significantly increase their aqueous solubility, modify their tissue distribution profile and enhance their plasma circulation half-life. An important attribute of colloidal systems is their hydrodynamic diameter, which are typically about 3–20 nm for polymer–drug conjugates (35) and between 10 and 200 nm for colloidal particles such as micelles or liposomes. The colloidal nature or size of these vehicles can facilitate their retention within the circulation for prolonged periods, in comparison to low molecular weight small molecules. One major difference between polymer–drug conjugates and delivery systems that contain physically entrapped drug (e.g., micelles and liposomes) is that the drug is chemically conjugated to the polymer and therefore these systems qualify as new chemical entities (NCE). Classification as an NCE is often accompanied by additional development and regulatory hurdles that must be met in order to receive approval. Over the last decade, polymer-conjugate technology has proven to be a viable formulation strategy. There have been reports (36 – 38) of bioconjugation of protein and peptide to PEG been able to significantly improve the efficacy of these macro- molecular drugs by increasing their stability in the presence of proteases and decreasing their immunogenicity. Studies have also shown that by using PEG in a specific molecular weight range, the fast renal clearance and mononuclear phagocytic system uptake of the drugs can be prevented or delayed leading to a prolonged plasma half-life for the conjugated molecules. Successful applications have led to several FDA- approved products e.g. Neulasta®. The first practical use of polymer therapeutics that resulted in an FDA-approved anti-cancer treatment was the introduction of PEG-L-asparaginase (Oncaspar1) in 1994. This conjugate is composed of PEG polymer (MW ~ 5 kD) attached to the enzyme, L-asparaginase, and is used for the treatment of acute lymphoblastic leukemia (39). In fact, polymer–drug conjugate itself can be considered as a nanovehicle. Various conjugates have been developed and clinically tested. Recent advances in polymer–drug conjugates are well described in reviews (Duncan, 2006; Duncan, Vicent, Greco, & Nicholson, 2005). One of the major advantages of polymer–drug conjugates is prolonged circulation in the blood stream by retarding degradation/metabolism/excretion rates of the conjugated drugs. Many peptide and protein drugs cannot be delivered by oral administration because of their large molecular weights. Even when administered directly into the blood stream, they do not remain in the blood for a long time due to fast degradation and metabolism, limiting the clinical applications. The circulation times of these drugs have increased substantially by conjugation with polymers, such as PEG. A good example is the glucagon-like peptide-1, which regulates food uptake and insulin release. The peptide is a very useful therapeutic agent for diabetic patients, but it is liable to degradation by a plasma enzyme, dipeptidyl dipeptidase IV, but by introducing one PEG chain, Lee et al (40) showed that its half-life could be increased up to 40 folds over the natural form. Very often, low molecular weight drugs with high hydrophobicity are used for conjugation with attendant reduction in the degradation/clearance rate as well as the toxicity of the conjugated drug. The therapeutic effect is achieved upon hydrolysis inside the target cells to release the original drug. The polymers used in conjugation usually have stimuli-responsiveness, imparting unique properties into the conjugated drug such that, its activities can be turned on or off by external signals. For example, Shimoboji et al, (41, 42) reported that, the catalytic activity endoglucanase 12A upon conjugation could be turned on by application of UV light or high temperature because, it was conjugated with either photo-sensitive or thermo-sensitive polymers. The active site of the enzyme was exposed by collapsing the conjugated long polymer chain by external stimuli. Once visible light was turned on or the temperature was lowered, the enzyme activity vanished due to the blocking of the active site by the extended polymer chain. (43, 44)

2.3. Multifunctional drug carriers

A multifunctional drug delivery system (MDDS) refers to drug carrier that has multiple properties of prolonged blood circulation, passive or active localization at specific disease site, stimuli-sensitivity, ability to deliver drug into intracellular target organelles, and/or imaging ability (45). Technically therefore, it has two or more functions, infact, SDDS and polymer–drug conjugates discussed above can be considered MDDS. In addition to delivering drugs, MDDS can carry out the second function, such as stimuli-responsiveness or hydrolysis inside cells. Some reported MDDS include the biotin-tagged pH-sensitive polymeric micelles based on a mixture of PLA-b-PEG-b-PHis-biotin (PLA=poly (L-lactic acid)) and PEG-b-PHis block copolymers by Lee et al (46) in which the targeting moiety, biotin, was masked until the carrier was exposed to an expected environment of pH 7.0. Once the nanocarrier was internalized to cancer cells by ligand– receptor interactions, lowered pH (< 6.5) destabilized the carrier resulting in a burst release of the loaded drug and that of Lukyanov et al (47), where a pH-degradable PEG-b-phosphatidylethanolamine (PE) liposome had anti-myosin monoclonal antibody as well as TAT or biotin attached on its surface.

2.4. Organic/inorganic composites

An inorganic-organic composite usually comprises an inorganic phase and a film forming organic phase. A typical green approach to developing an inorganic-organic composite involves the selection of film forming organic phase from starches having a degree of polymerization; degree of substitution and viscosity such that the substituted starches are insoluble in water during mixing but dissolve at a higher processing temperature during forming, setting or drying of the composite. Thus, excessive migration of the starch is prevented and the composite is substantially strengthened. There has also been reports on the lab-on-a-chip approach (48 – 54), which embodies micron- or nano-sized machines composed of sophisticated circuits. Small devices have many advantages including portability/disposability, low cost, high reproducibility, high-throughput screening, and multiple functionalities in a single device. Recently, combined with other technologies such as optics, single molecular imaging, or cell/protein-based assay systems, biomedical lab-on-a-chip devices have become an important part of drug discovery and diagnosis, but its application in drug delivery systems based on are just beginning to appear (55 – 57).

As rightly noted by several authors, to release a drug from a nanodevice is more complicated than to perform assay or screening drug candidates, this is because, successful drug delivery requires at least four components namely; drug reservoir, pump, valve, and sensor (58). Drugs can be placed either in a fabricated reservoir or in conventional micro-/nanoparticles. Other important organic/inorganic composites are metal nanoparticles, such as silver, iron oxide, or gold nanoparticles, coated with hydrophilic polymers. Their major application has been as theranostics. Only recently, Hirsch et al, (59) developed gold nanoshell, which provided tunable emission light for bioimaging. Importantly, is the fact that, gold nanoparticles can be detected by X-ray and emit thermal energy by excitation making it very useful for medical imaging and thermal therapy (theranostics). In a related report, Corot et al, (60) developed super paramagnetic iron oxide nanoparticles for magnetic resonance imaging (MRI) of the whole body. Mechanistically, these nanoparticles are primarily engulfed by monocyte or macrophage after intravenous administration. However, uptake of super paramagnetic iron oxide by macrophage does not induce activation of nearby cells making it suitable for diagnosis of inflammatory or degenerative diseases.

3. Nanoparticulate drug delivery systems

3.1. Liposomes

Use of micro and nano particles in biomedicine and especially in drug delivery has a great deal of advantages over conventional systems such as: the enhanced delivery, high performance characteristics of the product, use of lesser amounts of expensive drugs in the delivery systems, extension of the bioactivity of the drug by protecting it from environmental effects in biological media, more effective treatment with minimal side effects. In addition, research for the design of more effective delivery systems is more economical for the discovery of a new bioactive molecule. Micro and nano colloidal drug delivery systems such as emulsions, suspensions and liposomes have been used for decades for this purpose and recently, nanosized systems with dimension of less than 100 nm gained significant attention. Nanotechnology promises to generate a library of sophisticated drug delivery systems that integrate molecular recognition, diagnostic and feedback. Nanotechnology is expected to create lots of innovations and play a critical role in various biomedical applications including the design of drug and gene delivery systems, molecular imaging, biomarkers and biosensors. By understanding the signaling and interaction between the molecules at nano levels, it would be possible to mimic biological systems.

Liposomes are small spherical vesicles (Fig. 2) in which one or more aqueous compartments are completely enclosed by molecules that have hydrophilic and hydrophobic functionality. Liposomes vary with composition, size, surface charge and method of preparation. They can be single or in multiple bilayers. Those containing one bilayer membrane are termed small unilamellar vesicles or large unilamellar vesicles based on their sizes (61). If more than one bilayer is present then they are called multilamellar vesicles. Liposomes are commonly used as model cells or carriers for various bioactive agents including drugs, vaccines, cosmetics and nutraceuticals. Drugs associated with liposomes have markedly altered pharmacokinetic properties compared to free drugs in solution. Liposomes are also effective in reducing systemic toxicity and preventing early degradation of the encapsulated drug after administration. They can be covered with polymers such as polyethylene glycol (PEG) – in which case they are called pegylated or stealth liposomes, in this form, they usually will exhibit prolonged half-life in blood circulation. Liposomes can also be conjugated to antibodies or ligands to in order enhance target-specificity. For example, Visser et al (62) studied pegylated horse –radish-peroxidase loaded liposomes, tagged with transferrin to the blood-brain barrier. The authors showed an effective targeting of liposomes loaded with protein or peptides to the brain capillary endothelial cells and suggested that the system could be an attractive approach for targeting drug delivery to brain. In another report, Lopez-Pinto and coworkers (63) examined the dermal delivery of a lipophilic drug, minoxidil, from ethosomes versus classic liposomes by applying the vesicles non-occlusively on rat skin, yet in a separate study, Ozden and Hasirci (64) prepared small unilamellar vesicles composed of phosphatidyl- choline, dicetyl phosphate and cholesterol and entrapped glucose oxidase in them. Liposomes are also studied as carriers for cells, genes or DNA fragments. Ito et al (65) studied the effect of magnetite cationic liposomes which have positive surface charge to enrich and proliferate Mesenchymal stem cells (MSCs) in vitro. Kunisawa et al (66) established a protocol for the encapsulation of nanoparticles in liposomes, which were further fused with ultra violet-inactivated Sendai virus to compose fusogenic liposomes and observed that fusogenic liposome demonstrated a high ability to deliver nanoparticles containing DNA into cytoplasm.

Foco et al (67) studied the delivery of sodium ascorbyl phosphate (SAP), an effective oxygen species scavenger to prevent the degenerative effects of UV radiation on skin. SAP was encapsulated into liposomes to improve its penetration through the stratum corneum into the deeper layers of the skin. Sinico et al (68) studied transdermal delivery of tretinoin and examined the influence of liposome composition, size, lamellarity and charge on transdermal delivery. They studied positively or negatively charged liposomes of different types. It was reported that negatively charged liposomes strongly improved newborn pig skin hydration and tretinoin retention. Arcon et al (69) encapsulated an anticancer agent, cisplatin, in sterically stabilized liposomes and studied the systems with extended X-ray absorption fine structure method, and concluded that the liposome-encapsulated drug is chemically stable and does not hydrolyze.

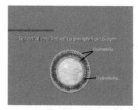

Figure 2. Spherical vesicles with a phospholipid bilayer

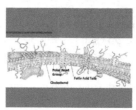

Figure 3. Cell Membrane

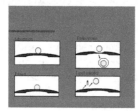

Figure 4. Modes of Liposome/Cell Interaction

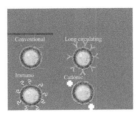

Figure 5. Classes of Liposomes

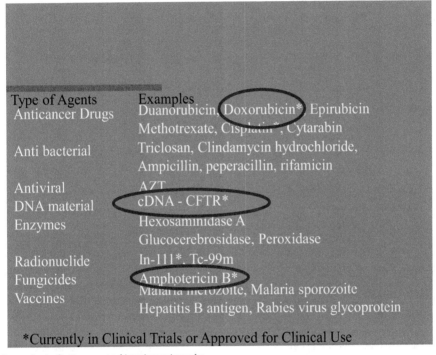

Type of Agents	Examples
Anticancer Drugs	Duanorubicin, Doxorubicin*, Epirubicin Methotrexate, Cisplatin*, Cytarabin
Anti bacterial	Triclosan, Clindamycin hydrochloride, Ampicillin, peperacillin, rifamicin
Antiviral	AZT
DNA material	cDNA - CFTR*
Enzymes	Hexosaminidase A Glucocerebrosidase, Peroxidase
Radionuclide	In-111*, Tc-99m
Fungicides	Amphotericin B*
Vaccines	Malaria merozoite, Malaria sporozoite Hepatitis B antigen, Rabies virus glycoprotein

*Currently in Clinical Trials or Approved for Clinical Use

Source: Jessica Scott, www.nanobiotec.iqm.unicamp.br

Table 1. Current liposomal drug preparations

3.2. Microemulsions

Microemulsions are isotropic, thermodynamically stable systems composed of oil, water, and surfactant. Thermodynamic stability rather than size, is the defining hallmark of a microemulsion, although the droplet sizes are still below 100 nm (and many times much smaller) (70). Be that as it may, what is critical about microemulsions is that, they contain two phases consisting of two immiscible liquids that are mixed together and stabilized with the aid of a surfactant with or without a co-surfactant. They may have droplets in the range

Liposome Utility	Current Applications	Disease States Treated
Solubilization	Amphotericin B, minoxidil	Fungal infections
Site-Avoidance	Amphotericin B – reduced nephrotoxicity doxorubicin – decreased cardiotoxicity	Fungal infections, cancer
Sustained-Release	Systemic antineoplastic drugs, hormones, corticosteroids, drug depot in the lungs	Cancer, biotherapeutics
Drug protection	Cytosine arabinoside, interleukins	Cancer, etc.
RES Targeting	Immunomodulators,vaccines, antimalarials,macophage-located diseases	Cancer, MAI, tropical parasites
Specific Targeting	Cells bearing specific antigens	Wide therapeutic applicability
Extravasation	Leaky vasculature of tumors, inflammations, infections	Cancer, bacterial infections
Accumulation	Prostaglandins	Cardiovascular diseases

Source: Handbook of Biological Physics Volume 1, (ed. R. Lipowsky and E. Sackmann). Elsevier Science B. V.

Table 2. Some applications of liposomes in the pharmaceutical industry

of 5–100 nm. The difference between microemulsions and emulsions is that, the later are opaque mixtures of two immiscible liquids, thermo- dynamically unstable and usually require the application of high torque mechanical mixing or homogenization to produce dispersed droplets in the range of 0.2–25 mm. Both types can be made as water-in-oil (w/o) or oil-in-water (o/w) (70). Choice of the dispersed and continuous phases for microemulsions formulations is based on the hydrophilicity of the model drug. Also, surfactants that have hydrophilic–lipophilic balances (HLB) of 3–6 tend to promote the formation of w/o microemulsions while those with HLB values of 8–10 tend to promote the formation of o/w microemulsions. It has been reported (70) that, the formation and stability of microemulsions are dependent on the interfacial tension between the dispersed and continuous phases. Microemulsion instability can lead to Oswald ripening leading to dissolution of the small droplets with a resultant increase in the size of the large droplets, therefore, stabilization against Ostwald ripening is very critical, this is because, the resultant change in the size of the droplets could lead to loss of physical stability of the dosage form. Choice of the components of microemulsions affects its stability (70). Safety is also another important factor that must be considered during component selection. Attwood, 1994 had opined that, the irritant and toxic properties of some alcohols (1-butanol and 2-butanol) could limit their potential use. Microemulsions have been proposed as drug delivery systems to enhance the absorption of drug across biological membranes (70). Some of the advantages of microemulsions include (i) Increased solubility and stability of drugs (ii) ease and economy of scale-up. Some of the disadvantages are; (a) premature leakage/release of incorporated drug (b) phase inversion (c) Many of the effective surfactants and/or co-surfactants do not have a pharmaceutically acceptable toxicity profile; and (d) microemulsion systems often require development of complex systems that may be time consuming.

Product	Developed	Applications
Rapamune®	Elan's	An immunosuppressant
Emend®	Elan's	Anti-nausea
Estrasorb®	Elan's	Topical estrogen therapy
Megace® ES	Elan's	Stimulate appetite
TriCor®	Elan's	Cholesterol-lowering
Abraxane®	APP	Breast cancer
Doxil®	Alza	Anti-cancer
Acticoat®	Smith & Nephew	Antimicrobial
SilvaGard	AcryMed, Inc.,	Antimicrobial

Source: B. K. Nanjwade, Department of Pharmaceutics, KLE University College of Pharmacy, BELGAUM-590010

Table 3. Some medical applications of liposomes

3.3. Nanoparticles

Nanoparticle drug delivery systems are nanometeric carriers used to deliver drugs or biomolecules. Generally, nanometeric carriers also comprise sub-micron particles with size below 1000 nm and with various morphologies, including nanospheres, nanocapsules, nano- micelles, nanoliposomes, and nanodrugs, etc. (71, 72). Nanoparticle drug delivery systems have outstanding advantages, some of which include; (1) they can pass through the smallest capillary vessels because of their ultra-tiny volume and avoid rapid clearance by phagocytes so that their duration in blood stream is greatly prolonged; (2) they can penetrate cells and tissue gap to arrive at target organs such as liver, spleen, lung, spinal cord and lymph; (3) they could show controlled- release properties due to the biodegradability, pH, ion and/or temperature sensibility of materials; (4) they can improve the utility of drugs and reduce toxic side effects. As drug delivery system, nanoparticles can entrap drugs or biomolecules into their interior structures and/or absorb drugs or biomolecules onto their exterior surfaces. Presently, nanoparticles have been widely used to deliver drugs, polypeptides, proteins, vaccines, nucleic acids, genes and so on. Over the years, nanoparticle drug delivery systems have shown huge potential in biological, medical and pharmaceutical applications (73). Currently, the researches on nanoparticle drug delivery system focus on: (1) the selectness and combination of carrier materials to obtain suitable drug release speed; (2) the surface modification of nanoparticles to improve their targeting ability; (3) the optimization of the preparation of nanoparticles to increase their drug delivery capability, their application in clinics and the possibility of industrial production; (4) the investigation of in vivo dynamic process to disclose the interaction of nanoparticles with blood and targeting tissues and organs, etc. One type of nanoparticle, which is differentiated from any of the above terms, is a solid lipid nanoparticle (SLN) with a lipid core that is solid at room temperature. During formation of SLNs the solid lipid is first melted, then emulsified as a liquid to form an o/w emulsion, and cooled to allow the lipid to solidify. Due to the similarity in formation and content, these particles have been referred to as "emulsions with solid fat globules".

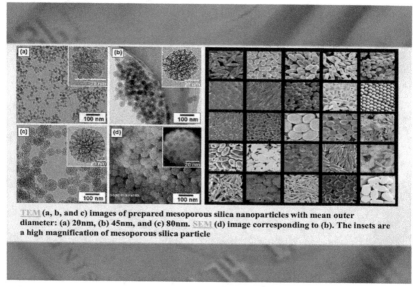

TEM (a, b, and c) images of prepared mesoporous silica nanoparticles with mean outer diameter: (a) 20nm, (b) 45nm, and (c) 80nm. SEM (d) image corresponding to (b). The insets are a high magnification of mesoporous silica particle

Source: B. K. Nanjwade *api.ning.com/.../DevelopmentofNanotechnologyBasedDrugsanditsGu*

Figure 6. Transmission and electron micrographs of silica nanopartcles

Nanoparticles are solid colloidal particles, ranging in size from 1 to 1000 nm, consisting of various macromolecules in which the therapeutic drugs can be adsorbed, entrapped or covalently attached. The distinct advantages offered by solid nanoparticles in drug development can be ascribed to their physical stability and the possibility of modifying the formulating materials in order to achieve controlled release characteristics. The ability to formulate nanoparticles to achieve sustained release offers an opportunity for product life cycle management by developing formulations with decreased dosing frequency for drugs that are going off patent. There has been a variety of materials used to engineer solid nanoparticles both with and without surface functionality. Perhaps the most widely used are the aliphatic polyesters such as poly (lactic acid) (PLA), the more hydrophilic poly (glycolic acid) (PGA) and their copolymers poly (lactide-coglycolide) (PLGA). The degradation rate of these polymers and often the corresponding drug release rate can vary from days (PGA) to months (PLA). The effectiveness of nanoparticles in drug delivery can be attributed to many factors such as physical and biological stability, good tolerability of the components, simplicity of the manufacturing process, possibility of facile scale-up of the manufacturing process, amenability to freeze drying and sterilization.

4. Some natural polymers in nanodrug delivery

4.1. Starch

Starch is a common polysaccharide. It occurs majorly in plants where they act as storage materials. Chemically, it is composed of recurring units of glycopyranose in an alpha D-(1, 4) linkage and on hydrolysis yields the monosaccharide, glucose (Heller et al., 1990). The use of starch in pharmaceutics is extensive. It is used as co-polymer and excipient in controlled drug delivery (74 – 76) as drug carriers in tissue engineering scaffolds (77) as Hydrogels (78) and as solubility enhancers (79).

Santander-Ortega et al. (80) investigated the potential of starch nano-particles as a transdermal drug delivery system (TDDS). The challenge faced in delivering drug through these systems is that the skin acts as an effective barrier to drug passage and must therefore be overcome for effective drug delivery. Nano-particles were shown to facilitate drug delivery without interference to the skin's integrity. The method used to prepare the nano-particles was emulsification-diffusion due to its reproducibility, higher yields, ease of scale-up and control over size of particles and degree of polydispersity. Maize starch modified and un-modified (by the addition of propyl groups) was used as polymeric material to formulate 2 different types of nano-particles. The modified starch nano-particles were shown to be non-toxic using LDH (Lactose dehydrogenase) and MTT assay and resulted in particles of uniform size distribution while the nano- particles formulated from the native starch was not observable. Flufenamic acid, caffeine and testosterone were used as model drugs and their delivery across the skin was analyzed using excised skin from female Caucasian patients who had undergone abdominal plastic surgery. Permeation data obtained for caffeine and testosterone were similar for nano-encapsulated and free drugs while the delivery of flufenamic acid using the nano-particles was enhanced by about ten-fold.

Starch nano-particles have been employed to deliver insulin via non-invasive routes; Makham (81) investigated the use of chitosan cross linked starch polymers as carriers for oral insulin delivery, manipulating the bio-adhesive and not so adhesive properties of chitosan and carboxymethyl starch to formulate hydrogels loaded with insulin. The authors however noted that, Insulin delivered by this method however faces the challenge of being broken down by proteases.

The nasal route can also be considered as an alternative to the subcutaneous route of administration because it is highly vascularised and is of great benefit in drug delivery as drugs given through this route are not subject to first-pass metabolism. However for effective delivery through this route, it is crucial that barriers to nasal drug delivery which include the lipophilic epithelium and muco-ciliary clearance must be overcome. Jain et al., (82) reports a size dependent insulin release in rats from starch nano-particles. Potato starch was used to prepare 2 differents types of nano-particles by cross-linking with epichlorohydrin and phosphoryl chloride (POCl₃) using both the gel and emulsion methods. These methods however led to the production of polydispersed nano-particles. There were statistically significant differences in mean sizes except in emulsion prepared epichlorohydrin cross linked particles which were smaller and of uniform distribution. In-vitro studies showed that drug release followed first order kinetics and was diffusion controlled along with burst effect, due to the presence of left-over insulin on the surface of the nanopartices after entrapment. Emulsion cross-linked particles released their drug faster than gel cross linked particles with 85-90% and 81% release in 12 hrs respectively. These differences were attributed to the diffusion path length of the drug within the particles. The smaller the particle size the less distance the drug will travel to be released. Tests carried out on the diabetes induced rats showed a 50-65% reduction in blood glucose by nano-particles compared to plain insulin formulation which served as control and this lasted for about 6hrs. Permeation enhancers modulated the hypoglycaemic effect and bioavailability of nano-particles, Plasma insulin levels of small sized nano-particles were also found to be significantly higher. Conclusions obtained from the study however recommend that further work would be needed in order to produce a more efficient carrier system.

Simi and Abraham (83) note that the presence of hydroxyl groups on starch enhances its hydrophilicity and confers on it low moisture resistance. This property poses a major constraint in drug delivery as a result of which it is often necessary to modify the polymer before it is made into nano particles as observed above. In their study, starch extracted from cassava tuber was modified by graft co-polymerization using long chain fatty acids before the resulting polymer was made into nano-particles (83). The nano-particles were prepared by dialysis and subsequently crosslinked using sodium tripolyphosphate. Oleic acid and stearic acid were both used as fatty acids while indomethacin was used as model drug. Findings showed that drug release from both types of nano-particles was effectively controlled. It is however not clear whether there was a significant difference between drug releases in both types of nano-particles. No attempts were also made to formulate the un-modified starch granules into nano-particles though this may have been due to results obtained from differential scanning calorimetry which showed that native starch was less processable than grafted starch.

In addition, magnetised iron-oxide nano-particles coated with starch were used by Cole et al. (84) as a means of targeting brain tumours. Magnetic resonance imaging and histological reports showed that surface modification with polyethylene oxide improved delivery to tumour cells resulting in a greater accumulation of particles in the glioma compared to the rest of the brain.

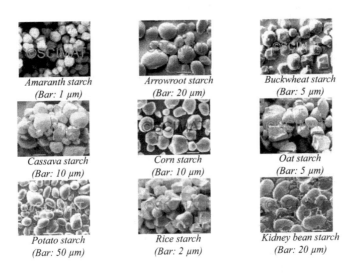

Amaranth starch *(Bar: 1 μm)*	*Arrowroot starch* *(Bar: 20 μm)*	*Buckwheat starch* *(Bar: 5 μm)*
Cassava starch *(Bar: 10 μm)*	*Corn starch* *(Bar: 10 μm)*	*Oat starch* *(Bar: 5 μm)*
Potato starch *(Bar: 50 μm)*	*Rice starch* *(Bar: 2 μm)*	*Kidney bean starch* *(Bar: 20 μm)*

Figure 7. Granule structure of some common native starches

4.2. Chitosan

This polymer is obtained from the partial N-deacetylation of chitin found in the shells of crustacean. It is composed of glucosamine and N-acetyl glucosamine linked by β 1-4 glucosidic bonds and is one of the most widely studied natural polymers for nano-drug delivery. The deacetylation of chitin is both concentration and temperature dependent with optimal yields achieved at temperatures between 60°C- 80°C using 50%w/w alkali (85).

Park et al.,(86) in a review on chitosan describes its numerous applications in delivering low molecular weight drugs and summarises the reason for its choice being in its physiochemical and biological properties, enabling chemical modification and enhanced residence time respectively. It has been used   as both a composite membrane with collagen (87) and a cross linked polymer for transdermal delivery of   propranolol (88).

Nano-particles fabricated with chitosan as co-polymer was used to by Dev et al., (89) to investigate the controlled release of anti-retroviral drug, lamivudine. The nano-particles were prepared by emulsion and solvent evaporation technique and characterised using dynamic light scattering. The use of this method resulted in monodispersed particles with a size range of 300-350nm. Two formulations with differences in percentage drug weight (3% and 6%) were made, of which drug release rate was higher from the nano-particles with higher drug loading, though both were able to control drug release fairly well. Drug release kinetics showed that the mechanism of drug release was by diffusion. Conclusions reached suggested that the nano-particles could be applied for gastrointestinal drug delivery because drug release was relatively slower at neutral pH compared to acidic pH and also slower in the acidic pH compare to the alkaline pH.

Chitosan combination was also used by Menon et al. (90) for therapeutic drug delivery. Nano-complexes of chitosan and polyoxometalates (POM) were tested as anti-cancer preparation. Since POM's though toxic have shown promise in being used as anti- viral and anti-tumour agent, the role of chitosan was to minimise the toxicity associated with POM, by modifying its surface properties. Mono-dispersed particles with size 200nm were produced using ionotropic gelation technique and the use of probe sonication was shown to control particle size and distribution compared to ultrasonication. In-vitro studies showed that the nano-complex was able to sustain drug release with enhanced anti-tumour activity at much lesser doses than the POM alone.

Similarly as with starch nano particles, Luo et al. (91) used chitosan oligosaccharides (COS) to coat lipid based carriers in order to enhance ocular drug delivery. This material is obtained from the decomposition of chitosan, but it is more soluble in water than chitin and chitosan. Drug introduced into the eye have minimal residence times as they are quickly washed away and have to be re-administered regularly. But in this study, COS enhanced permeation and adhesion of the cornea. There was a 7.7 fold and 2.8 fold retention of the model drug, flubiprofen by the COS coated nano lipid carriers compared to the phosphate buffer solution and uncoated nanolipid carriers which were attributed to the mucoadhesive properties of COS. The use of COS was also found to be non-irritating to the eye, a property which is of utmost importance in the choice of a suitable eye formulation.

4.3. Gelatin

Gelatin is obtained from the breakdown and hydrolysis of collagen, obtained from the connective tissues, bones and skins of animals. It is a known matrixing agent drug delivery. Bajpai and Shoubey (92) describes a process for the controlled release of sulphamethoxazole using 2 different gelatin nano-particles {Type A (porcine skin) and type B gelatin(bovine skin)} and cross linked with gluteraldehyde; Nano-particles of varying gelatin concentrations were prepared by solvent evaporation techniques and drug release kinetics evaluated using appropriate kinetic models. Findings from this system suggest that this system could be of use in targeted drug delivery such as colon drug delivery where pH is an important consideration. Drug release was found to increase following increased swelling of the nanoparticles. In addition, swelling was further enhanced by an increase in pH with greater drug release occuring at pH 7.5 than at pH 1.8. The nano particles were also not degraded in simulated gastric fluid thereby showing their stability under acidic conditions. An increase in concentration of the cross linker led to an increase in swelling and drug release up until a certain concentration(10.6mM) when swelling began to decline. This relationship between the amount of cross linker and the polymer has also been reported by Das et al. (93); In their case, nano-particles composed of gelatin blended with montmorillonite (MMT) were loaded with the anti-cancer agent paclitaxel. These nano-particles were prepared by the same method of solvent evaporation and produced similar results. Increase in gluteraldehyde concentrations was reported to increase swelling and consequently drug release up until a certain point, when further increases in concentration of the cross linker led to decreased swelling and drug release. There was also a cumulative increase in drug release with increased pH. 80% of the drug was released within 8hrs at pH 7.4 while there was less than 44% drug release within 4 h at pH 1.2. Increasing concentration of the loaded drug also led to an increase in drug release.

The use of proteins as nano carriers is also employed in gene therapy. Viral and non-viral vectors are used for the transfection of DNA into cells, because, the injection of naked DNA into living tissue results in enzymatic degradation and reduced cellular uptake due to repulsion between the negatively charged DNA and cell membrane. In this domain, Coester et al., (94) used avidin modified gelatin nano-particles for the delivery of biotinylated PNA (Peptide nucleic acids) in other to investigate their use as anti-sense therapy. Zwiorek et al. (95) suggests that gelatin nano- particles have the potential to be used for effective non-viral gene delivery and are a safer alternative to the use of viral vectors. A 2 step desolvation process was used to prepare cationized particles of uniform size distribution and low polydispersity and comparisons between polyethyleneimine- DNA complexes and the gelatin particles showed that the latter is effective in facilitating gene expression, has less toxic and better tolerated.

Transfection with the aid of gelatin nanoparticles was also used by Xu et al. (96) for the delivery of DNA plasmids encoding for insulin growth like factor 1(IGF-1) into chrondrocytes. In order to incorporate the plasmids into the gelatin nano-particles, complex coacervation was employed because it is an easy, fast and particularly useful method for the incorporation of large molecules. The authors proved that, cationized gelatin particles were of smaller sizes than non- cationized particles, this they attributed to the condensation of the cationized particles. Fluorescence spectroscopy showed that the cationized gelatin nano-particles were successfully transfected and expressed the gene while the reverse was the case for the non-cationized gelatin particles. This is probably due to enhanced endocytosis, occurring as a result of interactions between the positive charge on the former and the negative charge on the cell membrane. A 5-fold increase in growth factor production was observed in cells containing these nano-particles. Findings also showed that over expression of the gene was maintained steadily for up to 2 weeks when they were grown in collagen (type II) -glycosaminoglycan scaffolds in 3D culture. Since a prolonged and localized release of IGF-1 was achieved in this study, and IGF-1 is known to promote growth in skeletal muscle, cartilage and bones and numerous other tissues in the body tissue, this approach shows potential applications in gene therapy and tissue engineering.

5. Properties of nanoparticles

Some of the properties of nanoparticles that are important for application in drug delivery include simple, affordable manufacturing process that is easy to scale up. The manufacturing process excludes organic solvents or potentially toxic ingredients. All the components of the formulation should be commercially available, safe, affordable, non-toxic and biodegradable. The nanoparticles should be stable with respect to size, surface morphology, size distribution and other important physical and chemical properties.

6. Preparation of nanoparticles

6.1. Nanosuspensions

Nanosuspension refers to production of sub-micron-sized particles by subjecting the combination of drug and a suitable emulsifier to the process of milling or high-pressure homogenization. Conventional milling and precipitation processes generally result in particles with sizes that are much greater than 1 mm. As such, a critical step in the nanosuspension preparation is the choice of the manufacturing procedure to ensure production of sub-micron particles. Nanosuspension formulations can be used to improve the solubility of poorly soluble drugs. A large number of new drug candidates emerging from drug discovery programs are water insoluble, and therefore poorly bioavailable, leading to abandoned development efforts. These can now be rescued by formulating them into crystalline nanosuspensions. Techniques such as media milling and high-pressure homogenization have been used commercially for producing nanosuspensions. The unique features of nanosuspensions have enabled their use in various dosage forms, including specialized delivery systems such as mucoadhesive hydrogels. Nanosuspensions can be delivered by parenteral, per- oral, ocular, and pulmonary routes. Currently, efforts are being directed to extending their applications in site-specific drug delivery. Various particle sizes of spironolactone, a model low solubility drug, have been formulated to yield micro- and nanosuspensions of the type solid lipid nanoparticles and DissoCubes. The DissoCubes nanosuspension yielded highly significant improvements in bioavailability. Particle size minimization is not the major determining factor in the bioavailability improvement. Rather, the type of surfactant used as stabilizer in the formulations is of greater importance. Improvement in drug solubility in the intestine as well as in dissolution rate of spironolactone is the most likely mechanisms responsible for the observed effect, although additional mechanisms such as permeability enhancement may also be involved.

Development of nanoparticle formulations for improved absorption of insoluble compounds and macromolecules enables improved bioavailability and release (97)

Particle size reduction to sizes below 1 mm is usually difficult due to possible particle aggregation and generation of high surface area materials. Milling techniques that have been used to generate nano-sized particles are ball milling or pearl milling that applies milling beads of sizes ranging from 0.4 to 3 mm and these beads may be composed of glass, ceramics or plastics (98). The time required for milling depends on the hardness and brittleness of the drug material in comparison to milling material and inertial forces set up within the mill. Some of the challenges that milling processes can pose in drug development are (i) undesirable erosion of the milling equipment components into the drug product; (ii) the process is usually time consuming, thereby prolonging drug development time; (iii) milling over a few days may bring the risk of microbiological problems or increases in the cost of production; also (iv) prolonged milling may induce the formation of amorphous domains in crystalline starting materials or may lead to changes in the polymorphic form of the drug. The generation of amorphous form of the drug is problematic because these forms may crystallize during the shelf life of the drug leading to changes in solubility and bioavailability of the drug. An example of the conversion of crystalline to amorphous form of the drug was observed in jet milling of albuterol sulfate. Also, the generation of high-energy surfaces that affected wettability was observed with acetylsalicylic acid. Some examples of nano-sized particles produced by milling as reviewed by Majuru and Oyewumi (70) are (i) naproxen nanoparticles approximately 200 nm in diameter and (ii) danazol particles of a mean size of 169 nm. The authors also reported that, there were four approved drug products in the USA that are based on NanoCrystal technology: (a) Rapamune (sirolimus) tablets by Wyeth; (b) Tricor (fenofibrate) tablets by Abbott; (c) Emend (aprepitant) capsules by Merck; and (d) Megace ES (megestrol) oral suspension by Par Pharmaceuticals (70). High pressure homogenization has also been recognized as an effective method of producing nanosuspensions (98). Again, Majuru and Oyewumi (70) reported that, high-pressure homogenization has been applied commercially with the development of some drug products, such as fenofibrate and paclitaxel. A typical procedure for preparing nanosuspension involves, preparing an aqueous suspension of drug in surfactant solution, this is then passed through a high pressure of typically 1500 bar at 3–20 homogenization cycles. The suspension is then passed through a small gap in the homogenizer of typical width 25 mm at 1500 bar. Due to built up cavitation forces that are created drug particles are broken down from micro to nanoparticles. An example is in the micro fluidization of atovaquone to obtain particles in the 100–300 nm size range Majuru and Oyewumi (70). It has been reported that, nanosuspension particles in most cases have an average size ranging from 40 to 500 nm with a small (0.1%) proportion of particles larger than 5 mm Majuru and Oyewumi (70). Experts have recognized that, a major challenge in the use of high-pressure homogenization is the possible changes in drug crystal structure that may cause batch-to-batch variation in crystallinity level, and have suggested that, application in drug delivery should include the desired specification by which the quality of each batch will be evaluated.

6.2. Polymeric nanoparticles

Polymeric nanoparticles can be identified as submicronic (size< 1μm) colloidal carriers. Compared to other colloidal carriers polymeric Nanoparticles hold significant promise for the advancement of treating diseases and disorders. They have attractive physicochemical properties such as size, surface potential, hydrophilic-hydrophobic balance and for this reason they have been recognized as potential drug carriers for bioactive ingredients such as anticancer drugs, vaccines, oligonucleotides , peptides, etc. Their widespread use for oral delivery also aims at improving the bioavailability of drugs with poor absorption characteristic, reducing GI mucosa irritation caused by drugs and assuring stability of drugs in the GI tract. Thus, all these and many more such characteristics of nanoparticles qualify them as a promising candidate in drug-delivery technology. Although various biodegradable nanoparticles of natural polymers such as starch, chitosan, liposomes etc, are largely in use as drug carriers in con- trolled Drug-delivery technology (99). Many FDA-approved biodegradable and biocompatible polymers have been used in nanoparticle preparation. These include polylactide-polyglycolide copolymers, polyacrylates and polycaprolactones. Nanoparticles can be prepared from polymerization of monomers or from preformed polymer with the possibility of performing many chemical modifications. The polymerization reaction in these systems generally occurs in two steps: a nucleation phase followed by a growth phase and the process can be carried out in two ways either as emulsion polymerization or as interfacial polymerization. When nanoparticle preparation involves polymerization, it is undesirable to have residual monomers and initiators in the final nanoparticle formulation. A critical step of the process is the purification and removal of residual monomers. It is also very important to separate free drugs from the drug loaded nanoparticle suspension. A potential challenge for polymeric nanoparticles is associated with residues from organic solvents and polymer toxicity. If the drug to be incorporated in nanoparticles is hydrophobic, the drug is dissolved or dispersed into the polymer solution. The polymer solution is then added to an aqueous solution, followed by high-speed homogenization or sonication to form an oil-in-water emulsion. Nanoparticle preparation is usually facilitated and stabilized with the aid of an emulsifier or stabilizer. If the drug to be incorporated in nanoparticles is hydrophilic, the drug is added to the aqueous phase and entrapped into nanoparticles through a double emulsification method to form water-in-oil-in-water emulsion Majuru and Oyewumi (70). Residual organic solvent can be removed by evaporation or a decreased pressure or under a vacuum environment with or without the aid of inert gas flow. Solid nanoparticles are cured from the suspension by centrifugation, filtration or freeze drying. Another method is based on particle precipitation upon addition of a non-solvent to polymer solution under mechanical stirring. This method allows the formation of nanoparticles without prior emulsification. Nanoparticle formation and characteristics are dependent on the choice of the polymer/solvent/non-solvent system that will ensure mutual miscibility of the solvent and non-solvent of the polymer, Majuru and Oyewumi (70). Nanoparticles can also be prepared from natural macromolecules using methods such as thermal denaturation of proteins (such as albumin) or gelification process such as in alginates. In general, the controlling factors in the nanoparticle formulation process, which are adjustable for an ideal design, are the polymer type and its molecular weight, the copolymer blend ratio, the type of organic solvent, the drug loading level, the emulsifier/stabilizer and oil–water phase ratio, the mechanical strength of mixing, the temperature and the pH. These authors have opined that, in production of a drug product it is important to set a limit for residual solvent in the formulation that is based on the acceptable daily intake and to develop analytical methods for testing of the solvent levels in the nanoparticles. Table 4 below shows some of the applications of polymeric materials in nanodrug delivery.

COLLOID BASED DELIVERY FOR THERAPEUTICS			
Delivery system type	Typical mean particle diameter (in micrometers)	Representative systems of each type	Characteristic applications
Microspheres, Hydrogels	0.5-20	Alginate, gelatin, chitosan, polymeric hydrogels	Sustained release of therapeutics
Microparticles	0.2-5	Polystyrene, polylactide microspheres.	Targeted delivery of therapeutics
Emulsions, Microemulsions	0.15-2	o/w, w/o, lipid emulsions, o/w microemulsions.	Control and targeted delivery of therapeutics
Liposomes	30-1000	Phospholipid and polymer based bilayer vesicles.	Targeted delivery of therapeutics
Micelles	3-80	Natural and synthetic surfactant micelles.	Targeted delivery of therapeutics
Nanoparticles	2-100	Lipid, Polymer, Inorganic nanoparticles.	Targeted delivery of therapeutics, in vivo navigational devices
Nanocrystals	2-100	Quantum dots	Imaging agents

Source: B. K. Nanjwade *api.ning.com/.../DevelopmentofNanotechnologyBasedDrugsanditsGu*

Table 4. Polymer colloids for nanodrug delivery

6.3. Polymers for gene delivery

The delivery of nucleic acid into cells in vitro and in vivo is a critical technique for the study of genes and development of potential gene therapies. To fully utilize this potential, safer and more efficient vectors for delivery of genes are required. Current nucleic acid delivery falls into two major categories, viral and nonviral. In nonviral gene delivery, cationic lipids or polymers are used to both protect nucleic acids from degradation and facilitate entry into the target cells. The resulting complexes self-assemble via electrostatic interactions to form stable aggregates. Recent reports have discussed the promise of lipid-DNA (lipoplex) and polycation-DNA complexes (polyplexes) (77) as potential therapeutics, including recent efforts to incorporate bioresponsive chemistries for increased effectiveness. Successful gene transfer requires sufficient stability of DNA during the extracellular delivery phase, transportation through cell membranes and cytoplasm, and eventual disassembly and nuclear delivery. A molecular architecture that achieves all the requirements will most likely consist of a virus like layered structure incorporating several components. Though nonviral gene vectors can be efficient in vitro and in vivo, their uncontrolled and often undefined interactions under physiological conditions still represent a major obstacle to their use in gene therapy. In particular, it has been shown that nonviral gene vectors or their constituents interact strongly with negatively charged serum proteins and other blood components. Such opsonization alters the physicochemical characteristics of vectors, may interfere with vector targeting, and is of concern if vectors are to be applied in humans. Consequently, one major objective in nonviral vector development is to devise vectors that are inert in the in vivo environment during the delivery phase. Poly (ethylene glycol) (PEG) has often been used to confer to these drug carriers the desired stability during the extracellular delivery phase. The incorporation of PEG to lipo- or polyplexes has been proven effective in reducing undesired effects such as immune response, unspecific interactions, and degradation. PEGylation can be implemented by using PEGylated components in the initial complex formation. Alternatively, PEG shielding can be applied to preformed complexes in a secondary processing step by using either electrostatic self-assembly or chemical grafting. While PEGylation is a necessity to improve extracellular stability and circulation half-life, it often decreases the transfection efficiency due to reduced specificity and inhibited cell association and uptake. Incorporating receptor targeting or using bioresponsive linkers to release PEG have proven useful to overcome these intracellular barriers to efficient delivery (100). Previous work (100) with a copolymer-protected gene vector (COPROG), consisting of a branched polyethylenimine (bPEI)/ DNA polyplex subsequently shielded with a copolymer consisting of both PEG and anionic peptides (P6YE5C), showed the presence of the copolymer, which provides steric stabilization, protection from opsonization, and allows freeze-drying of the vector with little loss of activity. COPROG particles have proven to be effective gene delivery vectors with decreased cellular toxicity without impairing gene transfer. The decreased toxicity of COPROG is likely a result of the removal of unbound polycation by the excess anionic copolymer emphasizing the potential role of binding stoichiometry in three-component complexes. Likely due to their stabilizing and opsonization- inhibiting properties, COPROGs have proven advantageous in promoting the tranfection capacity of polyplex-loaded sponges upon subcutaneous implantation, and when colyophilized with fibrinogen, are a simple means to achieve an injectable fibrin gene-activated matrix (100). At the level of research, many synthetic DNA particles have been prepared for transfection in cell cultures and in animal studies. However, several authors (70).are of the opinion that, certain issues must be addressed in the development of DNA particles with cationic polymers. These are (i) potential toxicity of cationic polymers especially when administered at high concentrations; (ii) instability of particles on storage; (iii) instability of DNA particle size and particle size distribution leading to undesirable particle aggregation; (iv) poor transfection efficiency; (v) poor stability in blood circulation; and (vi) high cost of scaling up the process to achieve reproducible product quality.

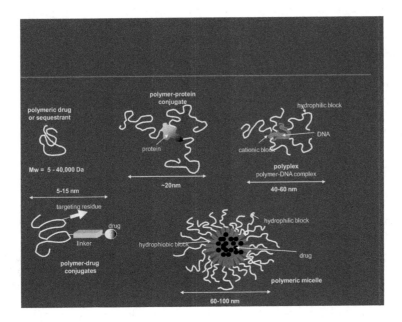

Figure 8. Nanosize medicines

6.4. Solid lipid nanoparticles

Solid lipid nanoparticles (SLN) are particles made from solid lipids with mean diameters ranging between 50–1000nm and represent an alternative to polymeric particulate carriers. The main advantage offered by lipid carriers in drug delivery is the use of physiological lipids or lipid molecules with a history of safe use in human medicine, which can decrease the danger of acute and chronic toxicity (101). Sufficient data are available for the use of drug-loaded lipid nano and microparticles for oral delivery, the main mechanism of lipid particulate materials translocation across the intestine being the uptake via Peyer's patches. Research reported in literature (102) shows that SLN constituted of stearic acid and phosphatidylcholine were evidenced in lymph and blood after duodenal administration to rats: the small diameters of SLN may facilitate their uptake by the lymphatics. Up until today, only a few methods are described in the literature for SLN preparation, including high pressure hot homogenization and cold homogenization techniques (101) microemulsion-based preparation and solvent emulsification/evaporation method. Particularly, the emulsification/evaporation method concerns the preparation of nanoparticles dispersions from O/W emulsions: the lipophilic material is dissolved in a water-immiscible organic solvent that is emulsified in an aqueous phase. Upon evaporation of the solvent, a nanoparticle dispersion is formed by precipitation of the lipid in the aqueous medium. Depending on the composition and the concentration of the lipid in the organic phase, very low particle sizes can be obtained, ranging from 30–100nm, but a clear disadvantage of this method is the use of organic solvents, whose toxicity cannot always be neglected. Recently, an emulsification–diffusion technique was developed using non-toxic and physiologically compatible solvents and monoglycerides or waxes as components of the disperse phase of oil-in-water emulsions obtained at 50 °C (103). The solvent-in-water emulsion–diffusion technique was before described in the literature mostly for the obtainment of polymeric micro- and nanoparticles and only a few authors proposed its application in the production of SLN (101). According to the moderate water solubility of the solvents employed, the dilution of the emulsions determined the diffusion of the organic solvent from the droplets to the continuous phase with the consequent instant solidification of lipophilic material. The emulsion compositions and process parameters used were the results of a formulative study aimed to develop optimized nanosphere formulations, whose mean sizes were below 200nm. In a separate report (104), the possibility of incorporating a peptide drug such as insulin in the SLN obtained with the developed method was considered, aiming to protect it from chemical and enzymatic degradation, as it is well-known that the incorporation of peptides in polymeric or non-polymeric particles should exert a certain protection of the drug against the proteolytic enzymes present in the gastrointestinal tract (101). Indeed, the use of lipids as matrix materials for sustained-release formulations for peptides and proteins has been reported only by few authors (101), owing to the hydrophobic nature of the lipid matrix that can be more appropriate to incorporate lipophilic drugs rather than hydrophilic proteins. An adequately high solubility of the drug in the lipid melt is therefore the pre-requisite to obtain a sufficient SLN loading capacity. Considering that the solubility of insulin in most commonly employed solvents and lipids is quite low, a specific solvent medium of the peptide was required. Isobutyric acid, a partially water-miscible solvent with low toxicity, revealed a totally unexpected high insulin-solubilization capacity at 50 °C, further increasing when the solvent was water-saturated (104). Solid lipid insulin-loaded microparticles were therefore produced using isobutyric acid as a solvent. Preliminary analysis of microparticles content after processing showed an insulin-high encapsulation efficiency; moreover, insulin in SLN did not undergo any chemical modification and its in vitro release from the microparticles was very low, with an initial burst effect of 20% of the dose.

Of recent, SLN has become a popular drug delivery system for ophthalmic application. It is gaining prominence as promising approach to improve the poor ocular bioavailability of biomolecules. In particular, solid lipid nanoparticles (SLN) and nanostructured lipid carriers (NLC), regarded as the first and second generation of lipid nanoparticles are currently being applied.(105, 106) NLC was developed due by combining the advantages of SLN and avoidance of their limitations such as low drug loading capacity, poor long-term stability and early drug expulsion caused by lipid polymorphism.(107, 108) NLC consist of a mixture of spacially different solid and liquid lipids molecules, resulting in a structure with more imperfections in crystal lattice to accommodate drugs.(109, 110) As drug delivery devices, NLC show great promise for the eye, due to their better biocompatibility, modified drug release kinetics, reduction of drug leakage during storage, avoidance of organic solvents during production process and feasibility of large scale production.(111, 112)

To prepare particles using the homogenization method, the drug is dissolved or solubilized in the lipid that has been melted and heated to a temperature approximately 5–10 ℃ above its melting point. For the hot homogenization technique, the drug dissolved in the lipid melt is dispersed under stirring in a hot aqueous surfactant solution of identical temperature. The obtained pre-emulsion is homogenized to produce nanoemulsions that are subsequently cooled to room temperature. Solid lipid nanoparticles are obtained upon lipid recrystallization at room temperature. Some of the process variables that will affect the particle size of nanoparticles as well as drug loading are (i) the type of homogenization technique; (ii) speed of homogenization; and (iii) rate of cooling in hot homogenization. Cold homogenization is applied for highly temperature-sensitive drugs and hydrophilic drugs. For the cold homogenization technique the drug containing lipid melt is cooled and ground to obtain lipid particles. The lipid particles are dispersed in a cold surfactant solution that is homogenized at or below room temperature. The process avoids or minimizes the melting of lipids and therefore minimizing the loss of hydrophilic drugs to the water surface. Solid lipid nanoparticles can also be prepared by using microemulsions as precursors.

7. Characterization of nanoparticles

Measurement of nanoparticles can be carried out by photon correlation spectroscopy (PCS) or dynamic light scattering (DLS). Photon correlation spectroscopy determines the hydrodynamic diameter of the nanoparticles by Brownian motion. In addition to the size, other important properties of nanoparticles include (i) density, molecular weight and crystallinity which can affect drug release and degradation; (ii) surface charge and hydrophobicity which may significantly influence nanoparticle behavior after administration. Zeta potential is also one of the properties of nanoparticles, and this is usually employed to measure the cell-surface charge density. The surface and bulk morphology are also important in determining the drug release kinetics of nanoparticles. Nanoparticles are usually visualized by scanning electron microscope (SEM) and atomic force microscopy (AFM). Thermal profile of nanoparticles can be studied using the differential scanning calorimetry (DSC), thermogravimetric analysis (TGA), while crystallinity can be monitored by x-ray crystallography. Other parameters which should normally be evaluated include; drug encapsulation efficiency; physical properties such as size, shape, stability of size, drug loading as well as drug release.

The common techniques for characterization as summarized by B. K. Nanjwade is shown in Tabs 5 – 8 below:

Morphology	
Properties	**Common Techniques**
Size (primary particle)	TEM, SEM, AFM, XRD
Size (primary/aggregate/agglomerate)	TEM, SEM, AFM, DLS, FFF, AUC, CHDF, XDC, HPLC, DMA(1)
Size distribution	EM, SEM, AFM, DLS, AUC, FFF, HPLC, SMA
Molecular weight	SLS, AUC, GPC
Structure/Shape	TEM, SEM, AFM, NMR
Stability (3D structure)	DLS, AUC, FFF, SEM, TEM

Source: B. K. Nanjwade *api.ning.com/.../Developmentof**Nanotechnology**BasedDrugsanditsGu*

Table 5.

Surface	
P roperties	**Common Techniques**
Surface area	BET
Surface charge	SPM, GE, Titration methods
Zeta potential	LDE, ESA, PALS
Surface coating composition	SPM, XPS, MS, RS, FTIR, NMR
Surface coating coverage	AFM, AUC, TGA
Surface reactivity	Varies with nanomaterial
Surface-core interaction	SPM, RS, ITC, AUC, GE
Topology	SEM, SPM, MS

Source: B. K. Nanjwade *api.ning.com/.../Developmentof**Nanotechnology**BasedDrugsanditsGu*

Table 6.

Chemical	
Properties	**Common Techniques**
Chemical composition (core, surface)	XPS, MS, AAS, ICP-MS, RS, FTIR, NMR
Purity	ICP-MS, AAS, AUC, HPLC, DSC
Stability (chemical)	MS, HPLC, RS, FTIR
Solubility (chemical)	Varies with nanomaterial
Structure (chemical)	NMR, XRD
Crystallinity	XRD, DSC
Catalytic activity	Varies with nanomaterial

Source: B. K. Nanjwade *api.ning.com/.../Developmentof**Nanotechnology**BasedDrugsanditsGu*

Table 7.

Other	
Properties	**Common Techniques**
Drug loading	MS, HPLC, UV-Vis, varies with nanomaterial
Drug potency/functionality	Varies with nanomaterial
In vitro release (detection)	UV-Vis, MS, HPLC, varies with nanomaterial
Deformability	AFM, DMA(2)

Source: B. K. Nanjwade *api.ning.com/.../DevelopmentofNanotechnologyBasedDrugsanditsGu*

Table 8.

8. Nanoparticle application in non-parenteral applications

8.1. Oral administration

For many reasons, oral drug delivery continues to be the preferred route of drug administration. It is the oldest and the commonest mode of drug administration as it is safer, more convenient, does not need assistance, non-invasive, often painless, the medicament need not be sterile and so is cheaper (113). However, the oral route is not suitable for drugs that are poorly permeable or easily degradable in the gastrointestinal tracts (GIT). For instance, delivery of proteins and peptides via the oral route will be greatly impacted by barriers such as (i) epithelial cell lining; (ii) the mucus layer; (iii) proteolytic enzymes in the gut lumen (such as pepsin, trypsin and chymotrypsin); and (iv) proteolytic enzymes (endopeptidases), at the brush border membrane. Drug loaded in nanoparticles will be protected from the enzymatic degradation along the GIT providing the potential benefit of enhanced absorption. It has been reported (70) that, particulate absorption takes place mainly at the intestinal lymphatic tissues (the Peyer's patches). The epithelial cell layer overlying the Peyer's patches contains Mcells. The differences between absorptive enterocytes and M cells are expressed in that M cells have (a) underdeveloped microvillous and glycocalyx structures, (b) apical microfolds, (c) increased intracellular vacuolization and (d) absence of mucus. The follicle-associated epithelia (FAE) are made up of the M cells and absorptive enterocytes (70). It has been reported that, the FAE and Mcells are predominantly responsible for particle uptake along the GIT. In this regard, nanotechnology is reportedly gaining attention in the development of proteins, peptides and DNA delivery systems (70).

8.2. Pulmonary administration

Micronization of drugs plays an important role in improving the drug dosage form and therapeutic efficiency today. If a drug is micronized into microspheres with suitable particle size, it can be addressed directly to the lung by the mechanical interception of capillary bed in the lungs. If a drug is prepared as microspheres in the size range of 7–25 μm, the microspheres can be concentrated in lung through i.v. administration (114). This technique can improve pulmonary drug concentration to maximize its effectiveness against some pulmonary infections such as mycoplasmal pneumonia and minimize the adverse side effects. The final nanoparticulate formulation may be administered either as a nebulizer (metered dose inhalers) or dry powder inhalers. Local delivery of drugs to the lung is desirable for many clinical conditions such as asthma; chronic pulmonary infections, lung cancer and cystic fibrosis. For both local and/or systemic delivery, the effectiveness of drug delivery by inhalation may be greatly imparted by mucociliary clearance (70). Studies have shown that nanoparticles may facilitate transport of drugs to the epithelium while avoiding undesirable mucociliary clearance. Other benefits of nanoparticle-based formulations are in the suitability for (i) sustained drug effect due to possible prolonged residence of drug at the site of action or absorption; (ii) controlled or targeted drug delivery. The small size of nanoparticles makes them highly suitable for pulmonary delivery because they can easily be air borne and delivered to the alveolus. It is important that the components of the nanoparticle formulation are biodegradable to avoid accumulation in the lungs and that they do not cause irritation of the air ways and lung tissue. The control of the particle size of the formulation during manufacture and the entire shelf life of the drug product is also very important for an acceptable product (70).

8.3. Topical administration

As noted by Majuru and Oyewumi (70) the feasibility of applying nanoparticles in topical/cosmetic preparations has been a subject of several commentaries. In any case, this dosage form utilizes the advantages of nanoparticles such as (a) protection of labile compounds; (b) controlled release of incorporated drugs; (c) ability of solid lipid nanoparticles to act as occlusive to increase the water content of the skin; and (d) ability of nanoparticles to serve as physical barriers on the skin for blocking UV light and, as such, for use in sunscreen formulations.

9. Conclusions

Drug Delivery scientists are searching for the ideal nanovehicle for the ideal nanodrug delivery system; one that would dramatically reduce drug dosage, such that, there is improvement in the absorption of the drug, so that the patient can take a smaller dose, and yet have the same benefit, Deliver the drug to the right place in the living system, Increase the local concentration of the drug at the desired site and limit or eliminate side effects. As it stands today, the scope of this emerging field seems to be limitless. However, considerable technological and financial obstacles still need to be properly addressed by both the private sector and governments before nanotechnology's full promise can be realized. Ranking highest among the challenges is the need to develop and perfect reliable techniques to produce nanoscale particles that does not just have the desirable particle sizes, but also minimal structural defects and acceptable purity levels. This is because these attributes can drastically alter the anticipated behavior of the nanoscale particles. Moving today's promising nanotechnology-related developments from laboratory- and pilot-scale demonstrations to full-scale commercialization is still a big challenge and nanotechnology scientists must gear up to these challenges. Nanotechnology, deals with the design, characterization, production and application of structures, devices and systems by controlling shape and size at the nanometer scale. Two principal factors cause the properties of nanomaterials to differ significantly from other materials: increased relative surface area, and quantum effects. These factors can change or enhance properties such as reactivity, strength, electrical characteristics as well as most of the biomedical properties. Nanotechnology in biomedical sciences is expected to create innovations and play a vital role, not only in drug delivery and gene therapy, but also in molecular imaging, biomarkers and biosensors. Today the application of nanotechnology in drug delivery is widely expected to change the landscape of pharmaceutical and biotechnology industries for the foreseeable future. Target-specific drug therapy and methods for early diagnosis of pathologies are the priority research areas where nanotechnology would play a prominent role. Using nanotechnology, it may be possible to achieve (1) improved delivery of poorly water-soluble drugs; (2) targeted delivery of drugs in a cell- or tissue-specific manner; (3) transcytosis of drugs across tight epithelial and endothelial barriers; (4) delivery of large macromolecule drugs to intracellular sites of action; (5) co-delivery of two or more drugs or therapeutic modality for combination therapy; (6) visualization of sites of drug delivery by combining therapeutic agents with imaging modalities; and (7) real-time read on the in vivo efficacy of a therapeutic agent. For example, with more than 10 million new cases every year, cancer has become one of the most devastating diseases worldwide, yet, the most common cancer treatments are limited to chemotherapy, radiation, and surgery. Although conventional treatment options such as chemotherapy and radiation have experienced many advances over the past decades, cancer therapy is still far from optimal. Frequent challenges encountered by the current cancer therapies include nonspecific systemic distribution of antitumor agents, inadequate drug concentrations reaching the tumor, and the limited ability to monitor therapeutic responses. Poor drug delivery to the target site leads to significant complications, such as multidrug resistance, here nanodrug delivery holds great promise. A large number of nanocarriers have been designed for delivery of peptides via liposomes, noisome, polymeric nanoparticles, solid lipid nanoparticles etc. Polymeric based nanoparticles have taken much attention for safe and effective delivery of proteins. Nanoparticles prepared, particularly in the size range from 10 nm to 100 nm, are considered optimal for cancer therapeutics. Thus multifunctional nanoparticles combining different functionalities like targeting, imaging and therapy into one system can be used for effective cancer treatment. Multifunctional nanoparticles hold great promise for the future of cancer treatment because they can detect the early onset of cancer in each individual patient and deliver suitable therapeutic agents to enhance therapeutic efficacy. The combination of tumor-targeted imaging and therapy in an all-in-one system provides a useful multimodal approach in the battle against debilitating health conditions like cancer. Despite the promise of many of the early nanotechnology-related breakthroughs, the ability to develop cost-effective, commercially and technically viable applications for these laboratory wonders will ultimately be predicated on the research community's ability to bridge the gap—some might say chasm—between the science involved and engineering required, particularly during scale up.

Author details

Martins Ochubiojo Emeje
Centre for Nanomedicine and Biophysical Drug Delivery,
National Institute for Pharmaceutical Research and Development,
Nigeria

Ifeoma Chinwude Obidike
National Institute for Pharmaceutical Research and Development,
Nigeria

Ekaete Ibanga Akpabio
University of Uyo, Akwa-Ibom State,
Nigeria

Sabinus Ifianyi Ofoefule
University of Nigeria, Nsukka,
Nigeria

10. References

[1] Maeda, H., Wu, J., Sawa, T., Matsumura, Y., and Hori, K. (2000) Tumor vascular permeability and the EPR effect in macromolecular therapeutics: a review. J. Controlled Release 65, 271-84.

[2] Palmer, T. N., Caride, V. J., Caldecourt, M. A., Twickler, J., and Abdullah, V. (1984) The mechanism of liposome accumulation in infarction. Biochim. Biophys. Acta 797, 363-8.

[3] Jaracz, S., Chen, J., Kuznetsova, L. V., and Ojima, I. (2005) Recent advances in tumor-targeting anticancer drug conjugates. Bioorg. Med. Chem. 13, 5043-54.

[4] Torchilin, V. P. (2004) Targeted polymeric micelles for delivery of poorly soluble drugs. Cell Mol. Life Sci. 61, 2549-59.

[5] Gabizon, A., Shmeeda, H., Horowitz, A. T., and Zalipsky, S. (2004) Tumor cell targeting of liposome-entrapped drugs with phospholipid- anchored folic acid-PEG conjugates. AdV. Drug DeliVery ReV.56, 1177-92.

[6] Widera, A., Norouziyan, F., and Shen, W. C. (2003) Mechanisms of TfR-mediated transcytosis and sorting in epithelial cells and applications toward drug delivery. AdV. Drug DeliVery ReV.55, 1439-66.

[7] Gupta, B., Levchenko, T. S., and Torchilin, V. P. (2005) Intracel- lular delivery of large molecules and small particles by cell- penetrating proteins and peptides. AdV. Drug DeliVery ReV.57, 637- 51.

[8] Lochmann, D., Jauk, E., and Zimmer, A. (2004) Drug delivery of oligonucleotides by peptides. Eur. J. Pharm. Biopharm. 58, 237- 51.

[9] Torchilin, V. P. (2005) Lipid-core micelles for targeted drug delivery. Curr. Drug DeliVery 2, 319-27.

[10] Torchilin, V. P. (2005) Recent advances with liposomes as pharmaceutical carriers. Nat. ReV. Drug DiscoVery 4, 145-60.

[11] Maheshwari, A., Mahato, R. I., McGregor, J., Han, S., Samlowski, W. E., Park, J. S., and Kim, S. W. (2000) Soluble biodegradable polymer-based cytokine gene delivery for cancer treatment. Mol. Ther. 2, 121-30.

[12] Tachibana, R., Harashima, H., Shono, M., Azumano, M., Niwa, M., Futaki, S., and Kiwada, H. (1998) Intracellular Regulation of Macromolecules Using pH-Sensitive Liposomes and Nuclear

[13] Lo- calization Signal: Qualitative and Quantitative Evaluation of Intra- cellular Trafficking. Biochem. Biophys. Res. Commun. 251, 538- 544.

[14] Torchilin, V. P., Rammohan, R., Weissig, V., and Levchenko, T. S. (2001) TAT peptide on the surface of liposomes affords their efficient intracellular delivery even at low temperature and in the presence of metabolic inhibitors. Proc. Natl. Acad Sci. U.S.A. 98, 8786-91.

[15] Wattiaux, R., Laurent, N., Wattiaux-De Coninck, S., and Jadot, M. (2000) Endosomes, lysosomes: their implication in gene transfer. AdV. Drug DeliVery ReV.41, 201- 208.

[16] Caron, N. J., Torrente, Y., Camirand, G., Bujold, M., Chapdelaine, P., Leriche, K., Bresolin, N., and Tremblay, J. P. (2001) Intracellular delivery of a Tat-eGFP fusion protein into muscle cells. Mol. Ther. 3, 310-8.

[17] Vives, E., Brodin, P., and Lebleu, B. (1997) A truncated HIV-1 Tat protein basic domain rapidly translocates through the plasma membrane and accumulates in the cell nucleus. J. Biol. Chem. 272, 16010-7.

[18] Fawell, S., Seery, J., Daikh, Y., Moore, C., Chen, L. L., Pepinsky, B., and Barsoum, J. (1994) Tat-mediated delivery of heterologous proteins into cells. Proc. Natl. Acad. Sci. U.S.A. 91, 664-8.

[19] Rudolph, C., Plank, C., Lausier, J., Schillinger, U., Muller, R. H., and Rosenecker, J. (2003) Oligomers of the arginine-rich motif of the HIV-1 TAT protein are capable of transferring plasmid DNA into cells. J. Biol. Chem. 278, 11411-8.

[20] Santra, S., Yang, H., Holloway, P. H., Stanley, J. T., and Mericle, R. A. (2005) Synthesis of water-dispersible fluorescent, radio-opaque, and paramagnetic CdS: Mn/ZnS quantum dots: a multifunctional probe for bioimaging. J. Am. Chem. Soc. 127, 1656-7.

[21] Schwarze, S. R., Ho, A., Vocero-Akbani, A., and Dowdy, S. F. (1999) In vivo protein transduction: delivery of a biologically active protein into the mouse. Science 285, 1569-72.

[22] Torchilin, V. P., Levchenko, T. S., Rammohan, R., Volodina, N., Papahadjopoulos-Sternberg, B., and D'Souza, G. G. (2003) Cell transfection in vitro and in vivo with nontoxic TAT peptide- liposome-DNA complexes. Proc. Natl. Acad. Sci. U.S.A. 100, 1972- 7.

[23] Zhao, M., Kircher, M. F., Josephson, L., and Weissleder, R. (2002) Differential conjugation of tat peptide to superparamagnetic nano- particles and its effect on cellular uptake. Bioconjugate Chem. 13, 840-4.

[24] Mai, J. C., Shen, H., Watkins, S. C., Cheng, T., and Robbins, P. D. (2002) Efficiency of protein transduction is cell type-dependent and is enhanced by dextran sulfate. J. Biol. Chem. 277, 30208-18.

[25] Vives, E., Richard, J. P., Rispal, C., and Lebleu, B. (2003) TAT peptide internalization: seeking the mechanism of entry. Curr. Protein Pept. Sci. 4, 125-32.

[26] Snyder, E. L., and Dowdy, S. F. (2004) Cell penetrating peptides in drug delivery. Pharm. Res. 21, 389-93.

[27] Wadia, J. S., Stan, R. V., and Dowdy, S. F. (2004) Transducible TAT-HA fusogenic peptide enhances escape of TAT-fusion proteins after lipid raft macropinocytosis. Nat. Med. 10, 310-5.

[28] Sawant, R. M. Hurley, J. P. Salmaso, S. Kale, A. Tolcheva, E. Levchenko, T. S. and Torchilin V. P. (2006). "SMART" Drug Delivery Systems: Double-Targeted pH-Responsive Pharmaceutical Nanocarriers. Bioconjugate Chem. 17, No. 4, 943–949

[29] Chu, L. Y., Liang, Y. J., Chen, W. M., Ju, X. J.,&Wang, H. D. (2004). Preparation of glucose-sensitive microcapsules with a porous membrane and functional gates. Colloids Surf. B: Biointerfaces, 37, 9–14.

[30] Kim, J. J., & Park, K. (2001). Modulated insulin delivery from glucose-sensitive hydrogel dosage forms. J. Control. Release, 77, 39–47.

[31] Lee, E. S., Shin, H. J., Na, K., & Bae, Y. H. (2003). Poly(L-histidine)-PEG block copolymer micelles and pH-induced destabilization. J. Control. Release, 90, 363–74.

[32] Lee, E. S., Na, K., & Bae, Y. H. (2005a).Doxorubicin loadedpH-sensitive polymeric micelles for reversal of resistant MCF-7 tumor. J. Control. Release, 103, 405–18.

[33] Hruby, M., Konak, C., & Ulbrich, K. (2005). Polymeric micellar pH-sensitive drug delivery system for doxorubicin. J. Control. Release, 103, 137–48.

[34] Ringsdorf, H. (1975). Structure and properties of pharmacologically active polymers. J. Polym. Sci. Polym. Sympo., 51, 135–153.

[35] Duncan, R. (2006). Polymer conjugates as anticancer nanomedicines. Nat. Rev. Cancer, 6, 688–701.

[36] Duncan, R.; Ringsdorf, H.; Satchi-Fainaro, R., Polymer therapeutics: Polymers as drugs, drug and protein conjugates and gene delivery systems: Past, present and future opportunities. Advances in Polymer Science 2006, 192, (1), 1–8.

[37] Ringsdorf, H., Structure and Properties of Pharmacologically Active Polymers. Journal of Polymer Science, Polymer Symposia 1975, (51), 135–153.

[38] Harris, J. M.; Chess, R. B., Effect of pegylation on pharmaceuticals. Nature Reviews Drug Discovery 2003, 2, (3), 214–21.

[39] Veronese, F. M.; Pasut, G., PEGylation, successful approach to drug delivery. Nature Reviews Drug Discovery 2005, 10, (21), 1451–8.

[40] Parveen, S.; Sahoo, S. K., Nanomedicine: Clinical applications of polyethylene glycol conjugated proteins and drugs. Clinical Pharmacokinetics 2006, 45, (10), 965–988.

[41] Graham, M. L., Pegaspargase:Areview of clinical studies. Advanced Drug Delivery Reviews 2003, 55, (10), 1293–1302.

[42] Lee, S., Youn, Y. S., Lee, S. H., Byun, Y., & Lee, K. C. (2006). PEGylated glucagon-like peptide-1 displays preserved effects on insulin release in isolated pancreatic islets and improved biological activity in db/db mice. Diabetologia, 49, 1608–11.

[43] Shimoboji, T., Larenas, E., Fowler, T., Kulkarni, S., Hoffman, A. S., & Stayton, P. S. (2002). Photoresponsive polymer-enzyme switches. Proc. Natl. Acad. Sci. U S A, 99, 16592–6.

[44] Shimoboji, T., Larenas, E., Fowler, T., Hoffman, A. S., & Stayton, P. S. (2003). Temperature-induced switching of enzyme activity with smart polymer-enzyme conjugates. Bioconjug. Chem., 14, 517–25.

[45] Lee, E. S., Na, K., & Bae, Y. H. (2005b). Super pH-sensitive multifunctional polymeric micelle. Nano. Lett., 5, 325–9.

[46] Torchilin, V. P. (2006). Multifunctional nanocarriers. Adv. Drug Deliv. Rev., 58, 1532–55.

[47] Lukyanov, A. N., Elbayoumi, T. A., Chakilam, A. R., & Torchilin, V. P. (2004). Tumor-targeted liposomes: doxorubicin-loaded long-circulating liposomes modified with anticancer antibody. J. Control. Release, 100, 135–44.

[48] Craighead, H. (2006). Future lab-on-a-chip technologies for interrogating individual molecules. Nature, 442, 387–93.

[49] Demello, A. J. (2006). Control and detection of chemical reactions in microfluidic systems. Nature, 442, 394–402.

[50] El-Ali, J., Sorger, P. K., & Jensen, K. F. (2006). Cells on chips. Nature, 442, 403–11.

[51] Janasek, D., Franzke, J., & Manz, A. (2006). Scaling and the design of miniaturized chemical-analysis systems. Nature, 442, 374–80.

[52] Psaltis, D., Quake, S. R., & Yang, C. (2006). Developing optofluidic technology through the fusion of microfluidics and optics. Nature, 442, 381–6.

[53] Whitesides, G. M. (2006). The origins and the future of microfluidics. Nature, 442, 368–73.

[54] Yager, P., Edwards, T., Fu, E., Helton, K., Nelson, K., Tam, M. R., &Weigl, B. H. (2006). Microfluidic diagnostic technologies for global public health. Nature, 442, 412–8.

[55] Li, Y., Ho Duc, H. L., Tyler, B., Williams, T., Tupper, M., Langer, R., Brem, H., & Cima, M. J. (2005). In vivo delivery of BCNU from a MEMS device to a tumor model. J. Control. Release, 106, 138–45.

[56] Maloney, J. M., Uhland, S. A., Polito, B. F., Sheppard, N. F., Jr., Pelta, C. M., & Santini, J. T., Jr. (2005). Electrothermally activated microchips for implantable drug delivery and biosensing. J. Control. Release, 109, 244–55.

[57] Tao, S. L., & Desai, T. A. (2005). Micromachined devices: the impact of controlled geometry from cell-targeting to bioavailability. J. Control. Release, 109, 127–38.

[58] Richards Grayson, A. C., Scheidt Shawgo, R., Li, Y., & Cima, M. J. (2004). Electronic MEMS for triggered delivery. Adv. Drug Deliv. Rev., 56, 173–84.

[59] Hirsch, L. R., Gobin, A.M., Lowery, A. R., Tam, F., Drezek, R. A., Halas, N. J., & West, J. L. (2006). Metal nanoshells. Ann. Biomed. Eng., 34, 15–22.

[60] Corot, C., Robert, P., Idee, J. M., & Port, M. (2006). Recent advances in iron oxide nanocrystal technology for medical imaging. Adv. Drug Deliv. Rev., 58,1471–504.

[61] Mozafari M R and Sahin N O, Manufacturing methods and mechanism of formation of lipid vesicles. In: Nanoliposomes: From Fundamentals to Recent Developments. MozafariMR& Mortazavi S M (Eds.), Trafford Publishing Ltd, Oxford, UK, pp 39–48, 2005

[62] Visser C C, Stevanovic S, Voorwinden L H, Bloois L V, Gaillard P J, Danhof M, Crommelin D J A and Boer A G, (2005).Targeting liposomes with protein drugs to the blood-brain barrier in vitro, European Journal of Pharmaceutical Sciences, 25, 299–305

[63] Lopez-Pinto J M, Gonzalez-Rodriguez M L and Rabasco A M, (2005). Effect of cholesterol and ethanol on dermal delivery from DPPC liposomes, International Journal of Pharmaceutics, 298, 1–12.

[64] Ozden M Y and Hasirci V N, (1991). Preparation and characterization of polymer coated small unilamellar vesicles, Biochimica et Biophysica Acta (BBA) – General Subjects, 1075, 102–108.

[65] Ito A, Hibino E, Honda H, Hata K, Kagami H, Ueda M and Kobayashi T, (2004). A new methodology of mesenchymal stem cell expansion using magnetic nanoparticles, Biochemical Engineering Journal, 20, 119–125.

[66] Kunisawa J, Masuda T, Katayama K, Yoshikawa T, Tsutsumi Y, Akashi M, Mayumi T and Nakagawa S, (2005). Fusogenic liposome delivers encapsulated nanoparticles for cytosolic controlled gene release, Journal of Controlled Release, 105, 344–353.

[67] Foco A, Gasperlin M and Kristl J, (2005). Investigation of liposomes as carriers of sodium ascorbyl phosphate for cutaneous photoprotection, International Journal of Pharmaceutics, 291, 21–29.

[68] Sinico C, Manconi M, Peppi M, Lai F, Valenti D and Fadda A M, (2005). Liposomes as carriers for dermal delivery of tretinoin: in vitro evaluation of drug permeation and vesicle–skin interaction, Journal of Controlled Release, 103, 123–136.

[69] Arcon I, Kodre A, Abra R M, Huang A, Vallner J J and Lasic D D, (2004). study of liposome- encapsulated cisplatin, Colloids and Surfaces B: Biointerfaces, 33, 199–204.

[70] Shingai Majuru and Moses O. Oyewumi. Nanotechnology in Drug Development and Life Cycle Management. M.M. de Villiers et al. (eds.), Nanotechnology in Drug Delivery, (2009). Chapter 20, Pp. 597 – 619

[71] T. Jung,W. Kamm, A. Breitenbach, E. Kaiserling, J.X. Xiao, T. Kissel, (2000). Biodegradable nanoparticles for oral delivery of peptides: is there a role for polymers to affect mucosal uptake? Eur. J. Pharm. Biopharm. 50 147–160.

[72] C. Pinto Reis, R.J. Neufeld, A.J. Ribeiro, F. Veiga, (2006). Nanoencapsulation I. Methods for preparation of drug-loaded polymeric nanoparticles, Nanomedicine 2 8–21.

[73] L. Illum, (2007). Nanoparticulate systems for nasal delivery of drugs: a real improvement over simple systems? J. Pharm. Sci. 96 473–483.

[74] Geresh, S., Gdalevsky, G.Y., Gilboa, I., Voorspoels, J., Remon, J.P., Kost, J (2004). Bioadhesive grafted starch copolymers as platforms for peroral drug delivery: a study of theophylline release. Journal of controlled release 94(2-3): 391-399.

[75] Levina, M., Rajabi-Siahboomi,A.R. (2004). The influence of excipients on drug release from hydroxypropylmethyl cellulose matrices. Journal of pharmaceutical sciences 93(11): 2746-2754.

[76] Yamini, K., Chalapathi, V., Lakshmi Narasimha Reddy, N., Lokesh, K.V., Praveen Kumar Reddy, S., Gopal,V. (2011). Formulation of diclofenac sodium tablets using tapioca starch powder- A promising binder. Journal of applied pharmaceutical sciences 1(3):125-127)

[77] Malafaya. B, P., Stappers, F., Reis, R.L. (2006). Starch-based microspheres produced by emulsion crosslinking with a potential media dependent responsive behavior to be used as drug delivery carriers. Journal of material science: Materials in medicine 17: 371-377.

[78] Heller J., P.S.H., Roskos K.V. (1990). Development of enzymatically degradable protective coatings for use in triggered drug delivery systems: derivatized starch hydrogels. Biomaterials 11(5)¬: 345-350

[79] Wu, C., Zhongyan, W., Zhi, Z., Jang, T., Zhang, J., Wang, S (2011). Development of biodegradable porous starch foam for improving oral delivery of poorly water soluble drugs. International journal of pharmaceutics 403: 162-169.

[80] Santander-Ortega, M.J., Stauner, T., Loretz, B., Ortega-Vinuesa, J.L., Bastos-González, D., Wenz, G., Schaefer U.F., Lehr, C.M. (2010). Nanoparticles made from novel starch derivatives for transdermal drug delivery. Journal of controlled release 141:85-92.

[81] Mahkam, M. (2010). Modified Chitosan Cross-linked Starch Polymers for Oral Insulin Delivery. Journal of Bioactive and Compatible polymers 25(4): 406-418

[82] Jain, A.K., Khar, R.K., Ahmed, F.J., Diwan. P.V (2008). Effective insulin delivery using starch nanoparticles as a potential trans-nasal mucoadhesive carrier.European Journal of Pharmaceutics and Biopharmaceutics 69 (2):426-435

[83] Simi, C.K., Abraham, T.E. (2007). Hydrophobic grafted and cross-linked starch nanoparticles for drug delivery. Bioprocess and biosystems engineering 30(3): 173-180

[84] Cole, A.J., David, A.E., Wang, J., Galbian, C., Yang, V.C. (2011). Magnetic brain tumor targeting and biodistribution of long-circulating PEG-modified, cross-linked starch-coated iron oxide nanoparticles. Biomaterials 32(26): 6291-6301

[85] Sabnis, S., Block, L (2000). Chitosan as an enabling excipient for drug delivery systems: 1.Molecular Modifications. International journal of biologicalmacromolecules 27(3): 181-186

[86] Park, J.H., Saravanakuma, G., Kwangmeyung, K., Kwon, I. (2010) Targeted delivery of low molecular drugs using chitosan and its derivatives. Advanced drug delivery reviews 62(1): 28-41

[87] Thacharodi, D., Panduranga Rao, K (1996) Collagen-Chitosan composite membranes controlled transdermal delivery of nifedipine and propranolol hydrochloride. International journal of pharmaceutics 134:239-241.

[88] Thacharodi, D., Panduranga Rao, K. (1995) Development and in-vitro evaluation of chitosan-based transdermal drug delivery systems for the controlled delivery of propranolol hydrochloride. Biomaterials 16: 145-148

[89] Dev, A., Binulal , N.S., Anitha, A., Nair, S.V., Furuike,T., Tamura, H., Jayakumar, R., (2010) Preparation of poly (lactic acid)/chitosan nanoparticles for anti-HIV drug delivery applications. Carbohydrate polymers 80: 833-838

[90] Menon, D., Thomas, R.T., Narayanan, S., Maya, S., Jayakumar, R., Hussain, F., Lakshmanana, V., Nair, S.V. (2011) A novel chitosan/polyoxometalate nano-complex for anti-cancer applications. Carbohydrate polymers 84:887-893

[91] Luo, Q., Zhao, J., Zhang, X., Pan, W (2011) Nanostructured lipid carrier (NLC) coated with chitosan oligosaccharides and its potential use in ocular drug delivery system. International journal of pharmaceutics 403(1-2): 185-191

[92] Bajpai, A.K., Choubey, J. (2005) Release study of sulphamethoxazole controlled by swelling of gelatin nanoparticles and drug-biopolymer interaction. Journal of macromolecular science 42:253-275.

[93] Das, P.R., Nanda, R.M., Behara, A., Nayak, P.R. (2011) Gelatin blended with nanoparticle cloisite30B (MMT) for control drug delivery of anticancer drug paclitaxel International research journal of biochemistry and bioinformatics 1(2):35-42.

[94] Coester, C., Kreuter, J., von Briesen, H., Langer. K. (2000) Preparation of avidin-labelled gelatin nanoparticles as carriers for biotinylated peptide nucleic acid (PNA). International journal of pharmaceutics 196:147-149

[95] Zwiorek, K., Kloeckner, J., Wagner, K,. Coeste. C. (2004) Gelatin nanoparticles as a new and simple gene delivery system. Journal of pharmacy and pharmaceutical sciences 7(4):22-28

[96] Xu, X., Capito, R.M.,Spector, M. (2008) Delivery of plasmid IGF-1 to chondrocytes via cationizedgelatin nanoparticles. Journal of Biomedical material research 84(1): 73-83

[97] K.K. Jain, Nanopharmaceuticals Chapter 4 In: *The Handbook of Nanomedicine*, 2008 Humana Press, Totowa, NJ pp 119 – 160

[98] Kipp, J.E. (2004) The role of solid nanoparticle technology in the parenteral delivery of poorly water-soluble drugs. Int. J. Pharm. 284, 109–122

[99] A. K. Bajpai, Jyoti Choubey. (2006). Design of gelatin nanoparticles as swelling controlled delivery system for chloroquine phosphate. J Mater Sci: Mater Med 17: 345–358

[100] Daniel Honig, Jason DeRouchey, Ralf Jungmann, Christian Koch, *Christian Plank* and Joachim O. Radler. Biophysical Characterization of Copolymer-Protected Gene Vectors. Biomacromolecules, *2010*, 11 *(7), pp 1802–1809*

[101] Luigi Battaglia, Michele Trotta, Marina Gallarate, M. Eugenia Carlotti, Gian Paolo Zara,& Alessandro Bargon. Solid lipid nanoparticles formed by solvent-in-water emulsion–diffusion technique: Development and influence on insulin stability. Journal of Microencapsulation, November 2007; 24(7): 672–684

[102] Bargoni A, Cavalli R, Caputo O, Fundaro A, Gasco MR, Zara GP. 1998. Solid lipid nanoparticles in lymph and plasma after duodenal administration to rats. Pharmaceutical Research 15:745–750.

[103] Trotta M, Debernardi F, Caputo O. 2003. Preparation of solid lipid nanoparticles by a solvent emulsification-diffusion technique. International Journal of Pharmaceutics 257:153–160.

[104] Trotta M, Cavalli R, Carlotti ME, Battaglia L, Debernardi F. 2005. Solid lipid microparticles carrying insulin formed by solvent-in-water emulsion-diffusion technique. International Journal of Pharmaceutics 288:281–288.

[105] Müller RH. Lipid nanoparticles: recent advances. Adv Drug Deliv Rev 2007;59:522-30.

[106] Joshi M, Müller RH. Lipid nanoparticles for parenteral delivery of actives. Eur J Pharm Biopharm 2009;71:161-72.

[107] Müller RH, Radtke M, Wissing SA. Nanostructured lipid matrices for improved microencapsulation of drugs. Int J Pharm 2002;242:121-8.

[108] Müller RH. Preparation, characterization and physico-chemical properties of solid lipid nanoparticles (SLN) and nanostructured lipid carriers (NLC): their benefits as colloidal drug carrier systems. Pharmazie 2006;61:375-86.

[109] Müller RH, Radtke M, Wissing SA. Solid lipid nanoparticles (SLN) and nanostructured lipid carriers (NLC) in cosmetic and dermatological preparations. Adv Drug Deliv Rev 2002;54:S131-55.

[110] Doktorovova S, Souto EB. Nanostructured lipid carriers-based hydrogel formulations for drug delivery: A comprehensive review. Expert Opin Drug Deliv 2009;6:165-76.

[111] Souto EB, Müller RH. Lipid nanoparticles: effect on bioavailability and pharmacokinetic changes. Handb Exp Pharmacol 2010;115-41.

[112] Souto EB. A special issue on lipid-based delivery systems (liposomes, lipid nanoparticles, lipid matrices and medicines). J Biomed Nanotechnol 2009;5:315-6.

[113] Martins Emeje; John-Africa, Lucy; Yetunde Isimi; Olobayo Kunle and Sabinus
      Ofoefule (2012). Eudraginated – polymer blends: a potential oral controlled drug
      delivery system for theophylline. Acta Pharmaceutica 62: 71 – 82.
[114] Lu B, Zhang JQ, Yang H. (2003). Lung-targeting microspheres of carboplatin. Int J
      Pharm, 265:1–11.

Chapter 5

Niosomes as Carrier in Dermal Drug Delivery

Yahya Rahimpour and Hamed Hamishehkar

Additional information is available at the end of the chapter

1. Introduction

Colloidal vesicular carriers such as liposomes or niosomes have been extensively applied in drug delivery systems due to unique advantages. These vesicles can act as drug reservoirs and the rate of drug release can be modified by changing of their composition. These lipid carriers can encapsulate both hydrophilic drugs (by loading in inner space) and hydrophobic drugs (in lipid area). Because of their potential to carry a variety of drugs, these lipid vesicles have been widely used in various drug delivery systems like drug targeting, controlled release and permeation enhancement of drugs (Akhilesh et al., 2011). Dermal (topical) delivery defines a targeting to the pathological sites within the skin with the least systemic absorption. Drug localization in this case is a crucial issue in the treatment of dermatological problems such as skin cancer, psoriasis, alopecia and acne, where the origin of disease is located in the skin (Brown et al., 2006). Topical drug administration has been initiated since long time to accomplish several functions on different skin levels (skin surface, epidermis, dermis and hypodermis). But, several limitations have been associated with the conventional topical preparations e.g. low percutaneous penetration because of the barrier function of the stratum corneum, the outermost layer of the skin, (Rubio et al., 2011) and absorption to the systemic circulation (Dubey et al., 2012). The scientific reports nowadays offer several systems that can be able to deliver drugs through the skin (Higaki et al., 2005). Recently niosomes are becoming popular in the field of topical drug delivery due to its outstanding characteristics like enhancing the penetration of drugs, providing a sustained pattern of drug release and ability to carry both hydrophilic and lipophilic drugs (Sathali et al., 2010). This chapter deals with the potential of niosome in topical delivery system focusing on its clinical approach. Skin represents a multilayered effective barricade to the penetration of drugs. The outer layer of skin, stratum corneum, provides a rate limiting step during percutaneous absorption of drug. Drug transfer across the stratum corneum is mainly a passive process, and thus the physicochemical properties of a permeant have a key role in its capability to penetrate and diffuse across the membrane. Compounds can penetrate through the stratum corneum via three routes: intercellular, transcellular (paracellular), and transappendageal (figure 1). Once it has transferred through the epidermis, a compound may be carried away by the dermal blood circulation or to be transported to deeper tissues. The relative significance of these penetration pathways will be largely dependent on the physicochemical characteristics of the drug molecules, particularly the partition and diffusion coefficients into the protein or lipid regions (Barry, 1991).

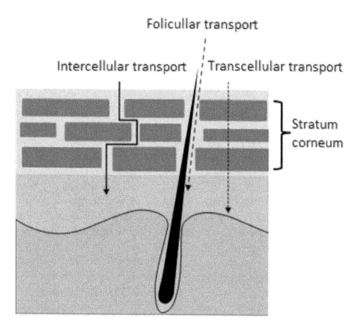

Figure 1. Possible pathways for delivery of compounds across the stratum corneum adapted from reference (Gašperlin et al., 2011).

For successful dermal or transdermal delivery, a reversible overcoming of skin barrier is required. Therefore, many strategies have been assessed to overcome the barrier function of the stratum corneum and to improve drug transport into the skin (Ghafourian et al., 2004; Rahimpour et al., 2012). Targeting of topically administered drugs to the different skin layers and appendages is becoming a main center of interest for many pharmaceutical research groups studying in dermatology (Nounou et al., 2008). The carrier is one of the most important entities required for successful targeted drug delivery (figure 2). Carriers will enable a drug to reach the desired pharmacological site of action at a controlled rate and to have a sustained duration of action. Consequently, as a vehicle for active substances and targeting to skin layers, surfactant based carriers such as niosomal systems are gaining more interest.

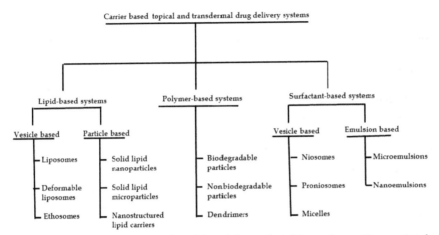

Figure 2. Carriers for topical and transdermal drug delivery adapted from reference (Venuganti et al., 2009).

2. Niosome

Niosomes are microscopic lamellar structures composed of non-ionic surfactants and cholesterol. The niosomes have amphiphillic bilayer structure in a way that polar region is oriented outside and inside the vesicles where the hydrophilic drug will be entrapped and non-polar region is formed within the bilayer where hydrophobic drug can be entrapped (Khan et al., 2011). The formation of vesicular system based on hydration of mixture of a single-alkyl chain nonionic surfactant and cholesterol was firstly reported in 1979 (Handjani-Vila et al., 1979). Niosomes might be produced by various types of nonionic surfactants including polyglycerol alkyl ethers, crown ethers, ester-linked surfactants, glucosyldialkyl ethers, polyoxyethylene alkyl ethers, Brij, Tweens and Spans. Nonionic surfactants used to prepare niosomes carry no charge and are relatively nontoxic and mild to use (Azeem et al., 2009).

2.1. Types of niosomes

2.1.1. Proniosomes

Proniosome is a dry granular product that can be able to form a niosome suspension after hydration (Hu et al., 2000). Proniosomes are developed to overcome the disadvantage of vesicular system. Proniosome are prepared based on the simple scheme that a mixture of surfactant/alcohol/aqueous phase can be used to prepare a concentrated proniosome gel, which can instinctively be converted to a stable niosomal dispersion by dilution with excess aqueous phase (Perrett et al., 1991).

Carrier + surfactant = Proniosomes

Proniosomes + water = Niosomes

2.1.2. *Aspasomes*

Mixture of acorbyl palmitate, cholesterol and highly charged lipid diacetyl phosphate leads to the construction of vesicles named aspasomes. Aspasomes are first hydrated with water/aqueous solution and then sonicated to attain the niosomes. Aspasomes are suggested to improve the transdermal permeation of drugs. Aspasomes have also been used to reduce disorders caused by reactive oxygen species due to its intrinsic antioxidant property (Gopinath et al., 2004; Rajera et al., 2011).

2.1.3. *Vesicles in water and oil system (v/w/o)*

In this system suspension of aqueous niosomes (v/w) are emulsified into the oily phase at 60°C to form vesicle in water in oil emulsion (v/w/o) (Yoshida et al., 1992; Hu et al., 2000). Cooling to room temperature forms vesicle in water in oil gel (v/w/o gel) (Yoshioka et al., 1992). The prepared v/w/o gel can entrap the hydrophilic active ingredients which are susceptible for enzymatic degradation such as proteins/proteinous drugs and also provide a controlled release pattern in drug delivery.

2.1.4. *Deformable niosomes*

Elastic niosomes are prepared of nonionic surfactants, ethanol and water. They show superior to conventional niosomes due to their capability to increase penetration efficiency of a compound through intact skin by passing through pores in the stratum corneum, which are smaller than the vesicles (figure 3). The flexibility of their structure allows them to pass through pores that are less than one-tenth of these vesicles (Cevc, 1996; Cevc et al., 1996).

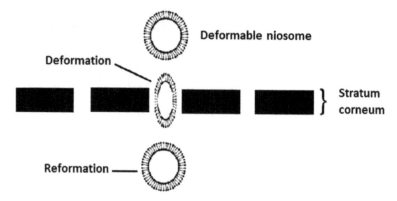

Figure 3. Mechanism of skin permeation of deformable niosome adapted from reference (Kumar et al., 2012)

2.2. Advantages of noisome

The major advantages of niosomes can be mentioned as: i) niosomes are biodegradable, biocompatible, non-toxic and non-immunogenic (Azeem et al., 2009); ii) niosomes are able to encapsulate large amount of materials in a small volume of vesicles (Nasr et al., 2008); iii) niosomes have better patient adherence and satisfication and also better effectiveness than conventional oily formulations (Jain et al., 2006); iv) niosomes can entrap wide range of chemicals (hydrophilic, lipophilic and amphiphilic drugs) due to its unique structure (Raja Naresh et al., 1994); v) the characteristics of niosome such as shape, fluidity and size can be easily controlled by changing in structural composition and method of production (Bayindir et al., 2010); vi) niosomes can be prescribed via different administration routes such as oral, parenteral and topical, etc. with different dosage forms such as semisolids, powders, suspensions (Malhotra et al., 1994) and vii) due to chemical stability of structural composition, the storage of the niosome is easy (Jain et al., 2006). In spite of several above mentioned merits, niosomes show some disadvantages. The aqueous suspensions of niosomes may undergo fusion, aggregation, leaking of entrapped drugs, and hydrolysis of encapsulated drugs, which lead to limited shelf life. The methods of preparation of multilamellar vesicles such as extrusion, sonication, are time consuming and may require specialized equipments for processing (Khan et al., 2011)

2.3. Application of niosome

Niosomes have been successfully used in drug targeting to various organs such as skin (Agarwal et al., 2001), brain (Abdelkader et al., 2012), liver (Baillie et al., 1986; Lala et al., 2004), lung (Desai et al., 2002; Abd-Elbary et al., 2008) ocular systems (Pugeat et al., 1991; Abdelkader et al., 2012), tumor (Ruckmani et al., 2000; Shi et al., 2005) etc. Niosomes show a higher bioavailability than conventional dosage forms (Raja Naresh et al., 1994). Controlled and sustained release of drugs have been achieved by niosomes (Bayindir et al., 2010). Permeation of drugs through the skin has been enhanced by niosomes (Pardakhty et al., 2007). Noisome, itself improves the stratum corneum properties both by reducing transepidermal water loss and skin condition by increasing smoothness via reloading lost skin lipids (Firthouse et al.). Niosomes can be applied for drug protection from biological enzymes and acid thereby increasing the drug stability (Jain et al., 2006).

2.4. Niosomes in comparison with liposomes

Niosomes and liposomes have similar application in drug delivery but chemically differ in structure units. Niosomes constitute of non-ionic surfactant whereas liposomes comprise of phospholipids (Khan et al., 2011). They are functionally the same, have the same physical properties and act as amphiphilic vesicules. Both can be used in targeted and sustained drug delivery system. Property of both depends upon composition of the bilayer and methods of their preparation (Verma et al., 2012). Studies have also shown that the function of niosomes in vivo is similar to that of liposomes (Hofland et al., 1994). In spite of these comparable characteristics, niosomes offer several advantages over liposomes: intrinsic skin penetration enhancing properties, higher chemical stability and lower costs (Nasr et al., 2008). Both of the last features make the niosome more attractive for industrial manufacturing (Hu et al., 2000). Also, niosomes do not require special conditions such as low temperature or inert atmosphere during preparation and storage (Verma et al., 2012). Although the niosome shows better chemical stability, the physical instability during dispersion may be comparable to that of the liposome. Both niosomes and liposomes are at risk of aggregation, fusion, drug leakage, or hydrolysis of entrapped drugs during storage (Hu et al., 2000; Rahimpour et al., 2012).

3. Mechanisms of niosomal skin delivery

Several mechanisms have been suggested to describe the ability of niosomes in transdermal and dermal drug delivery: i) niosomes diffuse from the stratum corneum layer of skin as a whole; ii) new smaller vesicles are formed in skin (re-formation of noisome vesicles). The water content of skin is crucial issue for interpreting and establishing this mechanism. Smaller diameter of lipid lamellar spaces of the stratum corneum than noisome vesicles makes this mechanism more meaningful (Sahin, 2007). iii) noisomes interact with stratum corneum with aggregation, fusion and adhesion to the cell surface which causes a high thermodynamic activity gradient of the drug at the vesicle-stratum corneum surface, which is the driving force for the penetration of lipophilic drugs across the stratum corneum (Ogiso et al., 1996). Scanning electron microscopy confirmed the fusion of niosome vesicles of estradiol on the surface of skin (Schreier et al., 1994) iv) niosomes may modify stratum corneum structure which makes the intercellular lipid barrier of stratum corneum looser and more permeable (Fang et al., 2001); v) non-ionic surfactant itself, the composing ingredient of niosome, acts as a permeation enhancer and might partly contribute to the improvement of drug permeation from niosomes (Javadzadeh et al., 2010). The type of surfactant plays an important role in modification of permeation using niosome vehicles. Niosomes fabricated from polyoxyethylene stearyl ether and existing in the gel state did not enhance estradiol permeation, and those prepared from polyoxyethylene lauryl ether and polyoxyethylene oleyl ether, both existing as liquid crystalline vesicles, considerably improved transport (Hofland et al., 1991).

4. Toxicity of niosomes

Surfactants are suspected to show toxicity but there are virtually not enough research about toxicity of niosomes (Yadav et al., 2011). A study on the toxicity effect of surfactant type of niosomal formulations on human keratocytes showed that the ester type surfactants are less toxic than ether type due to enzymatic degradation of ester bounds (Hofland et al., 1991). Hofland et al. studied the toxicity of CxEOy surfactants via ciliotoxicity model on nasal mucosa (which is important for intranasal administration) and on human kerationocytes (which is important for the transdermal application of vesicles). The results showed that increase in alkyl chain length of surfactant causes a reduction in toxicity, while, increase in the polyoxyethylne chain length enhances ciliotoxicity. The study supposed that ciliotoxicity related to liquid state formation with increasing in polyoxyethylene chain length, while increase in alkyl chain length of surfactant leads to formation of gel which is more safe than liquid state (Hofland et al., 1992). In another study, vincristine, a potent anti-tumor agent, was loaded into niosomes and administered intravenously. Result showed a significant increase in vincristine anti-tumor activity in S-180 sarcoma and Erlich ascites mouse models followed by reduction of its side effect such as diarrhea, neurological toxicity and alopecia compared with free drug (Parthasarathi et al., 1994). Toxicity effect of niosomes should be considered according to the intended route of delivery. For example, hemocompatibility studies should be carried out when the niosomes are meant to be delivered by intravenous route to evaluate their toxic potential (Uchegbu et al., 1997). The first in vivo experiment on drug delivery by means of synthetic non-ionic surfactant vesicles were carried out by Azmin et al. and reported that no unfavorable effects were observed in the performed experiment (Azmin et al., 1985). Rogerson et al. reported in vivo experiment over 70 male BALB/C mice and stated that no fatalities were related to niosomes. The drug associated toxicity were also reduced (Rogerson et al., 1987). Niosomes which have been prepared with Bola-surfactants showed a certain and encouraging safety and tolerability both in vitro on human keratinocyte cells up to an incubation time of 72 h for the different concentrations studied (0.01-10 μM) and in vivo on human volunteers that showed no skin erythema when topically treated with the drug free Bola-niosome formulation (Paolino et al., 2007).

5. Indications for niosomes as drug carriers in dermatology

Niosomes were formulated and patented for the dermatological purposes in 1975 for the first time and since then many of products were developed based on this technology and appeared in the market such as Lancome Noisome Plus as an anti-ageing formulation (Azeem et al., 2009). Recently, the topical delivery of certain drugs using niosome has been developed. Here, current attempts with a focus on clinical application were reviewed to prove the ability of niosomes as the superior topical carrier.

5.1. Local anesthesia

Dermatologists take benefit of topical anesthetics for decreasing pain relief prior to cutaneous procedures, pain associated with laser pulses, or soft tissue augmentation. Inefficient formulations of local anesthetics resulted in severe dermatitis, systemic toxicity, or inadequate local analgesia. Carafa et al. fabricated lidocaine and lidocaine hydrochloride-loaded non-ionic surfactant vesicles using Tween 20™ and cholesterol. The ability of drug to diffuse through a model lipophilic membrane (Silastic™) and through mouse skin were studied and compared with classical liposomes and Tween 20 micelles. Dicetylphosphate and N-cetylpyridinium chloride were also used to prepare negatively and positively charged vesicles, respectively to study the effect of vesicle charge on drug encapsulation efficiency. Diffusion experiments indicated that the flux of charged lidocaine (lidocaine hydrochloride) through Silastic™ membrane was possible only after the vesicle encapsulation. Permeation of lidocaine hydrochloride-loaded vesicles through mouse abdominal skin presented a higher flux and a shorter lag time with respect to classical liposome formulations, whereas lidocaine permeation rate was quite similar for niosomes and liposome formulations. Furthermore fluorescence quenching study showed that positive and negative charged vesicles had negligible entrapment efficiency of drug, at pH

5.5 compare with neutral vesicles (Tween 20 and cholesterol). The importance of non-ionic surfactant vesicles in dermal delivery of charged local anesthetics is concluded in this study (Carafa et al., 2002).

5.2. Psoriasis

Psoriasis is a chronic inflammatory condition of the skin which may drastically undermined the patient quality of life. Psoriasis, a T-lymphocyte-mediated autoimmune disease of the dermis and epidermis, is characterized by leukocyte infiltration into the skin and localized deregulated skin growth, which leads to the development of scaling erythematous plaques (Dubey et al., 2007). Although psoriasis is rarely life-threatening, it causes an unpleasant appearance that makes the patients to miss their confidence and suffer from itching, painful and disfiguring skin lesions. Methotrexate, anthralin, corticosteroids, coal tar, vitamin D3 analogs, tacrolimus and retinoids are administered topically for psoriasis treatment (Su et al., 2008). Topical therapy is the commonly used in patients, even though the use of topical formulations based on conventional excipients shows some disadvantages that limit considerably their use in therapy (Puglia et al., 2012). With the use of niosomes as carrier for topical drug delivery, the possibility to improve efficacy and safety of the topical products has improved manifold. Dithranol, one of the key medicines in the topical treatment of psoriasis, has staining, burning, irritating and necrotizing effects on the normal and also the diseased skin. Entrapment of dithranol in niosomal and liposomal systems could be achieved after optimizing the various process and formulation variables. These systems presented size stability and improved drug permeation properties. Although the in vitro study using laca mice abdominal skin shows higher skin penetration for vesicular systems compared with the cream base but niosomal vesicular systems had three times less percutaneous permeation of dithranol compared with liposomal formulation (Agarwal et al., 2001). Methotrexate is an antifolate class of anti-neoplastic medicine which is commonly used in the psoriasis therapy. The systemic administration of this drug causes several side effects such as hepatic toxicity. Dermal delivery of methotrexate offers a valuable alternative way to reduce its adverse effects (Javadzadeh et al., 2011). The double-blind placebo-controlled study of methotrexate-loaded niosomal vesicles in chitosan gel on healthy human volunteers and psoriasis patients carried out and its efficacy compared with marketed methotrexate gel. The irritation and skin sensitivity of formulations were assessed via human repeated insult patch test (HRIPT). The HRIPT method did not yield any significant sensitization or irritation on healthy human volunteers. The severity of the lesions of psoriasis was assessed via Psoriasis Area Severity Index (PASI). The global score used to assess the outcome of therapy (on a scale of 0-5), where score of 5 indicates the worsening of lesion and score 0 indicates complete clearance of lesion. There was a three times reduction in PASI scores after 12 weeks of niosomal methotrexate gel. The results of study offer niosomal formulation of methotrexate for dermal treatment of psoriasis due to its better clinical efficacy, tolerability and patient compliance (Lakshmi et al., 2007). Urea is an emollient topically used for the non-surgical removal of dystrophic nails in cases of fungal infections for decades and used as a penetration enhancer for the topical corticosteroid treatment of hyperkeratotic psoriatic plaques (Draelos, 2008). Urea may increase ability of skin to retain water due to hygroscopic effect. The same group in another study encapsulated urea into niosomes and prepared a gel using chitosan polymer, to test the same on healthy human volunteers to check the irritation on the skin and to study its clinical effectives on psoriasis patients. Niosomes prepared using span 60 showed a better entrapment than other spans. Better diffusion of drug through the human skin and skin drug deposition were concluded from niosomal gel in comparison to plain gel. The niosomal urea gel and plain gel did not produce any irritation of the human skin. The gels were assessed on psoriasis patients with less than 25% severity of any types of psoriasis. The niosomal gel showed a significant decrease in the lesion (p<0.05) than plain urea gel. It is suggested that chitosan gel can be used as an adjuvant in the treatment of psoriasis due to antifungal and anti-inflammatory effect of chitosan that supported the action of urea (Lakshmi et al., 2011).

5.3. Whitening effect

The attractiveness of pigment-lightening cosmeceuticals comes from the desire to not only fade pigmentation but also to even lighten skin tone (Choi et al., 2006). N-acetyl glucosamine (NAG), which is an amino sugar that occurs widely in nature and essential component of dermal tissues, is well-known for its role as a precursor of hyaluronic acid, a key structural composition of skin. NAG shown to inhibit melanin production in melanocyte culture, thus has a potential to reduce hyperpigmentation by topical administration (Bissett et al., 2007). To improve NAG penetration into the skin Shatalebi et al. encapsulated it into niosomes and investigated its flux across excised rat skin using Franz diffusion cells. All formulations significantly enhanced the drug localization in the skin, as compared to NAG hydroalcoholic solution. Application of negatively charged dicetyl phosphate was suggested the reason for relatively high amount of entrapment of the very water soluble NAG. This study showed the potential of niosomes for improved NAG localization in the skin, as needed in hyperpigmentation disorders (Shatalebi et al., 2010). Ellagic acid, a polyphenol widely found in plants such as pomegranates, inhibits tyrosinase by its copper chelation. It may selectively inhibit melanin synthesis only in UV-activated melanocytes (Choi et al., 2006). A niosomal formulation of ellagic acid was developed from the mixture of Span 60 and Tween 60 for its dermal delivery. Skin distribution study revealed that the ellagic acid-loaded niosomes showed more efficient delivery of ellagic acid through human epidermis and dermis than ellagic acid solution. The results pointed out that the Span 60 and Tween 60 niosomes may be a potential carrier for dermal delivery of ellagic acid (Junyaprasert et al., 2011).

5.4. Vitiligo

Vitiligo is an acquired idiopathic, dermatological disorder described by well-circumscribed milky white macules in which melanocytes in the skin are damaged. Although vitiligo is not a life threatening issue but it might have an important negative impaction on the quality of life, even leading to attempted suicide in some cases (Nogueira et al., 2009; Bhawna et al., 2010). Application of novel dermal drug delivery systems can play a key role in vitiligo treatment because side-effects or poor efficacy of conventional topical dosage forms affect their utility and patient compliance (Bhawna et al., 2010). Human tyrosinase gene is responsible for the production of tyrosinase, an enzyme implicates in melanogenesis. The defect of tyrosinase gene is one of the reasons for depigmented skin or vitiligo (Zhang et al., 2005; Kingo et al., 2007). Manosroi et al. prepared elastic cationic niosomes (Tween 61/Cholesterol/ dimethyl dioctadecyl ammonium bromide at 1:1:0.5 molar ratio) for the effective dermal delivery of pMEL34 (tyrosinase encoding plasmid). Percutaneous absorption of formulation was investigated through exercised rat skin by Franz diffusion cells during 6 hours. The flux of pMEL34-loaded elastic niosomes was more than non-elastic niosomes in viable epidermis and dermis, while only pMEL34 loaded in elastic cationic noisome was observed in the receiver solution. By application of pMEL34-loaded elastic cationic niosomes in melanoma cell lines showed about four times higher tyrosinase gene expression than the free and the loaded plasmid in nonelastic niosomes means higher tyrosinase activity for efficient topical delivery in vitiligo therapy (Manosroi et al., 2010). In another study, luciferase plasmid (pLuc) was encapsulated in non-elastic and elastic cationic nanovesicles (niosomes and liposomes) and its transdermal absorption was investigated through rat skin follow by stratum corneum stripping or iontophoresis techniques. Free pLuc with or without the stratum corneum stripping and iontophoresis techniques and pLuc-loaded in nonelastic vesicles without the application techniques could not penetrate skin. Though, the elastic vesicles even without any application techniques can increase the transdermal absorption of pLuc. In case of elastic vesicles, the pLuc-loaded niosomes provided higher pLuc flux than that in liposomes. After 6 hours, pLuc encapsulated in nanovesicles with the iontophoresis application was still intact, but the free pLuc was degraded. Result of this study has showed the superior delivery of pLuc thorough skin by loading in niosomes, together with the application of iontophoresis, which can be used as a novel method to deliver genetic materials via dermal administration in gene therapy. Specifically, elastic cationic niosomes appeared to be a more promising approach since no additional equipment is required (Manosroi et al., 2009). Both mentioned studies demonstrated the potential application of elastic cationic niosomes as an efficient topical delivery for the purpose of gene therapy.

5.5. Cutaneous inflammation

5.5.1. Non - steroidal anti-inflammatory drugs (NSAIDs)

Celecoxib, a selective COX–2 inhibitor and most commonly used drug in the treatment of arthritis was embedded in niosomal gel for the purpose of sustained and site-specific delivery. In vitro, ex-vivo and in vivo studies were carried out through albino rats to compare the efficiency of formulation with carbopol gel as control formulation. Niosomal gel showed 6.5 times higher drug deposition in deep skin layer and muscle compare with carbopol gel indicating better drug localization with niosomal gel. A significant reduction of rat paw edema was resulted after administration of niosomal formulation compared to that after application of conventional gel confirming better skin permeation and deposition of celecoxib from niosomes. The authors concluded that niosomal gel formulation has great potential for improving site specific delivery, skin accumulation and prolonging release of celecoxib (Kaur et al., 2007). Multilamellar liposomes and niosomes of aceclofenac, a potent analgesic, anti-pyretic and anti-inflammatory agent were prepared and a comparative study was done between them through evaluation of entrapment efficiency, particle size, shape, differential scanning calorimetry, in vitro drug release and 3 months stability study. Results proved that niosomes have better stability than liposomes. Both vesicular systems showed considerable sustained anti-inflammatory activity compared with the commercial product, however niosomes being superior to liposomes as clearly showed by both oedema rate and inhibition rate percentages assessed by the rat paw oedema technique (Nasr et al., 2008). Proniosomal formulation of gugulipid (anti-inflamatory agent) was fabricated and characterized through in vitro drug release study and invivo anti-inflammatory activity via carrageenan-induced rat hind-paw method. In vitro study of proniosomal gel throught semi-permeable membrane exhibit the initial faster release followed by slow sustained release of gugulipid for 8 h. Gugulipid incoporated proniosomal gel showed good anti-inflammatory activity but not as good as commercial product diclofenac (Voveran®Emulgel). The authors state that proniosome formulation improve anti-inflammatory activity of gugulipids comparable to topical NSAIDs (Goyal et al., 2011). A niosome based transdermal drug delivery of nimesulide was prepared by lipid film hydration technique using different nonionic surfactants, Tweens® and Spans® and optimized for highest percent drug entrapment. Formulations were extensively characterized and evaluated in-vitro performance followed by in-vivo evaluation in rats by carrageenan induced rat paw edema method. The results were compared with plain drug gel, niosomally entrapment drug in carbopol gel base and marketed formulation. The percentage of edema inhibition was the highest for niosomal nimesulide gel after 24 hours more than five and three times than plain drug gel and market formulation, respectively. The results of this research suggest that niosomal formulation can offer consistent and prolonged anti-inflammatory effect and may improve therapeutic index of the formulation and is also expected to minimize the side effect due to drug localization at the site of action (Shahiwala et al., 2002).

5.5.2. Glucocorticosteroids

Topical corticosteroids are administered for the variety of dermatological disorders. Application of corticosteroid in proper carrier may help to prolonged action, subsequently less frequent administration and reduction of adverse effects. In a study, clobetasol propionate, a potent corticosteroid acts as an anti-inflammatory and anti-pruritic, was loaded in niosomal gel and its performance was compare with marketed gel and pure drug in term of in vitro drug release and in vivo pharmacodynamic studies. The results showed that the niosomal gel formulation provided a prolonged action due to the entrapment of clobetasol in vesicles (Lingan et al., 2011).

5.5.3. Antihistamines

Hence antihistamines are frequently administered as first line treatment to reduce the symptoms of urticaria pigmentosa because histamine is the single most important mediator involved (Osvaldo et al., 2010). The conventional oral administration of hydroxyzine hydrochloride (an antihistamine) causes CNS sedation, dry mouth and tachycardia whereas topical use in the form of semisolid dosage forms would lead to systemic side effects (Elzainy et al., 2003). A modified proniosomal gel of hydroxyzine hydrochloride was prepared by coacervation phase separation technique with different combination of non-ionic surfactants (Tweens and Spans) with phospholipids. Statistical experimental design was applied to optimize the various formulation variables. The optimized formulations were evaluated in vitro, ex vivo permeation, skin deposition, skin irritation and stability studies. The three months stability at refrigeration temperature and quite high encapsulation efficiency (95%) and drug deposition in the stratum corneum in 24 h (90%) were found for optimized formulation. The results indicated that modified proniosomal formulations of hydroxyzine hydrochloride were appropriate for topical drug delivery system for the treatment of localized urticarial (Rita et al., 2012). This formulation potentially improves drug penetration into the stratum corneum and localizes the drug within the dermoepidermal layers which would offer prompt onset and prolonged duration of action due to maintenance of effective concentrations in the skin, while systemic serum concentrations would be low (Carafa et al., 1998; Kirjavainen et al., 1999; Elzainy et al., 2003). Chlorpheniramine maleate is one of the most commonly used antihistamines and topically administered for skin disorders such as sunburns, urticaria, angioedema, pruritus, and insect bites. The proniosomes containing Span 40/lecithin/cholestrol formulated by ethanol showed optimum stability, loading efficiency, and particle size and appropriate release kinetic for percutaneous delivery of chlorpheniramine maleate. Ease of preparation and use of proniosomes were introduced as the greatest advantages provided by these types of dosage forms (Varshosaz et al., 2005).

5.6. Hair loss - Alopecia

The pilosebaceous unit including sebaceous gland, hair follicle and hair shaft has a unique biochemistry, metabolism and immunology. Targeted drug delivery may improve current therapeutic approaches to treat diseases of follicular origin (Weiner, 1998). In an increasing amount of topical studies, niosomes have been revealed to target drug delivery to the pilosebaceous unit. Androgenic alopecia (male pattern hair loss) is the most common reason of hair loss in men and characterized by the progressive hair thinning in genetically susceptible men (Jung et al., 2006). Semi-purified fraction of Oryza sativa contains the unsaturated fatty acids such as gamma-linolenic acid, linoleic acid and oleic acid have been proved to have anti-hair loss activity by inhibition of 5a-reductase type 1 (a key enzyme of androgenic alopecia) in DU-145 cell lines (Ruksiriwanich et al., 2011). Manosroi et al. prepared cationic niosomes (for higher stability) encapsulated with this extract and investigated physicochemical characteristics and transfollicular penetration of niosomes through porcine skin using follicular closing technique by Franz diffusion cells. The result of this study confirmed efficient transfollicular delivery of unsaturated fatty acids using cationic niosomes as well as the advantage of low systemic effect than the neutral niosomes (Manosroi et al., 2012). Thai Lanna medicinal plants have been reported to improve hair growth and reduce hair loss owing to increase the blood circulation, anti-fungal, anti-bacterial, and anti-oxidation of the hair roots. But, the extracts of these plants are naturally not stable and are problematic to be absorbed through hair follicles. Niosomal formulation containing the Thai Lanna plant extracts, such as turmeric, chili, ginger and Tong-Pan-Chang extract incorporated in gel was fabricated and tested in 20 human volunteers (9 males and 11 females). Results showed a significant increase in hair density and a decrease in hair loss without any irritation in all subjects from the 8-week application ($p<0.01$) in non-heredity alopecia volunteers, with non-differences in male and female volunteers. This in vivo study confirms potential of niosomes carrier for topical application of Thai Lanna medicinal plants for anti-hair loss (Manosroi et al., 2008). The enzyme 5a-reductase, responsible for production of dihydrotestosterone from testosterone in hair follicles, which is supposed to be the reason of androgenetic alopecia, can be inhibited by finasteride. Finasteride shows several unwanted systemic adverse effects which will be reduced if it acts locally in the hair follicles (Javadzadeh et al., 2010). Tabbakhian et al. studied dermal application of finasteride-containing vesicles (niosomes and liposomes) for increasing drug concentration at the pilosebaceous units, as compared with finasteride hydroalcoholic solution. Both in vitro permeation of 3H-finasteride through hamster flank skin and in vivo deposition studies in hamster ear demonstrated the potentials of liquid-state niosomes and liposomes for successful delivery of finasteride to the pilosebaceous units compared with hydroalcoholic solution while optimized niosomal formulation also showed higher targeting ration than liposomal vesicles (Tabbakhian et al., 2006). Minoxidil, the most commonly used medicine for the treatment of androgenic alopecia with unknown mechanism of action on hair follicles (Messenger et al., 2004) were encapsulated into noisome and liposome vesicles. The percutaneous absorption study was carried out in vitro using vertical diffusion Franz cells using human skin and the results compared with dissolved minoxidil in propylene glycol–water–ethanol solution as a control. Although penetration of niosomal minoxidil in epidermal and dermal layers was greater than control solution but lower than liposomal formulations. These differences suggested to be attributed to the smaller size and the greater potential targeting to skin and skin appendages of liposomal carriers, which enhanced globally the skin drug delivery. This work generally suggests that niosomes and liposomes have a proper potential for drug dermal targeting and could be considered as a reasonable and practicable therapeutic approach to skin diseases such as hair loss (Mura et al., 2007). In a another study the effects of niosomal minoxidil formulation on the drug penetration in hairless mouse skin were investigated by in vitro permeation experiments, and the results compared with control minoxidil hydroalcoholic solution and a leading commercial topical formulation "Minoxyl™" containing 5% minoxidil and 1% dexpentanol. The result of study showed niosomal formulations increased the percentage of dose accumulated in the skin (1.03 ± 0.18 to $19.41\pm4.04\%$) compared with control and commercial formulations (0.48 ± 0.17 and 0.11 ± 0.03 %, respectively). Physical stability of niosomal formulations which was evaluated for three month at refrigerator temperature (2–8 °C) have shown a fairly high retention of minoxidil inside the vesicles (80%). The authors finally proposed that these niosomal formulations could be used as a feasible cargo carrier for the dermal delivery of minoxidil and promising approach in treatment alopecia (Balakrishnan et al., 2009). Recently minoxidil-loaded niosomes were prepared with series of surfactant and cholesterol in different molar ratio by ethanol injection method. Surfactant screening exhibited that only Span 20, Span 60 and Tween 20 with cholesterol have ability of nano size vesicle formation and Span 60 was shown to be a better surfactant for niosomal stable form with maximum entrapment efficiency (31.27±1.5 %) and minimal particle size (approx. 219 nm). The in vitro skin permeation and deposition study of minoxidil-loaded niosomal gel formulation prepared with 1:2 ratio of Span 60 and cholesterol showed significant improvement in skin accumulation (more than eightfold) as compared with plain minoxidil gel (17.21±3.2 and 2.26±1.3 %, respectively). Result of study demonstrates an increase in cholesterol concentration in niosome vesicles enhance minoxidil skin retention and effect on entrapment efficiency as well as size of niosomes to better cutaneous treatment. It was also concluded that the developed niosomal formulation could be a suitable option for cutaneous targeting of minoxidil (Mali et al., 2012).

5.7. Acne

Acne is the most common skin disease of multifactorial origin with an incidence of 70 - 80% in adolescence. While topical therapy has an important role in acne treatment, side effects associated with several topical antiacne agents affect their efficacy and patient satisfaction. Niosomes, capable of great features for skin administration, can play an essential role in improving the dermal delivery of antiacne agents by increasing their topical localization with an associated reduction in their adverse effects (Maibach et al., 2005). Benzoyl peroxide is a macrolide antibiotic generally applied for the management of acne either alone or in combination with other antiacne agents. Dermal administration of benzoyl peroxide causes side effects such as skin redness, itching, irritation and edema which lead to discomfort and ignorance of therapy and outcomes in no profit or emergence of resistant to microorganisms. In a study, niosomal benzoyl peroxide incorporated into HPMC gel designed and optimized by partial factorial design. Ex vivo release study on human cadaver skin showed increase in drug skin retention, extended drug release and improved permeation of drug across the skin which in turn will reduce the toxicity of drug and enhance the therapeutic efficacy (Vyas et al., 2011). Gallidermin is mainly promising for the dermal and cosmetic treatment of acne in human medicines because of its greatly active against *Propionibacterium acnes* and treatment of multidrug resistant *Staphylococcus Aureus* strains, which is a snowballing problem especially in the hospitals (Kempf et al., 1999). Gallidermin has limited absorption through skin and chemical instability due to its large molecular structure and peptide nature, respectively (Manosroi et al., 2005). Anionic niosomal gallidermin composed of tween 61/cholesterol /dicetylphosphate prepared and antibacterial activity of formulations against *Propionibacterium acnes* and *Staphylococcus Aureus* assayed with macrodilution method to determine the minimal concentration of the sample necessary to inhibit or kill the microorganisms. Result of study demonstrates gallidermin loaded in niosomes offered lower antibacterial activity against tested microeorganisms compare with unloaded gallidermin due to the niosomes protecting role and making a sustained release of drug. Niosomal furmulation of gallidermin in gel showed more chemically stable at high temperatures and two fold higher cumulative amounts in viable epidermis and dermis of rat skin than aqueous solution of gallidermin. This study suggests that anionic niosomes of gallidermin can be considered as a superior topical antibacterial formulation because of chemical stability and high skin localization with no threat of systemic effect (Manosroi et al., 2010). Trans-retinoic acid or tretinoin, a vitamin A metabolite, is widely used in the topical treatment of various skin diseases such as acne, psoriasis and photoaging. But, high chemical instability and skin irritation strongly limited its administration for topical delivery (Ridolfi et al., 2011). Transdermal delivery of tretinoin-loaded niosomal and liposomal formulation was studied through the newborn pig skin using Franz diffusion cells and compared with commercial formulation (RetinA®). The effect of charge on the performance niosomes was studied by the preparation of niosomes with either stearylamine and dicetylphosphate as a positive and negative charge inducer, respectively. Small unilamellar negatively charged niosomal formulations saturated with tretinoin showed more upper cutaneous drug retention than both commercial and liposomal formulation. Result of this study demonstrates cutaneous delivery of tretinoin is powerfully affected by vesicle morphology, composition and thermodynamic activity of the drug (Manconi et al., 2006). The ability of niosomes as topical carriers capable of improving the stability of photosensitive drugs was studied by comparing the chemical stability of tretinoin in methanol and in vesicular suspensions exposed both to UV and artificial daylight conditions. Liposomes were also prepared and compared with niosomes. In order to evaluate the influence of vesicle structure on the photostability of tretinoin, tretinoin-loaded vesicles were prepared by the film hydration method, extrusion technique and sonication. Methanol dissolved tretinoin degraded immediately after UV irradiation while the loaded drug into vesicles showed a considerable reduction of the photodegradation process. The photoprotection provided by vesicles varied depending on the vesicle structure and composition. In addition, unilamellar vesicles showed a higher protection of tretinoin than the multilamellar ones. Unilamellar niosomes made from Brij®30 were the formulations with the highest protection of tretinoin (Manconi et al., 2003). In another study, the antiacne activity of the mixture of aromatic volatile oil extracted from Thai medicinal plants enhanced with encapsulating into nano sized niosomal vesicles (Manosroi et al., 2008). Slow penetration of drug through skin is the main disadvantage of transdermal route of delivery. An increase in the penetration rate has been achieved by transdermal delivery of erythromycin incorporated in niosomes for acne therapy (Jayaraman et al., 1996).

6. Conclusion

Niosomal drug delivery systems have been demonstrated to be promising controlled drug delivery systems for percutaneous administration. Niosomes also offer successful drug localization in skin which are relatively non-toxic and stable. This advantage of niosomes has the potential of strengthening the efficacy of the drug accompanying with reducing its adverse effects associated with drug systemic absorption. Drug-associated challenges such as physical and chemical instability is also can be protected by vesicular carriers. Niosomes appeared to be a well preferred drug delivery system over liposome as niosomes being stable and cost-effective. Hence, many topical drugs may be developed using niosomal systems. But there are still some challenges in this area. Although some new approaches have been developed to overcome the problem of drug loading, it is still remain to be addressed. The researchers should be more alert in the selection of suitable surfactant for noisome preparation due to this fact that the type of surfactant is the main parameter affecting the formation of the vesicles, their toxicity and stability.

Author details

Yahya Rahimpour
Biotechnology Research Center and Student Research Committee,
Tabriz University of Medical Sciences, Tabriz, Iran

Hamed Hamishehkar
Pharmaceutical Technology Laboratory, Drug Applied Research Center,
Tabriz University of Medical Sciences, Tabriz, Iran

7. References

Abd-Elbary, A.; El-laithy, H.M. & Tadros, M.I., (2008). Sucrose stearate-based proniosome-derived niosomes for the nebulisable delivery of cromolyn sodium. *Int J Pharm*, Vol. 357, No. 1-2, pp. 189-198, ISSN: 0378-5173.

Abdelkader, H.; Ismail, S.; Hussein, A.; Wu, Z.; Al-Kassas, R. & Alany, R.G., (2012). Conjunctival and corneal tolerability assessment of ocular naltrexone niosomes and their ingredients on the hen's egg chorioallantoic membrane and excised bovine cornea models. *Int J Pharm*, Vol. 432, No. 1-2, pp. 1-10, ISSN: 0378-5173.

Abdelkader, H.; Wu, Z.; Al-Kassas, R. & Alany, R.G., (2012). Niosomes and discomes for ocular delivery of naltrexone hydrochloride: morphological, rheological, spreading properties and photo-protective effects. Int J Pharm, Vol. 433, No. 1-2, pp. 142-148, ISSN: 0378-5173.

Agarwal, R.; Katare, O.P. & Vyas, S.P., (2001). Preparation and in vitro evaluation of liposomal/niosomal delivery systems for antipsoriatic drug dithranol. *Int J Pharm*, Vol. 228, No. 1, pp. 43-52, ISSN: 0378-5173.

Akhilesh, D.; Hazel, G. & Kamath, J.V., (2011). Proniosomes – A propitious provesicular drug carrier *International Journal of Pharmacy and Pharmaceutical Science Research*, Vol. 1, No. 3, pp. 98-103, ISSN: 2249-0337

Azeem, A.; Anwer, M.K. & Talegaonkar, S., (2009). Niosomes in sustained and targeted drug delivery: some recent advances. *J Drug Target*, Vol. 17, No. 9, pp. 671-689, ISSN: 1061-186X.

Azmin, M.N.; Florence, A.T. & Handjani-Vila, R.M., (1985). The effect of non-ionic surfactant vesicle (niosome) entrapment on the absorption and distribution of methotrexate in mice. *J Pharm Pharmacol*, Vol. 37, No. 4, pp. 237-242, ISSN: 0022-3573

Baillie, A.J.; Coombs, G.H.; Dolan, T.F. & Laurie, J., (1986). Non-ionic surfactant vesicles, niosomes, as a delivery system for the anti-leishmanial drug, sodium stibogluconate. *J Pharm Pharmacol*, Vol. 38, No. 7, pp. 502-505, ISSN: 0022-3573.

Balakrishnan, P.; Shanmugam, S.; Lee, W.S.; Lee, W.M.; Kim, J.O.; Oh, D.H.; Kim, D.D.; Kim, J.S.; Yoo, B.K. & Choi, H.G., (2009). Formulation and in vitro assessment of minoxidil niosomes for enhanced skin delivery. *Int J Pharm*, Vol. 377, No. 1, pp. 1-8, ISSN: 0378-5173.

Barry, B.W., (1991). Lipid-Protein-Partitioning theory of skin penetration enhancement. *J Control Release*, Vol. 15, No. 3, pp. 237-248, ISSN: 0168-3659.

Bayindir, Z.S. & Yuksel, N., (2010). Characterization of niosomes prepared with various nonionic surfactants for paclitaxel oral delivery. *J Pharm Sci*, Vol. 99, No. 4, pp. 2049-2060, ISSN: 1520-6017.

Bhawna, G.; Abir, S.; Amit, B. & Om, K., (2010). Topical treatment in vitiligo and the potential uses of new drug delivery systems. *Indian J Dermatol Venereol Leprol*, Vol. 76, ISSN: 0378-6323.

Bissett, D.L.; Robinson, L.R.; Raleigh, P.S.; Miyamoto, K.; Hakozaki, T.; Li, J. & Kelm, G.R., (2007). Reduction in the appearance of facial hyperpigmentation by topical N-acetyl glucosamine. *J Cosmet Dermatol*, Vol. 6, No. 1, pp. 20-26, ISSN: 1473-2165.

Brown, M.B.; Martin, G.P.; Jones, S.A. & Akomeah, F.K., (2006). Dermal and transdermal drug delivery systems: current and future prospects. *Drug Deliv*, Vol. 13, No. 3, pp. 175-187, ISSN: 1071-7544.

Carafa, M.; Santucci, E.; Alhaique, F.; Coviello, T.; Murtas, E.; Riccieri, F.; Lucania, G. & Torrisi, M.R., (1998). Preparation and properties of new unilamellar non-ionic/ionic surfactant vesicles. *Int J Pharm*, Vol. 160, No. 1, pp. 51-59, ISSN: 0378-5173.

Carafa, M.; Santucci, E. & Lucania, G., (2002). Lidocaine-loaded non-ionic surfactant vesicles: characterization and in vitro permeation studies. *Int J Pharm*, Vol. 231, No. 1, pp. 21-32, ISSN: 0378-5173.

Cevc, G., (1996). Transfersomes, liposomes and other lipid suspensions on the skin: permeation enhancement, vesicle penetration, and transdermal drug delivery. *Crit Rev Ther Drug Carrier Syst*, Vol. 13, No. 3-4, pp. 257, ISSN: 0743-4863.

Cevc, G.; Blume, G.; Schätzlein, A.; Gebauer, D. & Paul, A., (1996). The skin: a pathway for systemic treatment with patches and lipid-based agent carriers. *Adv Drug Deliv Rev*, Vol. 18, No. 3, pp. 349-378, ISSN: 0169-409X.

Choi, C.M. & Berson, D.S., (2006). Cosmeceuticals. *Semin Cutan Med Surg*, Vol. 25, pp.163-168, ISSN: 1085-5629

Desai, T.R. & Finlay, W.H., (2002). Nebulization of niosomal all-trans-retinoic acid: An inexpensive alternative to conventional liposomes. *Int J Pharm*, Vol. 241, No. 2, pp. 311-317, ISSN: 0378-5173.

Draelos, Z.D., (2008). New channels for old cosmeceuticals: aquaporin modulation. *Journal of cosmetic dermatology*, Vol. 7, No. 2, pp. 83-83, ISSN: 1473-2165.

Dubey, A.; Prabhu, P. & Kamath, J., (2012). Nano Structured lipid carriers: A Novel Topical drug delivery system. *Int J PharmTech Res*, Vol. 4, No. 2, pp. 705-714, ISSN: 0974-4304.

Dubey, V.; Mishra, D.; Dutta, T.; Nahar, M.; Saraf, D.K. & Jain, N.K., (2007). Dermal and transdermal delivery of an anti-psoriatic agent via ethanolic liposomes. *J Control Release*, Vol. 123, No. 2, pp. 148-154, ISSN: 0168-3659.

Elzainy, A.A.W.; Gu, X.; Simons, F.E.R. & Simons, K.J., (2003). Hydroxyzine from topical phospholipid liposomal formulations: Evaluation of peripheral antihistaminic activity and systemic absorption in a rabbit model. *The AAPS Journal*, Vol. 5, No. 4, pp. 41-48,

Fang, J.Y.; Hong, C.T.; Chiu, W.T. & Wang, Y.Y., (2001). Effect of liposomes and niosomes on skin permeation of enoxacin. *Int J Pharm*, Vol. 219, No. 1-2, pp. 61-72, ISSN: 0378-5173.

Firthouse, P.U.M.; Halith, S.M.; Wahab, S.U.; Sirajudeen, M. & Mohideen, S.K., (2011). Formulation and evaluation of miconazole niosomes. *Int J PharmTech Res*, Vol. 3, No. 2, pp. 1019-1022, ISSN: 0974-4304.

Gašperlin, M. & Gosenca, M., (2011). Main approaches for delivering antioxidant vitamins through the skin to prevent skin ageing. *Expert Opin Drug Del*, Vol. 8, No. 7, pp. 905-919, ISSN: 1742-5247.

Ghafourian, T.; Zandasrar, P.; Hamishekar, H. & Nokhodchi, A., (2004). The effect of penetration enhancers on drug delivery through skin: a QSAR study. *J Control Release*, Vol. 99, No. 1, pp. 113-125, ISSN: 0168-3659.

Gopinath, D.; Ravi, D.; Rao, B.R.; Apte, S.S.; Renuka, D. & Rambhau, D., (2004). Ascorbyl palmitate vesicles (Aspasomes): formation, characterization and applications. *Int J Pharm*, Vol. 271, No. 1-2, pp. 95-113, ISSN: 0378-5173.

Goyal, C.; Ahuja, M. & Sharma, S.K., (2011). Preparation and evaluation of anti-inflammatory activity of gugulipid-loaded proniosomal gel. *Acta Pol Pharm*, Vol. 68, No. 1, pp. 147-150, ISSN: 0001-6837.

Handjani-Vila, R.M.; Ribier, A.; Rondot, B. & Vanlerberghe, G., (1979). Dispersions of lamellar phases of non-ionic lipids in cosmetic products. *Int J Cosmetic Sci*, Vol. 1, pp. 303-314,

Higaki, K.; Nakayama, K.; Suyama, T.; Amnuaikit, C.; Ogawara, K. & Kimura, T., (2005). Enhancement of topical delivery of drugs via direct penetration by reducing blood flow rate in skin. *Int J Pharm*, Vol. 288, No. 2, pp. 227-233, ISSN: 0378-5173.

Hofland, H.; Bowuwstra, J.A.; Ponec, M. Boddé, H.E.; Spies, F.; Coos Verhoef, J.; Junginger H.E., (1991). Interactions of non-ionic surfactant vesicles with cultured keratinocytes and human skin in vitro: a survey of toxicological aspects and ultrastructural changes in stratum corneum. *J Control Release*, Vol. 16, No. 1, pp. 155-167, ISSN: 0168-3659.

Hofland, H.E.J.; Bouwstra, J.A.; Spies, F. & Bodde, H.E., (1992). Safety aspect of nonionic surfactant vesicles- a toxicity study related to the physicochemical characteristics of nonionic surfactants. *J Pharm Pharmacol*, Vol. 44, pp. 287-292, ISSN: 0022-3573

Hofland, H.E.J.; van der Geest, R.; Bodde, H.E.; Junginger, H.E. & Bouwstra, J.A., (1994). Estradiol permeation from nonionic surfactant vesicles through human stratum corneum in vitro. *Pharm Res*, Vol. 11, No. 5, pp. 659-664, ISSN: 0724-8741.

Hu, C. & Rhodes, D.G., (2000). Proniosomes: a novel drug carrier preparation. *Int J Pharm* Vol. 206, pp. 110-122, ISSN: 0378-5173.

Jain, C.P.; Vyas, S.P. & Dixit, V.K., (2006). Niosomal system for delivery of rifampicin to lymphatics. *Indian J Pharm Sci*, Vol. 68, No. 5, pp. 575, ISSN: 0250-474X.

Javadzadeh, Y. & Hamishehkar, H., (2011). Enhancing percutaneous delivery of methotrexate using different types of surfactants. *Colloid Surface B*, Vol. 82, No. 2, pp. 422-426, ISSN: 0927-7765.

Javadzadeh, Y.; Shokri, J.; Hallaj-Nezhadi, S.; Hamishehkar, H. & Nokhodchi, A., (2010). Enhancement of percutaneous absorption of Finasteride by cosolvents, cosurfactant and surfactants. *Pharm Dev Technol*, Vol. 15, No. 6, pp. 619-625, ISSN: 1083-7450.

Jayaraman, S.C.; Ramachandran, C. & Weiner, N., (1996). Topical delivery of erythromycin from various formulations: An in vivo hairless mouse study. *J Pharm Sci*, Vol. 85, No. 10, pp. 1082-1084, ISSN: 1520-6017.

Jung, S.; Otberg, N.; Thiede, G.; Richter, H.; Sterry, W.; Panzner, S. & Lademann, J., (2006). Innovative liposomes as a transfollicular drug delivery system: penetration into porcine hair follicles. *J Invest Dermatol*, Vol. 126, No. 8, pp. 1728-1732, ISSN: 0022-202X.

Junyaprasert, V.B.; Singhsa, P.; Suksiriworapong, J. & Chantasart, D., (2011). Physicochemical properties and skin permeation of span 60/tween 60 niosomes of ellagic acid. *Int J Pharm*, Vol. doi:10.1016/j.ijpharm.2011.11.032, ISSN: 0378-5173.

Kaur, K.; Jain, S.; Sapra, B. & Tiwary, A.K., (2007). Niosomal gel for site-specific sustained delivery of anti-arthritic drug: in vitro-in vivo evaluation. *Curr Drug Deliv*, Vol. 4, No. 4, pp. 276-282, ISSN: 1567-2018.

Kempf, M.; Theobald, U. & Fiedler, H.P., (1999). Economic improvement of the fermentative production of gallidermin by Staphylococcus gallinarum. *Biotechnol lett*, Vol. 21, No. 8, pp. 663-667, ISSN: 0141-5492.

Khan, A.; Sharma, P.K.; Visht, S. & Malviya, R., (2011). Niosomes as colloidal drug delivery system: A review. *Journal of Chronotherapy and Drug Delivery*, Vol. 2, No. 1, pp. 15-21,

Kingo, K.; Aunin, E.; Karelson, M.; Philips, M.A.; Rätsep, R.; Silm, H.; Vasar, E.; Soomets, U. & Kõks, S., (2007). Gene expression analysis of melanocortin system in vitiligo. *J Dermatol Sci*, Vol. 48, No. 2, pp. 113-122, ISSN: 0923-1811.

Kirjavainen, M.; Mönkkönen, J.; Saukkosaari, M.; Valjakka-Koskela, R.; Kiesvaara, J. & Urtti, A., (1999). Phospholipids affect stratum corneum lipid bilayer fluidity and drug partitioning into the bilayers. *J Control Release*, Vol. 58, No. 2, pp. 207-214, ISSN: 0168-3659.

Kumar, G.P. & Rao, P.R., (2012). Ultra deformable niosomes for improved transdermal drug delivery: The future scenario. *Asian Journal of Pharmaceutical Sciences*, Vol. 7, No. 2, pp. 96-109, ISSN: 0974-2441

Lakshmi, P.K. & Bhaskaran, S., (2011). Phase II study of topical niosomal urea gel - an adjuvant in the treatment of psoriasis. *International Journal of Pharmaceutical Sciences Review and Research*, Vol. 7, No. 1, pp. 1-7, ISSN: 0976 – 044X

Lakshmi, P.K.; Devi, G.S.; Bhaskaran, S. & Sacchidanand, S., (2007). Niosomal methotrexate gel in the treatment of localized psoriasis: Phase I and phase II studies. *Indian J Dermatol Venereol Leprol*, Vol. 73, No. 3, pp. 157, ISSN: 0378-6323.

Lala, S.; Pramanick, S.; Mukhopadhyay, S.; Bandyopadhyay, S. & Basu, M.K., (2004). Harmine: Evaluation of its antileishmanial properties in various vesicular delivery systems. *J Drug Target*, Vol. 12, No. 3, pp. 165-175, ISSN: 1061-186X.

Lingan, M.A.; Sathali, A.A.H.; Kumar, M.R.V. & Gokila, A., (2011). Formulation and evaluation of topical drug delivery system containing clobetasol propionate niosomes. *Sci Revs Chem Commun*, Vol. 1, No. 1, pp. 7-17,

Maibach, H.I. & Choi, M.J., (2005). Liposomes and niosomes as topical drug delivery systems. *Skin Pharmacol Physiol*, Vol. 18, pp. 209-219, ISSN: 1660-5527.

Malhotra, M. & Jain, N.K., (1994). Niosomes as drug carriers. *Ind Drugs*, Vol. 31, No. 3, pp. 81-86,

Mali, N.; Darandale, S. & Vavia, P., (2012). Niosomes as a vesicular carrier for topical administration of minoxidil: formulation and in vitro assessment. *Drug Deliv Transl Res*, pp. 1-6, ISSN: 2190-393X.

Manconi, M.; Sinico, C.; Valenti, D.; Lai, F. & Fadda, A.M., (2006). Niosomes as carriers for tretinoin: III. A study into the in vitro cutaneous delivery of vesicle-incorporated tretinoin. *Int J Pharm*, Vol. 311, No. 1-2, pp. 11-19, ISSN: 0378-5173.

Manconi, M.; Valenti, D.; Sinico, C.; Lai, F.; Loy, G. & Fadda, A.M., (2003). Niosomes as carriers for tretinoin: II. Influence of vesicular incorporation on tretinoin photostability. *Int J Pharm*, Vol. 260, No. 2, pp. 261-272, ISSN: 0378-5173.

Manosroi, A.; Khanrin, P.; Lohcharoenkal, W.; Werner, R.G.; Götz, F.; Manosroi, W. & Manosroi, J., (2010). Transdermal absorption enhancement through rat skin of gallidermin loaded in niosomes. *Int J Pharm*, Vol. 392, No. 1, pp. 304-310, ISSN: 0378-5173.

Manosroi, A.; Khositsuntiwong, N.; Götz, F.; Werner, R.G. & Manosroi, J., (2009). Transdermal enhancement through rat skin of luciferase plasmid DNA loaded in elastic nanovesicles. *J Liposome Res*, Vol. 19, No. 2, pp. 91-98, ISSN: 0898-2104.

Manosroi, A.; Ruksiriwanich, W.; Abe, M.; Manosroi, W. & Manosroi, J., (2012). Transfollicular enhancement of gel containing cationic niosomes loaded with unsaturated fatty acids in rice (Oryza sativa) bran semi-purified fraction. *Eur J Pharm Biopharm*, Vol. 81, No. 2, pp. 303-313, ISSN: 0939-6411.

Manosroi, A.; Sritapunya, T.; Jainonthee, P. & Manosroi, J., (2008). Anti P. acne activity of cream containing aromatic volatile oil from Thai medicinal plants entrapped in niosomes for acne treatment.

Manosroi, A.; Wongtrakul, P.; Manosroi, J.; Midorikawa, U.; Hanyu, Y.; Yuasa, M.; Sugawara, F.; Sakai, H. & Abe, M., (2005). The entrapment of kojic oleate in bilayer vesicles. *Int J Pharm*, Vol. 298, No. 1, pp. 13-25, ISSN: 0378-5173.

Manosroi, J.; Khositsuntiwong, N. & Manosroi, A., (2008). Performance test of gel containing extracts from Thai Lanna medicinal plants entrapped in niosomes for hair loss treatment.

Manosroi, J.; Khositsuntiwong, N.; Manosroi, W.; Götz, F.; Werner, R.G. & Manosroi, A., (2010). Enhancement of transdermal absorption, gene expression and stability of tyrosinase plasmid (pMEL34)-loaded elastic cationic niosomes: Potential application in vitiligo treatment. *J Pharm Sci*, Vol. 99, No. 8, pp. 3533-3541, ISSN: 1520-6017.

Messenger, A. & Rundegren, J., (2004). Minoxidil: mechanisms of action on hair growth. *Brit J Dermatol*, Vol. 150, No. 2, pp. 186-194, ISSN: 0007-0963.

Mura, S.; Pirot, F.; Manconi, M.; Falson, F. & Fadda, A.M., (2007). Liposomes and niosomes as potential carriers for dermal delivery of minoxidil. *J Drug Target*, Vol. 15, No. 2, pp. 101-108, ISSN: 1061-186X.

Nasr, M.; Mansour, S.; Mortada, N.D. & Elshamy, A.A., (2008). Vesicular aceclofenac systems: A comparative study between liposomes and niosomes. *J Microencapsul*, Vol. 25, No. 7, pp. 499-512, ISSN: 0265-2048.

Nogueira, L.S.; Zancanaro, P.C. & Azambuja, R.D., (2009). [Vitiligo and emotions]. *An Bras Dermatol*, Vol. 84, No. 1, pp. 41-45, ISSN: 1806-4841

Nounou, M.M.; El-Khordagui, L.K.; Khalafallah, N.A. & Khalil, S.A., (2008). Liposomal formulation for dermal and transdermal drug delivery: past, present and future. *Recent Pat Drug Deliv Formul*, Vol. 2, No. 1, pp. 9-18, ISSN: 1872-2113.

Ogiso, T.; Niinaka, N. & Iwaki, M., (1996). Mechanism for enhancement effect of lipid disperse system on percutaneous absorption. *J Pharm Sci*, Vol. 85, pp. 57-64, ISSN: 1520-6017.

Osvaldo, C.; Duarte, A.F.; Paula, Q.; Rosa, A. & Luis, D., (2010). Cutaneous mastocytosis: Two pediatric cases treated with topical pimecrolimus. *Dermatol Online J*, Vol. 16, No. 5, pp. 8, ISSN: 1087-2108

Paolino, D.; Muzzalupo, R.; Ricciardi, A.; Celia, C.; Picci, N. & Fresta, M., (2007). In vitro and in vivo evaluation of Bola-surfactant containing niosomes for transdermal delivery. *Biomed Microdevices*, Vol. 9, No. 4, pp. 421-433, ISSN: 1387-2176.

Pardakhty, A.; Varshosaz, J. & Roulholamini, A., (2007). In vitro study of polyoxyethylene alkyl ether niosomes for delivery of insulin. *Int J Pharm*, Vol. 328, pp. 130-141, ISSN: 0378-5173.

Parthasarathi, G.; Udupa, N.; Umadevi, P. & Pillai, G.K., (1994). Niosome encapsulated of vincristine sulfate: Improved anticancer activity with reduced toxicity in mice. *J Drug Target*, Vol. 2, No. 2, pp. 173-182, ISSN: 1061-186X.

Perrett, S.; Golding, M. & Williams, W.P., (1991). A simple method for the preparation of liposomes for pharmaceutical application and characterization of liposomes. *J Pharm Pharmacol*, Vol. 43, pp. 154-161, ISSN: 2042-7158.

Pugeat, M.; Nicolas, M.H.; Dechaud, H. & Elmidani, M., (1991). Combination of cyproterone acetate and natural estrogens in the treatment of hirsutism]. *J Gynecol Obst Bior R*, Vol. 20, No. 8, pp. 1057, ISSN: 0368-2315.

Puglia, C. & Bonina, F., (2012). Lipid nanoparticles as novel delivery systems for cosmetics and dermal pharmaceuticals. *Expert Opin Drug Del*, Vol. 9, No. 4, pp. 429-441, ISSN: 1742-5247.

Rahimpour, Y. & Hamishehkar, H., (2012). Liposomes in cosmeceutics. *Expert Opin Drug Del*, Vol. 9, No. 4, pp. 443-455, ISSN: 1742-5247.

Raja Naresh, R.A.; Pillai, G.K.; Udupa, N. & Chandrashekar, G., (1994). Antiinflammatory activity of niosome encapsulated diclofenac sodium in arthitic rats. *Indian J Pharmacol*, Vol. 26, pp. 46-48, ISSN: 0253-7613.

Rajera, R.; Nagpal, K.; Singh, S.K. & Mishra, D.N., (2011). Niosomes: A controlled and novel drug delivery system. *Bio Pharm Bull*, Vol. 34, No. 7, pp. 945-953, ISSN: 0918-6158.

Ridolfi, D.M.; Marcato, P.D.; Justo, G.Z.; Cordi, L.; Machado, D. & Durán, N., (2011). Chitosan-solid lipid nanoparticles as carriers for topical delivery of Tretinoin. *Colloid Surface B*, ISSN: 0927-7765.

Rita, B. & Lakshmi, P.K., (2012). Preparation and evaluation of modified proniosomal gel for localised urticaria and optimisation by statistical method. *Journal of Applied Pharmaceutical Science*, Vol. 2, No. 03, pp. 85-91,

Rogerson, A.; Cummings, J. & Florence, A.T., (1987). Adriamycin-loaded niosomes: drug entrapment, stability and release. *J Microencapsul*, Vol. 4, No. 4, pp. 321-328, ISSN: 0265-2048.

Rubio, L.; Alonso, C.; López, O.; Rodríguez, G.; Coderch, L.; Notario, J.; de la Maza, A. & Parra, J.L., (2011). Barrier function of intact and impaired skin: percutaneous penetration of caffeine and salicylic acid. *Int J Dermatol*, Vol. 50, No. 7, pp. 881-889, ISSN: 1365-4632.

Ruckmani, K.; Jayakar, B. & Ghosal, S.K., (2000). Nonionic surfactant vesicles (niosomes) of cytarabine hydrochloride for effective treatment of leukemias: Encapsulation, storage, and in vitro release. *Drug Dev Ind Pharm*, Vol. 26, No. 2, pp. 217-222, ISSN: 0363-9045.

Ruksiriwanich, W.; Manosroi, J.; Abe, M.; Manosroi, W. & Manosroi, A., (2011). 5 [alpha]-Reductase type 1 inhibition of Oryza sativa bran extract prepared by supercritical carbon dioxide fluid. *J Supercrit Fluid*, ISSN: 0896-8446.

Sahin, N.O. Niosomes as nanocarrier systems. Nanomaterials and nanosystems for biomedical applications2007. p. 67-81.

Sathali, A.A.H. & Rajalakshmi, G., (2010). Evaluation of transdermal targeted niosomal drug delivery of terbinafine hydrochloride. *Int J PharmTech Res*, Vol. 2, No. 3, pp. 2081-2089, ISSN: 0974-4304.

Schreier, H. & Bouwstra, J., (1994). Liposomes and niosomes as topical drug carriers: dermal and transdermal drug delivery. *J Control Release*, Vol. 30, No. 1, pp. 1-15, ISSN: 0168-3659.

Shahiwala, A. & Misra, A., (2002). Studies in topical application of niosomally entrapped nimesulide. *J Pharm Pharm Sci*, Vol. 5, No. 3, pp. 220, ISSN: 1482-1826.

Shatalebi, M.A.; Mostafavi, S.A. & Moghaddas, A., (2010). Niosome as a drug carrier for topical delivery of N-acetyl glucosamine. *Res Pharm Sci*, Vol. 5, No. 2, pp. 107, ISSN: 1735-5362.

Shi, B.; Fang, C.; You, M.X. & Pei, Y.Y., (2005). Influence of PEG chain length on in vitro drug release and in vivo pharmacokinetics of hydroxycamptothecin (HCPT) loaded PEG-PHDCA niosomes. *Chinese Pharmaceutical Journal*, Vol. 40, No. 21, pp. 1643-1646,

Su, Y.H. & Fang, J.Y., (2008). Drug delivery and formulations for the topical treatment of psoriasis. *Expert Opin Drug Del*, Vol. 5, No. 2, pp. 235-249, ISSN: 1742-5247.

Tabbakhian, M.; Tavakoli, N.; Jaafari, M.R. & Daneshamouz, S., (2006). Enhancement of follicular delivery of finasteride by liposomes and niosomes:: 1. In vitro permeation and in vivo deposition studies using hamster flank and ear models. *Int J Pharm*, Vol. 323, No. 1-2, pp. 1-10, ISSN: 0378-5173.

Uchegbu, I.F. & Duncan, R., (1997). Niosomes containing N-(2-hydroxypropyl) methacrylamide copolymer-doxorubicin (PK1): effect of method of preparation and choice of surfactant on niosome characteristics and a preliminary study of body distribution. *Int J Pharm*, Vol. 155, No. 1, pp. 7-17, ISSN: 0378-5173.

Varshosaz, J.; Pardakhty, A.; Mohsen, S. & Baharanchi, H., (2005). Sorbitan monopalmitate-based proniosomes for transdermal delivery of chlorpheniramine maleate. *Drug Deliv*, Vol. 12, No. 2, pp. 75-82, ISSN: 1071-7544.

Venuganti, V.V. & Perumal, O.P. Nanosystems for dermal and transdermal drug delivery. In: Pathak Y, Thassu D, editors. Drug delivery nanoparticles formulation and characterization. New York: Informa Healthcare USA, Inc; 2009. p. 126-155.

Verma, A.K. & Bindal, M., (2012). A review on niosomes: an ultimate controlled and novel drug delivery carrier. *Int J Nanoparticles* Vol. 5, No. 1, pp. 73-87,

Vyas, J.; Vyas, P.; Raval, D. & Paghdar, P., (2011). Development of topical niosomal gel of benzoyl peroxide. *ISRN Nanotechnology*, Vol. 2011, ISSN: 2090-6064.

Weiner, N., (1998). Targeted follicular delivery of macromolecules via liposomes. *Int J Pharm*, Vol. 162, No. 1-2, pp. 29-38, ISSN: 0378-5173.

Yadav, J.D.; Kulkarni, P.R.; Vaidya, K.A. & Shelke, G.T., (2011). Niosomes: a review. *J Pharm Res*, Vol. 4, pp. 632-636, ISSN: 0974-6943.

Yoshida, H.; Lehr, C.M.; Kok, W.; Junginger, H.E.; Verhoef, J.C. & Bouwstra, J.A., (1992). Niosomes for oral delivery of peptide drugs. *J Control Release*, Vol. 21, No. 1-3, pp. 145-153, ISSN: 0168-3659.

Yoshioka, T.; Sternberg, M.; Moody, M. & Florence, A.T., (1992). Niosomes from Span surfactants: Relations between structure and form. *J Pharm Pharmacol*, Vol. 44, pp. 1044-1044, ISSN: 0022-3573.

Zhang, X.J.; Chen, J.J. & Liu, J.B., (2005). The genetic concept of vitiligo. *J Dermatol Sci*, Vol. 39, No. 3, pp. 137-146, ISSN: 0923-1811.

Chapter 6

Lipid Nanoparticulate Drug Delivery Systems: A Revolution in Dosage Form Design and Development

Anthony A. Attama, Mumuni A. Momoh and Philip F. Builders

Additional information is available at the end of the chapter

1. Introduction

Nanoparticulate drug delivery systems (DDS) have attracted a lot of attention because of their size-dependent properties. Among the array of nanoparticles being currently investigated by pharmaceutical scientists, lipid nanoparticles have taken the lead because of obvious advantages of higher degree of biocompatibility and versatility. These systems are commercially viable to formulate pharmaceuticals for topical, oral, pulmonary or parenteral delivery. Lipid nano formulations can be tailored to meet a wide range of product requirements dictated by disease condition, route of administration and considerations of cost, product stability, toxicity and efficacy. The proven safety and efficacy of lipid-based carriers make them attractive candidates for the formulation of pharmaceuticals, as well as vaccines, diagnostics and nutraceuticals [1].

The most frequent role of lipid-based formulations has traditionally been to improve the solubility of sparingly water soluble drugs especially Biopharmaceutics Classification System (BCS) Classes II & IV drugs. However, the spectrum of applications for lipid-based formulations has widened as the nature and type of active drugs under investigation vary. Lipid-based formulations may also protect active compounds from biological degradation or transformation, that in turn can lead to an enhancement of drug potency. In addition, lipid-based particulate DDS have been shown to reduce the toxicity of various drugs by changing the biodistribution of the drug away from sensitive organs. This reduction in toxicity may allow for more drug to be administered and forms the basis for the current success of several marketed lipid-based formulations of amphotericin B (Ambisome®, Abelcet®) and doxorubicin (Doxil®, Myocet®) [1].

Rapid advances in the ability to produce nanoparticles of uniform size, shape, and composition have started a revolution in science. The development of lipid-based drug carriers has attracted increased attention over the last decade. Lipid nanoparticles (e.g. solid lipid nanoparticles, SLNs) are at the forefront of the rapidly developing field of nanotechnology with several potential applications in drug delivery, clinical medicine and research, as well as in other varied sciences. Due to their size-dependent properties, lipid nanoparticles offer the possibility to develop new therapeutics that could be used for secondary and tertiary level of drug targeting. Hence, lipid nanoparticles hold great promise for reaching the goal of controlled and site specific drug delivery and has attracted wide attention of researchers.

At the turn of the millennium, modifications of SLN, nanostructured lipid carriers (NLC) and lipid drug conjugate (LDC)-nanoparticles were introduced [2, 3] in addition to liquid crystal DDS. These carrier systems overcome observed limitations of conventional SLN and more fluid lipid DDS. Compared to liposomes and emulsions, solid particles possess some advantages, e.g. protection of incorporated active compounds against chemical degradation and more flexibility in modulating the release of the compound. This paper focuses on the different lipid based nano systems, their structure and associated features, stability, production methods, drug incorporation and other issues related to their formulation and use in drug delivery. The following advantages among others, could be ascribed to lipid based nanocarriers:

- ability to control and target drug release.
- ability to improve stability of pharmaceuticals.
- ability to encapsulate high drug content (compared to other carrier systems e.g. polymeric nanoparticles).
- the feasibility of carrying both lipophilic and hydrophilic drugs.
- most of the lipids used are biodegradable, and as such they have excellent biocompatibility, are non-toxic, non-allergenic and non-irritating.
- they can be formulated by water-based technologies and thus can avoid organic solvents.
- they are easy to scale-up and sterilize.
- they are less expensive than polymeric/surfactant based carriers.
- they are easy to validate.

2. Drug delivery systems

A drug delivery system is defined as a formulation or a device that enables the introduction of a therapeutic substance in the body and improves its efficacy and safety by controlling the rate, time, and place of release of drugs in the body. The process of drug delivery includes the administration of the therapeutic product, the release of the active ingredients by the product, and the subsequent transport of the active ingredients across the biological membranes to the site of action. DDS interface between the patient and the drug. It may be a formulation of the drug or a device used to deliver the drug [4].

3. Lipids

The carboxylic acid group of a fatty acid molecule provides a convenient place for linking the fatty acid to an alcohol, via an ester linkage. If the fatty acid becomes attached to an alcohol with a long carbon chain, the resultant substance is called a wax. When glycerol and a fatty acid molecule are combined, the fatty acid portion of the resultant compound is called an acyl group, and the glycerol portion is referred to as a glyceride. A triacylglyceride thus has three fatty acids attached to a single glycerol molecule. Sometimes, this name is shortened to triglyceride. Triglyceride substances are commonly referred to as fats or oils, depending on whether they are solid or liquid at room temperature [5]. A lipid is thus a fatty or waxy organic compound that is readily soluble in non-polar solvents (e.g. ether), but not in polar solvent (e.g. water). Examples of lipids are waxes, oils, sterols, cholesterol, fat-soluble vitamins, monoglycerides, diglycerides, triglycerides (fats), and phospholipids. Fatty acids (including fats) are a subgroup of lipids, hence, it will be inaccurate to consider the terms synonymous.

3.1. Classification of solid lipids for delivery of bioactives

Lipids can be grouped into the following categories based upon their chemical composition.

3.1.1. Homolipids

Homolipids are esters of fatty acids with alcohols. They are lipids containing only carbon (C), hydrogen (H), and oxygen (O), and as such are referred to as simple lipids. The principal materials of interest for oral delivery vehicle are long chain and medium chain fatty acids linked to a glycerol molecule, known as triacylglycerols. The long-chain fatty acids ranging from C14 to C24 appear widely in common fat while the medium chain fatty acids ranging from C6 to C12 are typical components of coconut oil or palm kernel oil [6]. Examples of homolipids include: cerides (waxes e.g. beeswax, carnauba wax etc.), glycerides (e.g. fats and oils) and sterides (e.g. the esters of cholesterol with fatty acids).

3.1.2. Heterolipids

Heterolipids are lipids containing nitrogen (N) and phosphorus (P) atoms in addition to the usual C, H and O e.g. phospholipids, glycolipids and sulfolipids. They are also known as compound lipids. The emphasis here will be on the phospholipids only. Two main classes of phospholipids occur naturally in qualities sufficient for pharmaceutical applications. These are the phosphoglycerides and phosphosphingolipids. Some phosphosphingolipids such as ceramide are used mainly in topical dosage forms. Phospholipids can be obtained from all types of biomass because they are essential structural components in all kinds of membranes of living organisms [6].

3.1.3. Complex lipids

The more complex lipids occur closely linked with proteins in cell membranes and subcellular particles. More active tissues generally have a higher complex lipid content. They may also contain phospholipids. Complex lipids in this context include lipoproteins, chylomicrons, etc. Lipoproteins are spherical lipid-protein complexes that are responsible for the transport of cholesterol and other lipids within the body. Structurally, lipoprotein consists of an apolar core composed of cholesterol esters or triacylglycerols, surrounded by monolayer of phospholipid in which cholesterol and one or more specific apoproteins are embedded e.g. chylomicrons and lipoproteins

3.2. Lipid drug delivery systems

Lipid-based DDS are an accepted, proven, commercially viable strategy to formulate pharmaceuticals for topical, oral, pulmonary or parenteral delivery. Lipid formulations can be tailored to meet a wide range of product requirements. One of the earliest lipid DDS-liposomes have been used to improve drug solubility. Currently, some companies have established manufacturing processes for the preparation of large scale batches of sparingly soluble compounds, often at drug concentrations several orders of magnitude higher than the nominal aqueous solubility because of the introduction of novel lipid-based DDS [1].

3.3. Lipid nanoparticulate drug delivery systems

Lipid nanoparticles show interesting nanoscale properties necessary for therapeutic application. Lipid nanoparticles are attractive for medical purposes due to their important and unique features, such as their surface to mass ratio that is much larger than that of other colloidal particles and their ability to bind or adsorb and carry other compounds. Lipid nano formulations produce fine dispersions of poorly water soluble drugs and can reduce the inherent limitations of slow and incomplete dissolution of poorly water soluble drugs (e.g. BCS II & IV drugs), and facilitate formation of solubilised phases from which drug absorption occurs. In any vehicle mediated delivery system (whether the vehicle is an emulsion, liposome, noisome or other lipidic systems), the rate and mode of drug release from the system is important in relation to the movement of the delivery system *in vivo*.

Lipid particulate DDS abound depending on their architecture and particle size. Due to the large number of administration routes available, these delivery systems perform differently depending on the formulation type and route of administration. Figure 1 shows some of the different lipid particulate DDS available.

3.3.1. Solid lipid nanoparticles (SLN)

SLN are particulates structurally related to polymeric nanoparticles. However, in contrast to polymeric systems, SLN can be composed of biocompatible lipids that are physiologically well tolerated when administered *in vivo* and may also be prepared without organic solvents. The lipid matrices can be composed of fats or waxes (homolipids) that provide protection to the incorporated bioactive from chemical and physical degradation, in addition to modification of drug release profile. Typical formulations utilize lipids such as paraffin wax or biodegradable glycerides (e.g. Compritol 888 ATO) as the structural base of the particle [7].

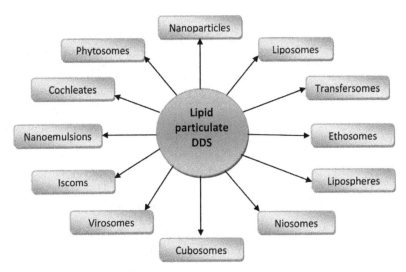

Figure 1. Lipid particulate drug delivery systems

SLN were developed in the 1990s as an alternative carrier system to the existing traditional carriers, such as emulsions, liposomes and polymeric nanoparticles. SLN are prepared either with physiological lipids or lipids with generally regarded as safe (GRAS) status. Under optimized conditions they can incorporate lipophilic or hydrophilic drugs and seem to fulfil the requirements for an optimum particulate carrier system [8]. SLN have a potential wide application spectrum- parenteral administration and brain delivery, ocular delivery, rectal delivery, oral delivery, topical delivery and vaccine delivery systems etc., in addition to improved bioavailability, protection of sensitive drug molecules from the outer environment and even controlled release characteristics. Common disadvantages of SLN are particle growth, unpredictable gelation tendency, unexpected dynamics of polymorphic transitions and inherent low incorporation rate due to the crystalline structure of the solid lipid [9].

3.3.2. Nanostructured lipid carriers (NLC)

NLC are colloidal carriers characterized by a solid lipid core consisting of a mixture of solid and liquid lipids, and having a mean particle size in the nanometer range. They consist of a lipid matrix with a special nanostructure [10]. This nanostructure improves drug loading and firmly retains the drug during storage. NLC system minimizes some problems associated with SLN such as low payload for some drugs; drug expulsion on storage and high water content of SLN dispersions.

The conventional method for the production of NLC involves mixing of spatially very different lipid molecules, i.e. blending solid lipids with liquid lipids (oils). The resulting matrix of the lipid particles shows a melting point depression compared with the original solid lipid but the matrix is still solid at body temperature. Depending on the method of production and the composition of the lipid blend, different types of NLC are obtained. The basic idea is that by giving the lipid matrix a certain nanostructure, the payload for active compounds is increased and expulsion of the compound during storage is avoided. Ability to trigger and even control drug release should be considered while mixing lipids to produce NLC. Newer methods of generating NLC are being developed.

3.3.3. Lipid drug conjugates (LDC)-nanoparticles

A major problem of SLN is the low capacity to load hydrophilic drugs due to partitioning effects during the production process. Only highly potent low dose hydrophilic drugs may be suitably incorporated in the solid lipid matrix [11]. In order to overcome this limitation, LDC nanoparticles with drug loading capacities of up to 33% were developed [8]. An insoluble drug-lipid conjugate bulk is first prepared either by salt formation (e.g. with a fatty acid) or by covalent linking (e.g. to ester or ethers). The obtained LDC is then processed with an aqueous surfactant solution to nanoparticle formulation by high pressure homogenization (HPH). Such nanoparticles may have potential application in brain targeting of hydrophilic drugs in serious protozoal infections [12].

3.3.4. Liposomes

Liposomes are closed vesicular structures formed by bilayers of hydrated phospholipids. The bilayers are separated from one another by aqueous domains and enclose an aqueous core. As a consequence of this alternating hydrophilic and hydrophobic structure, liposomes have the capacity to entrap compounds of different solubilities. Additionally, the basic liposome structure of hydrated phospholipid bilayers is amenable to extensive modification or 'tailoring' with respect to the physical and chemical composition of the vesicle. This versatility has resulted in extensive investigation into the use of liposomes for various applications such as in radiology, cosmetology and vaccinology.

Liposomes used in drug delivery typically range from 25 nm to several micrometers and are usually dispersed in an aqueous medium. There are various nomenclatures for defining liposome subtypes based either on structural parameters or the method of vesicle preparation. These classification systems are not particularly rigid and a variation exists in use the of these terms, particularly with respect to size ranges. Liposomes are often distinguished according to their number of lamellae and size. Small unilamellar vesicles (SUV), large unilamellar vesicles and large multilamellar vesicles or multivesicular vesicles are differentiated. SUVs with low particle sizes in the nanometer range are of interest as liposomal nanocarriers for drug and antigen delivery [13, 14].

3.3.5. Transfersomes

Transfersome technology was developed with the intention of providing a vehicle to allow delivery of bioactive molecules through the dermal barrier. Transfersomes are essentially ultra-deformable liposomes, composed of phospholipids and additional 'edge active' amphiphiles such as bile salts that enable extreme distortion of the vesicle shape. The vesicle diameter is in the order of 100 nm when dispersed in buffer [15]. These flexible vesicles are thought to permeate intact through the intact dermis under the forces of the hydrostatic gradient that exists in the skin [16]. Drug or antigen may be incorporated into these vesicles in a manner similar to liposomes.

3.3.6. Niosomes

Niosomes are vesicles composed mainly of non-ionic bilayer forming surfactants [17]. They are structurally analogous to liposomes, but the synthetic surfactants used have advantages over phospholipids in that they are significantly less costly and have higher chemical stability than their naturally occurring phospholipid counterparts [18]. Niosomes are obtained on hydration of synthetic non-ionic surfactants, with or without incorporation of cholesterol or other lipids. Niosomes are similar to liposomes in functionality and also increase the bioavailability of the drug and reduce the clearance like liposomes. Niosomes can also be used for targeted drug delivery, similar to liposomes. As with liposomes, the properties of the niosomes depend both on the composition of the bilayer and the method of production. Antigen and small molecules have also been delivered using niosomes [19, 20].

3.3.7. Liquid crystal drug delivery systems

The spontaneous self assembly of some lipids to form liquid crystalline structures offers a potential new class of sustained release matrix. The nanostructured liquid crystalline materials are highly stable to dilution. This means that they can persist as a reservoir for slow drug release in excess fluids such as the gastrointestinal tract (GIT) or subcutaneous space, or be dispersed into nanoparticle form, while retaining the 'parent' liquid crystalline structure. The rate of drug release is directly related to the nanostructure of the matrix. Lyotropic liquid crystal systems that commonly consist of amphiphilic molecules and solvents can be classified into lamellar (L_α), cubic, hexagonal mesophases, etc. In recent years, lyotropic liquid crystal systems have received considerable attention because of their excellent potential as drug delivery vehicles [21]. Among these systems, reversed cubic (Q_{II}) and hexagonal mesophases (H_{II}) are the most important and have been extensively investigated for their ability to sustain the release of a wide range of bioactives from low molecular weight drugs to proteins, peptides and nucleic acids.

3.3.8. Nanoemulsions

Lipid-based formulations present a large range of optional delivery systems such as solutions, suspensions, self-emulsifying systems and nanoemulsions. Among these approaches, oral nanoemulsions offer a very good alternative because nanoemulsions can improve the bioavailability by increasing the solubility of hydrophobic drugs and are now widely used for the administration of BCS class II and class IV drugs. Oral nanoemulsions use safe edible materials (e.g., food-grade oils and GRAS-grade excipients) for formulation of the delivery system. Nanoemulsions possess outstanding ability to encapsulate active compounds due to their small droplet size and high kinetic stability [22, 23]. Nanoemulsions have sizes below 1 μm and have been extensively investigated as novel lipid based DDS [22] together with microemulsions.

3.4. Functional properties of lipids used in formulating lipid drug delivery systems

3.4.1. Crystallinity and polymorphism of lipids

Many pharmaceutical solids exist in different physical forms. It is well recognised that drug substances and excipients can be amorphous, crystalline or anhydrous, at various degrees of hydration or solvated with other entrapped solvent molecules, as well as varying in crystal hardness, shape and size. Amorphous solids consist of disordered arrangements of molecules and do not possess a distinguishable crystal lattice. In the crystalline state (polymorphs, solvates/hydrates, co-crystals), the constituent molecules are arranged into a fixed repeating array built of unit cells, which is known as lattice. Possession of adequate crystallinity is a prerequisite for a good lipid particulate DDS.

Triglycerides, which are mainly used as lipid matrices crystallize in different polymorphic forms. The most important forms are the α and β forms. Since the formulation of lipid particulate DDS may involve melting at some point, recrystallization from the melt results in the metastable α-polymorph, which subsequently undergoes a polymorphic transition into the stable β-form via a metastable intermediate form (β') [24]. The β-polymorph especially consists of a highly ordered, rigid structure with low loading capacity for drugs. The formation of all these polymorphic forms has been proved amongst solid triglyceride nanoparticles [25].

3.4.2. Melting characteristics of lipid matrices

A pure triacylglycerol has a single melting point that occurs at a specific temperature. Nevertheless, certain lipids contain a wide variety of different triacylglycerols, with different melting points and as a result, they melt over a wide range of temperatures, producing a wide endothermic transition in differential scanning calorimeter. High purity lipids with sharp melting transitions exclude drugs on recrystallization. In addition to the solidity or melting point of each individual triglyceride, in drug delivery, we are interested and concerned with the combination of triglycerides throughout the fat mixture. This impacts the plasticity and the melting point range. In the development of lipid nanoparticles, lipids with melting points well above the body temperature are preferred. This will enable among others, sustained release of the encapsulated drug.

3.5. Crystallinity and polymorphism vs drug loading capacity and drug release

Crystallinity and polymorphism have a lot of influence on some properties of lipid matrices used in lipid DDS. Parameters like drug loading capacity and drug release depend highly on the crystallinity and the polymorphic form of the lipids. The crystalline order and density increase from α to β forms and are highest for the β-forms of polymorphic lipids [24]. An increasing crystalline order has a great impact on the drug loading capacity, since an increase in order reduces the ability to incorporate different molecules including drugs [24]. Hence, the drug loading capacity of the poorly organized polymorphic forms is high [26]. However, this advantage goes along with the particles being in a metastable form which are able to transform into the stable β-polymorph upon storage. As a consequence of this transformation, often drug expulsion occurs. The increasing order of the matrix also reduces the diffusion rate of a drug molecule within the particle and hence reduces the rate of drug release.

3.6. Strategies to improve drug loading in lipid particulate drug delivery systems

The high crystallinity of SLN leads to a rather low drug loading capacity for many drugs, a problem still being addressed. However, for lipophilic drugs the incorporation into the particles is much easier and often results in rather high drug loading. In order to overcome the disadvantage of low loading capacity, many investigations have been done. Müller *et al.* [10] introduced NLC. In these formulations, lipids of highly ordered crystalline structure are combined with chemically different lipids of amorphous structure, giving rise to structured matrices that accommodate more drug.

Friedrich *et al* [27] reported a different method to increase the drug payload by incorporating amphiphilic phospholipids into the lipid matrix. This resulted in a much higher solubility of the drug in the matrix, which was attributed to the formation of a solidified reverse micellar solution within the matrix. In this case, the nanoparticles were prepared by cold homogenization which may have prevented a redistribution of the lecithin to the surface of the particles or into the aqueous phase. Such a behaviour could be observed for a similar system after high pressure homogenization of the molten lipids [28].

Another mechanism of increasing the drug loading capacity of SLN has been recently developed [29-32]. In these works, the researchers used mixtures of solid lipids of natural origin possessing fatty acids of different chain lengths. In the analytical characterization of the lipid mixtures using differential scanning calorimetry (DSC), X-ray diffraction and isothermal microcalorimetery, it was observed that the mixtures were able to form matrices of imperfect structure composed of mixed crystals and mixtures of crystals, which enhanced drug incorporation compared with the single lipids.

3.7. Ingredients used in the formulation of lipid based particulate drug delivery systems

3.7.1. Emulsifiers

Emulsifiers are essential to stabilize lipid nanoparticle dispersions and prevent particle agglomeration. The choice of the ideal surfactant for a particular lipid matrix is based on the surfactant properties such as charge, molecular weight, chemical structure, and respective hydrophile-lipophile balance (HLB). The HLB of an emulsifier is given by the balance between the size and strength of the hydrophilic and the lipophilic groups. Table 1 shows some of the emulsifiers employed in the production of lipid nanoparticles. The choice of the emulsifiers depends on the route of administration of the formulation, for e.g. for parenteral formulations, there are limits of the emulsifiers to be used [33]. For topical and ocular route the issue of skin sensitization has to be considered, while for oral route, the emulsifier should not produce any physiological effect at the use concentration. Emulsifiers could be used in combination to produce synergistic effect and better stabilize the formulation [22].

Emulsifiers/coemulsifiers	HLB	References
Lecithin	4-9	[9]
Poloxamer 188	29	[34]
Poloxamer 407	21.5	[35]
Polysorbate 20	16.7	[36]
Polysorbate 65	10.5	[7]
Polysorbate 80	15	[9]
Cremophor EL	12-14	[37]
Solutol HS 15	15	[28]

Table 1. Some emulsifiers used for the production of lipid nanoparticles

3.7.2. Lipids

The matrices for lipid nanoparticle preparation are natural, semi-synthetic or synthetic lipids which can be biodegradable, including triglyceride (tri-stearic acid, tri-palmitic acid, tri-lauric acid and long-chain fatty acid), steroid and waxes (e.g. beeswax, carnauba wax, etc) and phospholipids. They could be used singly or in combination. Lipids for the production of nanoparticles may be grouped into two: bilayer and non-bilayer lipids.

3.7.3. Bilayer lipids used in drug delivery

Some lipids are capable of adopting a certain orientation depending on the processing condition. Compounds that have approximately equal-sized heads and tails e.g. phospholipids (Figures 2 and 3) tend to form bilayers instead of micelles in aqueous system. In these structures, two monolayers of lipid molecules associate tail to tail, thus minimizing the contact of the hydrophobic portions with water and maximizing hydrophilic interactions [38] (Figure 3). The phospholipid molecules can move about in their half the bilayer, but there is a significant energy barrier preventing migration to the other side of the bilayer. Cholesterol can insert into the bilayer, and this helps to regulate the fluidity of the membrane. The self-assembled nature of lipid bilayers implies that they are normally in a tension-less state.

Tail 1   Head group

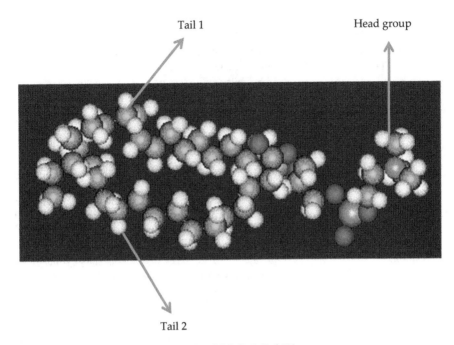

Tail 2

Figure 2. Structure of phospholipid (phosphatidylcholine) [Ref. 39].

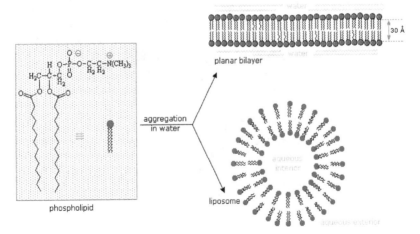

Figure 3. Interaction of phospholipid with water [38].

Phospholipids with certain head groups e.g. phosphatidylcholine (Figure 2) [39], can alter the surface chemistry of a lipid particle. The packing of phospholipid chains within the surface of the particle also affects its mechanical properties, including swelling, stretching, bending and deformability. Many of these properties have been taken advantage of in the design of novel lipid particulate DDS such as surface modification for improved drug loading capacity [31, 32, 40]. Deformability has been utilized in the development of ultra-deformable liposomes termed transfersomal DDS (transfersomes). Cholesterol strengthens the bilayer but decrease its permeability. Bilayer lipids when present in lipid particulate DDS may define the boundaries of the particle and its environment (aqueous), and are often involved in many complex processes occurring at the interface.

3.7.4. Non-bilayer lipids used in drug delivery

In many biological systems, the major lipids are non-bilayer lipids, which in purified form cannot be arranged in a lamellar structure in the presence of aqueous systems. The structural and functional roles of these lipids in drug delivery are mainly in their utilization as matrix-forming lipids. They include such lipids as homolipids e.g. triglycerides and waxes. Their functional properties in lipid nanotechnology differs depending partly on their melting points, crystallinity and polymorphic characteristics. However, they may have absorption promoting properties especially for lipophilic drugs. Table 2 shows some of the non-bilayer lipids used in the formulation of lipid micro- and nanoparticles.

Hard fats e.g.	Natural hard fats e.g.
Stearic acid [Ref. 41] Palmitic acid [Ref. 42] Behenic acid [Ref. 43]	Goat fat [Ref. 45] Theobroma oil [Ref. 53]
Triglycerides e.g.	**Waxes e.g.**
Trimyristin (Dynasan 114) [Ref. 44] Tripalmitin (Dynasan 116) [Ref. 45] Tristearin (Dynasan 118) [Ref. 44] Trilaurin [Ref. 46]	Beeswax [Ref. 9] Cetyl palmitate [Ref. 47] Carnauba wax [Ref. 89]
Mono, di and triglycerides mixtures e.g.	
Witepsol bases [Ref. 48] Glyceryl monostearate (Imwitor 900) [Ref. 49] Glyceryl behenate (Compritol 888 ATO) [Ref. 50] Glyceryl palmitostearate (Precirol ATO 5) [Ref. 51] Softisan 142 and Softisan 154 [Refs. 52, 27]	

Table 2. Some non-bilayer lipids used in the formulation of lipid nanoparticles

3.8. Characterization and selection of lipids for particulate drug delivery systems

There is an increasing interest in lipid-based DDS due to factors such as better characterization of lipidic excipients and formulation versatility and the choice of different DDS. Apart from the fatty acid profile of previously undefined lipids, many different analytical procedures are used to characterize lipids. These technologies provide different scales of analysis and may be used in combination to select the appropriate lipid matrix for use in formulation. DSC is the most widely used thermo-analytic technique for studying fats, oils and their mixtures. It gives information about the temperatures and energy associated with their fusion and crystallization, phase behaviour, polymorphic transformations, and data to estimate solid fat contents. DSC reports the destruction of structures in recordings obtained in a permanent out-of-equilibrium state. X-ray diffraction (small angle X-ray diffraction, SAXD and wide angle X-ray diffraction, WAXD) is also an essential tool for elucidating properties of fats and their mixtures. However, it complements DSC. XRD recordings provide both short and long spacings at a given temperature at which the sample is supposed to be in equilibrium. Since lipid systems are quite sensitive to their preparation history, only simultaneous recordings of SAXD, WAXD, and DSC circumvent the problem of reproducibility and guarantee identical conditions for all three measurements whatever may be the thermal treatment of the sample. Polarized light microscopy (PLM) is an analytical technique used in characterization of fats to observe the microstructures of the various polymorphic forms of fats. With a hot stage coupled, it is used to observe the microstructural changes in fats during melting, as the lipid passes from crystalline phase to isotropic phase, to visualize crystallization from isotropic melts and to visually detect undissolved drug crystals in the lipid matrix.

Isothermal microcalorimetry (IMC) is a recent and an important tool in studying the time dependent crystallization of lipids and lipid matrices. It has been applied in both pure and mixed systems. Isothermal crystallization kinetics studies of mixtures of lipids using IMC also address the question of how the crystallinity of one component affects the crystallization behaviour of the other [29, 52, 53]. Atomic force microscopy (AFM) can provide invaluable information about the physicochemical characteristics of the carriers that play an important role in determining the performance of the DDS. A lot of this information cannot be obtained from other characterization techniques due to the unique ability of the atomic force microscope to probe nanometer scale features at the molecular level.

3.9. Preparation of lipid nanoparticulate drug delivery systems

There many methods for the preparation of lipid nanoparticulate DDS. The method used is dictated by the type of drug especially its solubility and stability, the lipid matrix, route of administration, etc. Liposomal preparation follows a different method as described by Mozafari [54]. In this section, emphasis was laid on the production of SLN, NLC and LDC-nanoparticles, with methods that can also be applied to the formulation of liquid crystal DDS.

3.9.1. High pressure homogenization

High pressure homogenisation (HPH) is a suitable method for the preparation of SLN, NLC and LDC-nanoparticles and can be performed at elevated temperature (hot HPH technique) or at and below room temperature (cold HPH technique) [11, 55]. The particle size is decreased by impact, shear, cavitation and turbulence. Briefly, for the hot HPH, the lipid and drug are melted (approximately 10 °C above the melting point of the lipid) and combined with an aqueous surfactant solution at the same temperature. A hot pre-emulsion is formed by homogenisation (e.g. using Ultra-Turrax). The hot pre-emulsion is then processed in a temperature-controlled high pressure homogenizer at 500 bar (or more) and predetermined number of cycles. The obtained nanoemulsion recrystallizes upon cooling down to room temperature forming SLN, NLC or LDC-nanoparticles. The cold HPH is a suitable technique for processing heat-labile drugs or hydrophilic drugs. Here, lipid and drug are melted together and then rapidly ground under liquid nitrogen forming solid lipid microparticles. A pre-suspension is formed by homogenisation of the particles in a cold surfactant solution. This pre-suspension is then further homogenised in a HPH at or below room temperature at predetermined homogenisation conditions to produce SLN, NLC or LDC-nanoparticles. The possibility of a significant increase in temperature during cold homogenisation should be borne in mind. Both HPH techniques are suitable for processing lipid concentrations of up to 40% and generally yield very narrow particle size distributions [56]. A schematic representation of HPH method of lipid particle preparation is shown in Figure 4.

3.9.2. Production of SLN via microemulsions

Gasco [57] developed and optimised a suitable method for the preparation of SLN via microemulsions. In a typical process, a warm microemulsion is prepared and thereafter, dispersed under stirring in excess cold water (typical ratio about 1:50) using a specially developed thermostated syringe. The excess water is removed either by ultra-filtration or by lyophilisation in order to increase the particle concentration. Experimental process parameters such as microemulsion composition, dispersing device, effect of temperature and lyophilisation on size and structure of the obtained SLN should be optimized. The removal of excess water from the prepared SLN dispersion is a difficult task with regard to the particle size. Also, high concentrations of surfactants and cosurfactants (e.g. butanol) are necessary for the formulation, but less desirable with respect to regulatory purposes and application.

3.9.3. SLN prepared by solvent emulsification/evaporation

For the production of nanoparticle dispersions by solvent emulsification/evaporation, the lipophilic material is dissolved in water immiscible organic solvent (e.g. cyclohexane) that is emulsified in an aqueous phase [58]. Upon evaporation of the solvent, nanoparticle dispersion is formed by precipitation of the lipid in the aqueous medium. Siekmann and Westesen [59] produced cholesterol acetate nanoparticles with a mean size of 29 nm using solvent emulsification/evaporation technique.

Other methods of lipid nanoparticle preparation include phase inversion and supercritical fluid (SCF) technology.

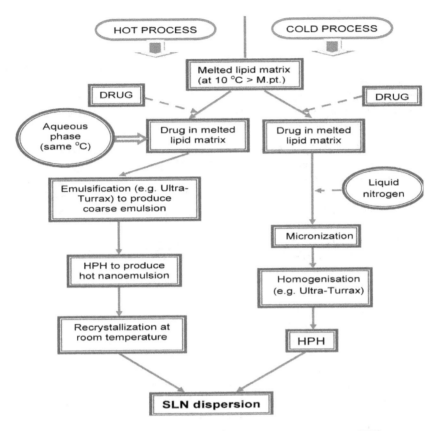

Figure 4. Production of lipid nanoparticles (SLN) by high pressure homogenisation (HPH)

3.10. Characterization of lipid nanoparticle quality

Quantitative analysis of particle characteristics such as morphological features can be very informative as biophysical properties are known to influence biological activity, biodistribution and toxicity. Several techniques are often used to assess nanoparticle characteristics such as lamellarity, size, shape and polydispersity [60]. Adequate and proper characterization of the lipid nanoparticles is necessary for quality control. However, characterization of lipid nanoparticles is a serious challenge due to the colloidal size of the particles and the complexity and dynamic nature of the delivery system.

The important parameters which need to be evaluated for the lipid nanoparticles are particle size, size distribution kinetics (zeta potential), degree of crystallinity and lipid modification (polymorphism), coexistence of additional colloidal structures (micelles, liposome, super cooled melts, drug nanoparticles), time scale of distribution processes, drug content (encapsulation efficiency and loading capacity), *in vitro* drug release and surface morphology.

Particle size and size-distribution may be studied using photon correlation spectroscopy (PCS) otherwise known as dynamic light scattering (DLS), static light scattering (SLS), transmission electron microscopy (TEM), scanning electron microscopy (SEM), atomic force microscopy (AFM), scanning tunneling microscopy (STM), freeze fracture electron microscopy (FFEM) or cryoelectron microscopy (Cryo-EM). These microscopy techniques are also used to study the morphology of nanoparticles.

Among the imaging techniques, AFM has been widely applied to obtain the size, shape and surface morphological information on nanoparticles. It is capable of resolving surface details down to 0.01 nm and producing a contrasted and three-dimensional image of the sample. X-ray diffraction and differential scanning calorimetric analysis give information on the crystalline state and polymorphic changes in the nanoparticles. Confocal laser scanning microscopy (CLSM) gives information on interaction of nanoparticles with cells. Nuclear magnetic resonance (NMR) can be used to determine both the size and the qualitative nature of nanoparticles. The selectivity afforded by chemical shift complements the sensitivity to molecular mobility to provide information on the physicochemical status of components within the nanoparticle.

An important characterization technique for lipid nanoparticles is determination of solid state properties. This is very important in order to detect the possible modifications in the physicochemical properties of the drug incorporated into the lipid nanoparticles or the lipid matrix. It has been proven that although particles were produced from crystalline raw materials, the presence of emulsifiers, preparation method and high shear encountered (e.g. HPH) may result in changes in the crystallinity of the matrix constituents compared with bulk materials. This may lead to liquid, amorphous or only partially crystallized metastable systems [61]. Polymorphic transformations may cause chemical and physical changes (e.g. shape, solubility, melting point) in the active and auxiliary substances. The solid state analysis of lipid nanoparticles is usually carried out using the following procedures: DSC, X-ray diffraction, hot stage microscopy, Raman spectroscopy and Fourier-transform infrared spectroscopy.

3.11. Drug incorporation and loading capacity

Many different drugs have been incorporated in lipid nanoparticles. A very important point to judge the suitability of a drug carrier system is its loading capacity. The loading capacity is generally expressed in percent related to the lipid phase (matrix lipid and drug). Westesen *et al.* [61] studied the incorporation of drugs using loading capacities of typically 1 - 5%, but for ubidecarenone loading capacities of up to 50% were reported. Different loading capacities were obtained for other drugs [62]. Factors determining the loading capacity of a drug in the lipid include among others, solubility of drug in melted lipid; miscibility of drug melt and lipid melt; chemical and physical structure of solid lipid matrix; and polymorphic state of lipid material.

The prerequisite to obtain a sufficient loading capacity is a sufficiently high solubility of the drug in the lipid melt. This is why it is necessary to determine the solubility of a drug in the lipid matrix as a preformulation strategy. Typically, the solubility should be higher than required because it decreases when cooling the melt and might even be lower in the solid lipid. Solubility of a drug in the lipid melt could be enhanced by the addition of solubilizers.

3.12. Drug release from lipid nanoparticles

There have been many studies dealing with drug incorporation, however, there are distinctly less data available about drug release, especially information about the release mechanisms. Drug release from lipid nanoparticles could be conducted using different models and biorelevant media. Generally, artificial membranes, tissue constructs or excised skin are used as barriers. A major problem encountered with lipid nanoparticles is the burst release observed with these systems, however, a prolonged drug release could also be obtained with these systems. It is possible to modify the release profiles as a function of lipid matrix, surfactant concentration and production parameters (e.g. temperature) and by surface modification [40].

The release profiles of drugs from lipid nanoparticles could be modulated to obtain prolonged release without burst effect, or to generate systems with tailored burst, followed by prolonged release. The burst can be exploited to deliver an initial dose when desired. It is important to note that the release profiles are not or only slightly affected by the particle size. Predominant factors for the shape of the release profiles are the production parameters (surfactant concentration, temperature) and the nature of the lipid matrix. During particle production of lipid nanoparticles by the hot homogenization technique, drug partitions from the liquid oil phase to the aqueous water phase. The amount of drug partitioning to the water phase will increase with the solubility of the drug in the water phase, that means with increasing temperature of the aqueous phase and increasing surfactant concentration as these two parameters directly affect the solubility of drugs in aqueous system.

It was reported that there was a decrease in release with decrease in temperature for a drug encapsulated in lipid nanocapsule [63]. This decrease in drug release with decreasing temperature was attributed to an increased microviscosity of the oil delaying the drug diffusion out of lipid nanocapsule core into the aqueous release medium. The effect of ambient temperature on viscosity, however, was not limited to the internal oily core material but applies also to the external aqueous phase.

Investigation of drug release from different wax matrix pellets using theophylline as a lipophilic drug showed that as the hydrophobicity of the wax increased, the drug release rate decreased. The more hydrophilic is the wax, the more it is susceptible to hydration by the release medium and therefore the faster the drug release. The drug release pattern was also highly dependent on the drug aqueous solubility. The release process was mainly affected by the relative affinity of the drug to the wax and the aqueous release medium [63]. Therefore, wax could be modified with compatible hydrophilic material to moderate drug release from lipid-based wax matrices. It was also found that minor temperature changes around 37 °C will not significantly influence the drug release from these lipid nanocapsules, which excluded the option of a temperature-dependent release under *in vivo* conditions. zur Mühlen *et al.* [64] reported that interactions between drug and lipid molecules plays important role in controlling the drug release. These interactions could affect the viscosity of the solid lipid matrix leading to different release rates for different drugs although having similar lipophilic properties. They demonstrated that the development of sustained release SLN is possible by the proper choice of the drug and the lipid and their degree of interaction.

3.13. Challenges of lipid nanoparticle drug delivery system

One major problem with the intravenous administration of colloidal particles is their interaction with the reticulo-endothelial system (RES). Nanoparticles for medical applications are frequently given via parenteral administration. As with any foreign material, the body mounts a biological response to an administered nanoparticle. This response is the result of a complex interplay of factors, not just the intrinsic characteristics of the nanoparticle. In particular, most materials, upon contact with biological matrices, are immediately coated by proteins, leading to a protein "corona" [65]. Protein coronas are complex and variable. Certain components of the nanoparticle corona, called opsonins, may enhance uptake of the coated material by cells of the RES. The presence of opsonins on the particle surface creates a "molecular signature" which is recognized by immune cells and determines the route of particle internalization. The route of internalization affects the eventual fate of the nanoparticle in the body (i.e. its rate of clearance from the bloodstream, volume of distribution, organ disposition, and rate and route of clearance from the body). The cells of RES are capable of mopping up particles that they do not recognise as self i.e. particles they recognise as foreign. The negative effect can however, be remedied by linking of polyethylene glycol molecules to the lipid nanoparticles, thus increasing their hydrophilicity and the residence time of these particles in circulation. Alternatively, the lipid nanoparticles could be engineered to evade these RES cells by limiting the particle sizes to about 200 nm or less. It is believed that these cells do not recognise low nanometer-sized particles as foreign. Several other varied and unrelated challenges are encountered in lipid nanoparticle technology. These challenges constitute a serious research question which current strategies are targeted to address.

3.13.1. Formation of perfect crystalline structure during storage

Triglycerides crystallize in different polymorphic forms such as α, γ, β', and β- forms. Recrystallization from the melt results in the metastable α-polymorph which subsequently undergoes a polymorphic transition into the stable β-form via a metastable intermediate. The β-polymorph especially consists of a highly ordered, rigid structure with low loading capacity of drugs. Transition to the β-form via a metastable intermediate form leads to drug expulsion and inability to protect or prolong the release of the encapsulated drug.

3.13.2. Physical stability

The stability of lipid particulate systems is influenced by the size of the nanoparticles. Lipid nanoparticles are prevented from sedimentation by Brownian motion, but other instabilities like Ostwald ripening and aggregation may occur. Since nanoparticles have a large specific surface area, stabilization of the surface with sufficient amounts of emulsifier(s) is necessary. The formulation of the colloidal carriers themselves is a difficult task due to many problems that arise from their colloidal state and specific pharmaceutical demands on such formulations. Stability in a pharmaceutical sense refers to a shelf life of usually 3-5 years. Shorter shelf lives will only be accepted in very special cases. However, for most systems of pharmaceutical interest the colloidal state is at its best metastable. The colloidal state may cause several additional instabilities, for example, due to the presence of large interfaces (adsorption-desorption processes, interactions in the stabilizer layer, higher risk of chemical instabilities, etc.). Since many colloidal administration systems are intended for intravenous use, stability is very crucial. Ability to be sterilized is also an added advantage.

3.13.3. Gel formation

The change in morphology of lipid nanoparticles from spheres to platelets is responsible for the gelation of solid lipid nanoparticle dispersions [66]. Depending on the composition, especially of the emulsifier(s) and the amount of lipid matrix, a gelation of the normally liquid dispersions can be observed on storage [66, 67]. By means of TEM and synchrotron measurements, the reason for the gelation was found. The gelation may derive from a reversible self-association of the particles due to a stacking of the platelets [68, 69]. This gel-like feature of highly concentrated dispersions favours application as dermal drug delivery system since the viscoelastic features resemble those of semisolid creams [56]. In contrast, the lipid nanoparticle formulations for intravenous and ocular administration have to remain fluid. Phase transitions that would lead to an unusual lamellar gel phase (L_β) should be investigated for in parenteral formulations.

3.13.4. High water content of dispersions

The high water content of lipid nanoparticles (70-95%) could lead to drug degradation and high cost of energy input during lyophilisation. During lyophilisation, the integrity of the nanoparticles could be affected if adequate croprotectant or lyoprotectant was not included in the formulation. Water free nanoparticles could be used in tablet production or the nanoparticle dispersion used as granulating fluid during production. SLN can be transformed into a powder by spray-drying. In any case, it is beneficial to have a higher solid content to avoid the need of having to remove too much water. For cost reasons, spray drying might be the preferred method for transforming SLN dispersions into powders, with the previous addition of a protectant [26].

3.13.5. Dosing problems

Selection of appropriate dosage form for lipid nanoparticle may be a problem. Outside injectables, there is need to package lipid nanoparticles in appropriate dosage units e.g. dispersible powders or hard/soft gelatine capsules especially for oral administration. Since the stomach acidic environment and its high ionic strength favour particle aggregation, aqueous dispersions of lipid nanoparticles might not be suitable to be administered orally as a dosage form. In addition, the presence of food will also have a high impact on their performance [70]. Packaging of SLN in a sachet for redispersion in water or juice prior to administration will allow an individual dosing by volume of the reconstituted SLN. This means additional step in packaging, which might result in introduction of additional technology and increase in the cost of the product.

3.13.6. Coexistence of other colloidal structures in the system (e.g. liposome and vesicles in SLN and NLC containing phospholipids)

Considerable amounts of emulsifiers are needed for the stabilization of lipid nanoparticles. If the emulsifiers redistribute from the particles into the aqueous phase, they can form colloidal structures like micelles or liposomes or other vesicular structures by self-assembly. Drugs can be solubilized within these structures, affecting drug release as well as drug loading capacity [70]. Hence the formation of additional colloidal structures has to be investigated for each formulation to enable further precautions to be taken to avoided it. The coexistence of liposomes and oil droplets was detected in an intravenous o/w nanoemulsion [71]. In solid lipid nanoparticle dispersion, additional liposomes were observed by means of cryo-TEM, although the amount was lower than in a corresponding emulsion [72]. In contrast to this, Schubert *et al.* [73] performed NMR, TEM and small angle X-ray scattering (SAXS) measurements and showed that no additional colloidal structures were formed. Drug nanocrystals could also be formed when the amount of the drug present far exceeds its solubility limit in the lipid matrix.

3.13.7. Supercooling of nanoparticles

Lipid nanoparticles prepared from triglycerides which are solid at room temperature may not necessarily crystallize on cooling to common storage temperatures. The particles can remain liquid for several months without crystallization (supercooled melt) [74]. Dispersions with lower melting points, in particular, monoacid triglycerides such as trilaurin or trimyristin, do not display melting transitions upon heating in differential scanning calorimeter or reflections due to crystalline nature in X-ray diffractometer after storage at room temperature. As confirmed by studies with quantitative ^{1}H NMR spectroscopy, the matrix of the dispersed particles consists of liquid triglycerides in such particles. The particles have a high tendency toward supercooling. The critical crystallization temperature is mainly dependent on the composition of the triglyceride matrix and can also be modified by incorporated drugs. The degree of supercooling is much higher in the nanoparticles than for the bulk triglyceride. This supercooling could be taken advantage of and utilized as a delivery system of its own but this has to be planned for *ab initio*.

3.14. Applications of lipid particulate drug delivery systems

During the last decade, different substances have been entrapped into lipid nanoparticles ranging from lipophilic to hydrophilic molecules and including difficult compounds such as proteins and peptides.

3.14.1. Lipid nanoparticles as carriers for oral drug delivery

Lipid nanoparticles such as SLN can be administered orally as dispersion, SLN-based tablet, pellets or capsules [70] or even as lyophilized unit dose powders for reconstitution for oral delivery. The stability of the particles in the GIT has to be thoroughly tested, since low pH and high ionic strength in the GIT may result in aggregation of the particles. In order to prove this, an investigation of the effect of artificial gastric fluids on different lipidic nanoparticle formulations was performed. The authors showed that a zeta potential of at least 8-9 mV in combination with a steric stabilization hinders aggregation under these conditions [75]. Additionally, for oral drug delivery, a release upon enzymatic degradation has to be taken into account [3, 76].

The routes for particle uptake after oral application are transcellular (via the M cells in the Peyer's patches or enterocytes) or paracellular (diffusion between the cells). However, the uptake via M cells is the major pathway, resulting in the transport of the particles to the lymph [77]. Uptake into the lymph and the blood was demonstrated by means of TEM and gamma counting of labelled SLN. It was found that uptake to the lymph was considerably higher than to the plasma [78], and as such, a reduced first pass effect concludes, as the transport via the portal vein to the liver is bypassed [79].

SLN containing the antituberculosis drugs rifampicin, isoniazid and pyrazinamide have been studied in animals model and it was found that administration every 10 days could be successful for the management of tuberculosis [80].

3.14.2. Lipid nanoparticles for parenteral drug delivery

Lipid nanoparticles can be formulated for subcutaneous, intramuscular or intravenous administration. For intravenous administration, the small particle size is a prerequisite as passage through the needle and possibility of embolism should be considered. SLN offer the opportunity of a controlled drug release and the possibility to incorporate poorly soluble drugs. Additionally, especially for intravenous application, drug targeting via modification of the particle surface is possible, and for SLN formulation with a controlled release, higher plasma concentrations over a prolonged period of time can be obtained. Such systems form an intravenous depot. Further studies with different drugs such as idarubicin, doxorubicin, tobramycin, clozapine or temozolomide also showed a sustained release as described in a review paper by Harms and Müller-Goymann [81].

3.14.3. Lipid nanoparticles as carriers for peptides and proteins drugs

Lipid nanoparticles have been extensively studied for the delivery of proteins and peptides [82]. Therapeutic application of peptides and proteins is restricted by their high molecular weight, hydrophilic character and limited chemical stability, which cause low bioavailability, poor transfer across biological membranes and low stability in the bloodstream. Most of the available peptides and proteins are delivered by injection, but their short half life demands repeated doses that are costly, painful and not well tolerated by patients. Lipid nanoparticles could be useful for peptide and protein delivery due to the stabilizing effect of lipids and to the absorption promoting effect of the lipidic material that constitute this kind of nanoparticles [83]. The use of niosomes and liposomes as adjuvants for the delivery of Newcastle disease virus to chicks has been reported [14].

3.14.4. Lipid nanocarriers for nasal vaccination

The use of lipid nanocarriers provides a suitable way for the nasal delivery of antigenic molecules. Besides improved protection and facilitated transport of the antigen, nanoparticulate delivery systems could also provide more effective antigen recognition by immune cells. These represent key factors in the optimal processing and presentation of the antigen, and therefore in the subsequent development of a suitable immune response. In this sense, the design of optimized vaccine nanocarriers offers a promising way for nasal mucosal vaccination [82].

3.14.5. Lipid nanoparticles as carriers in cosmetic and dermal preparation

Lipid nanoparticles can be incorporated into a cream, hydrogel or ointment to obtain semisolid systems for dermal applications. Another possibility is to increase the amount of lipid matrix in the formulation above a critical concentration, resulting in semisolid formulations [84]. The substances used for the preparation of dermal SLN are rather innocuous since they are mostly rated as GRAS and many of them are used in conventional dermal formulations. This resulted in the first dermal formulations containing SLN for cosmetic purposes entering the market [85].

Due to the adhesiveness of small particles, SLN adhere to the stratum corneum forming a film as this films have been shown to possess occlusive properties [86]. It was shown that the degree of crystallinity has a great impact on the extent of occlusion by the formulation. With increasing crystallinity the occlusion factor increases as well [87]. This explains why liquid nanoemulsions in contrast to SLN do not show an occlusive effect and why the extent of occlusion by NLC compared to SLN is reduced. Other parameters influencing the occlusion factor are the particle size and the number of particles. Whilst with increasing size the factor decreases, an increase in number results in an increase in the extent occlusion [88]. The occlusive effect leads to reduced water loss and increased skin hydration. Highly crystalline SLN can be used for physical sun protection due to scattering and reflection of the UV radiation by the particles. A high crystallinity was found to enhance the effectiveness and was also synergistic with UV absorbing substances used in conventional sunscreens [89]. Similarly synergism was observed on the sun protection factor and UV-A protection factor exhibited by the incorporation of the inorganic sunscreen, titanium-dioxide in NLC of carnauba wax and decyl oleate [90].

3.14.6. Lipid nanoparticles for ocular application

The eye possesses unique challenges with respect to drug delivery especially with respect to the posterior segment and treating vision threatening diseases. Poor bioavailability of drugs from ocular dosage form is mainly due to the pre-corneal loss factors which include tear dynamics, non-productive absorption, transient residence time in the cul-de-sac, and relative impermeability of the corneal epithelial membrane. Due to the adhesive nature of the small nanoparticles, these negative effects can be reduced. For ocularly administered SLN an increase in bioavailability was observed in rabbits by Cavalli *et al.* [91] using tobramycin ion pair as the model drug. Various *in vitro* studies show a prolonged and enhanced permeation when the drug is incorporated in lipid nanoparticles [39]. For systems containing phospholipids, a further improved permeation of diclofenac sodium was observed [31].

3.14.7. Pulmonary application of lipid nanoparticles

Pulmonary drug application offers the advantage of minimizing toxic side effects if a local impact is intended. Systemic delivery can be achieved through pulmonary delivery, offering the advantage of bypassing the first pass effect, as well as offering a large absorptive area, extensive vasculature, easily permeable membrane and low extracellular and intracellular enzyme activities [92]. A problem of this method of administration is the low bioavailability. SLN can easily be nebulized to form an aerosol of liquid droplets containing nanoparticles for inhalation [82]. *In vivo* studies showed that the administered drugs (rifampicin, isoniazid and pyrazinamide for the treatment of tuberculosis) resulted in a prolonged mean residence time and a higher bioavailability than the free drug [93, 94].

3.14.8. Application of liquid crystal drug delivery systems

The spontaneous self assembly of some lipids to form liquid crystalline structures offers a potential new class of sustained release matrix. The nanostructured liquid crystalline materials are highly stable to dilution. This means that they can persist as a reservoir for slow drug release in excess fluids such as the GIT or subcutaneous space, or be dispersed into nanoparticle form, while retaining the parent liquid crystalline structure. The rate of drug release is directly related to the nanostructure of the matrix. The particular geometry into which the lipids assemble can be manipulated through either the use of additives to modify the assembly process, or through modifying conditions such as temperature, thereby providing a means to control drug release.

Liquid crystal depot could be injected as a low-viscosity solution. Once in the body, it self-assembles and encapsulates the drug in a nanostructured, viscous liquid crystal gel. The drug substance is then released from the liquid crystal matrix over a time period, which can be tuned from days to months. The liquid crystal depot system is capable of providing *in vivo* sustained release of a wide range of therapeutic agents over controlled periods of time. Liquid crystal nanoparticles can be combined with controlled-release and targeting functionalities. The particles are designed to form *in situ* at a controlled rate, which enables an effective *in vivo* distribution of the drug. The system has been shown to give more stable plasma levels of peptides in comparison to competing microsphere and conventional oil-depot technologies [21, 95].

Oral liquid crystal DDS are designed to address the varied challenges in oral delivery of numerous promising compounds including poor aqueous solubility, poor absorption, and large molecular size. Compared with conventional lipid or non-lipid carriers, these show high drug carrier capacity for a range of sparingly water-soluble drugs. For drugs susceptible to *in vivo* degradation, such as peptides and proteins, liquid crystal nanoparticles protect the sensitive drug from enzymatic degradation. The system also addresses permeability limitations by exploiting the lipid-mediated absorption mechanism. For water-soluble peptides, typical bioavailability enhancements range from twenty to more than one hundred times. In an alternative application large proteins have been encapsulated for local activity in the GIT. Liquid crystal nanoparticle systems can be designed to be released at different absorption sites (e.g., in the upper or lower intestine) which is important for drugs that have narrow regional absorption windows.

With regards to topical application, liquid crystal systems form a thin surface film at mucosal surfaces consisting of a liquid crystal matrix, whose nanostructure can be controlled for achieving an optimal delivery profile. The system also provides good temporary protection for sore and sensitive skin. Their unique solubilizing, encapsulating, transporting, and protecting capacity is advantageously exploited in liquid and gel products used to increase transdermal and nasal bioavailability of small molecules and peptides.

3.15. Lipid nanoparticles in drug targeting

Nanoscale lipid materials containing drugs and diagnostics are being developed to image the distribution of tumour cells in the body, target and attach to cancerous cells, destroy unwanted cells via ablation or interference with cellular functions. Drug targeting might overcome the problem of repeated administration by facilitating the efficacy of drug administered systemically and attenuating side effects on healthy tissues. Ultimately, lipid nanoparticles represent versatile DDS, with the ability to overcome physiological barriers and guide the drug to specific cells or intracellular compartments by means of passive or ligand-mediated targeting mechanisms.

There are many research reports dealing with targeting of drugs to certain cellular targets in the organs using lipid nanoparticles. The knowledge of the pathophysiological/passive targeting approaches used in cancer chemotherapy is used to develop nanocarriers for targeting drug to appropriate cancer cells in the body. Small molecules administered systemically are easily eliminated through the kidney into the urine and distributed equally not only in the target tissue but also in other healthy tissues, resulting in less efficacy and more possible side effects [96]. On the other hand, large molecules have longer half-life in the blood and tend to be passively delivered to the lesions with highly permeable vessels in neovascularization and inflammation. This tendency is remarkable especially in solid tumors because of high density of neovascular vessels and immature lymph systems, and is termed enhanced permeability and retention (EPR) effect. Because of the successes being recorded from *in vitro* experiments, lipid nanoparticles have been subject of further investigation for drug targeting to the brain, several types of cancer, posterior segments of the eye, otic (inner ear) diseases, and delivery of nucleic acids and genes, utilizing the both active and passive targeting opportunities [97].

3.16. Scale up issues and ultimate dosage form development

Large scale production of lipid nanoparticles is possible using lines available in pharmaceutical plants. In spite of intensive research on colloidal drug carrier systems, in some cases for several decades (e.g., with lipid emulsions or liposomes), remarkably few have been introduced into the market [98, 99] as presented in Table 3 indicating that there seem to be problems either with the underlying concepts or with the formulation of adequate colloidal carriers, or both. Most of the products are cosmetic products. In this context, it has, of course, to be taken into account that the development and registration of a new type of administration system may take as long for a new drug or novel formulation thereof; that means up to 10 years or even more. Therefore, products will appear on the market only after considerable period of time when the concept has been successfully realized.

Product name	Producer	Market entry date	Main active ingredients
Cutanova Cream Nano Repair Q10	Dr. Rimpler	10/2005	Q 10, polypeptide, Hibiscus extract, ginger extract, ketosugar
Intensive Serum NanoRepair Q10		10/2005	Q 10, polypeptide, mafane extract
Cutanova Cream NanoVital Q10		06/2006	Q 10, TiO$_2$, polypeptide, ursolic acid, oleanolic acid, sunflower seed extract
SURMER Crème Legère Nano-Protection SURMER Crème Riche Nano-Restructurante SURMER Elixir du Beauté Nano- Vitalisant SURMER Masque Crème Nano-Hydratant	Isabelle Lancray	11/2006	Kukuinut oil, Monoi Tiare Tahiti®, pseudopeptide, milk extract from coconut, wild indigo, noni extract
NanoLipid Restore CLR	Chemisches Laboratorium Dr. Kurt Richter, (CLR)	04/2006	Black currant seed oil containing ω-3 and ω-6 unsaturated fatty acids
Nanolipid Q10 CLR		07/2006	coenzyme Q10 and black currant seed oil
Nanolipid Basic CLR		07/2006	caprylic/capric triglycerides
NanoLipid Repair CLR		02/2007	black currant seed oil and manuka oil
IOPE SuperVital - Cream - Serum - Eye cream	Amore Pacific	09/2006	coenzyme Q10, ω-3 und ω-6 unsaturated fatty acids

Product name	Producer	Market entry date	Main active ingredients
- Extra moist softener - Extra moist emulsion			
NLC Deep Effect Eye Serum NLC Deep Effect Repair Cream NLC Deep Effect Reconstruction Cream NLC Deep Effect Reconstruction Serum	Beate Johnen	12/2006	coenzyme Q10, highly active oligo saccharides Q10, TiO₂, highly active oligo saccharides Q10, Acetyl Hexapeptide-3, micronized plant collagen, high active oligosaccharides in polysaccharide matrix
Regenerationscreme Intensiv	Scholl	6/2007	Macadamia Ternifolia seed oil, Avocado oil, Urea, Black currant seed oil
Swiss Cellular White Illuminating Eye Essence Swiss Cellular White Intensive Ampoules	la prairie	1/2007	Glycoprotiens, Panax ginseng root extract, Equisetum Arvense extract, Camellia Sinensis leaf extract, Viola Tricolor Extract
SURMER Creme Contour Des Yeux Nano-Remodelante	Isabelle Lancray	03/2008	Kukuinut oil, Monoi Tiare Tahiti®, pseudopeptide, hydrolized wheet protien
Olivenöl Anti Falten Pflegekonzentrat Olivenöl Augenpflegebalsam	Dr. Theiss	02/2008	Olea Europaea Oil, Panthenol, Acacia Senegal, Tocopheryl Acetate Olea Europaea Oil, Prunus Amygdalus Dulcis Oil, Hydrolized Milk Protein, Tocopheryl Acetate, Rhodiola Rosea Root Extract, Caffeine

Table 3. Examples of cosmetic products currently on the market containing lipid nanoparticles (Adapted from [98, 99]).

4. Future prospects of novel lipid particulate drug delivery systems

Novel lipid based nanoparticles offer a highly versatile platform that should be considered when working with drugs that present solubility and/or bioavailability challenges. An increasing number of drugs under development are poorly water soluble and therefore have poor bioavailability. These are designated BCS class II and class IV drugs. Creative formulation techniques are required to produce finished drug products of these drugs that have acceptable pharmacokinetics. A common formulation approach with such compounds is to focus on creating and stabilizing very small particles of the drug in an attempt to increase the surface area available for dissolution *in vivo*, and hence the rate of dissolution, and consequently plasma or tissue levels of drug. Shelf-life stability and enzymatic degradation are two main areas of concern, and formulation design focuses on stabilizing the drug in storage and protecting it from endogenous enzyme degradation until it reaches its therapeutic target. These novel DDS are well suited for the formulation of these bioactives.

Lipid nanoparticle DDS can be employed for the delivery of phytomedicines intended for oral and topical administration, which are the main routes of administration of phytomedicinals. This application holds great promise in the development and use of phytomedicines considering the difficulties of their delivery owing to their physicochemical properties. Since many phytomedicines usually possess different pharmacological activities, the delivery can be targeted to specific part(s) of the body where action is desired by means of lipid nanoparticle technology [60]. Thus, undesired effects and wastage of materials would be avoided. The implication is that with efficiency of preparation, only required quantity is utilized for formulation and adequate dose is absorbed and successfully delivered to the target for the desired activity. Lipid nanoparticle formulation of phytomedicinals would find useful applications in nanomedicine especially where targeted delivery is important such as in the treatment of cancer.

5. Conclusions

The use of lipid particles as drug carrier systems has been favoured recently as result of the GRAS status of the excipients and their traditional use in other food and pharmaceutical products. Lipids and lipid nanoparticles are promising delivery systems for oral administration of small molecule drugs, proteins and peptides. Lipid formulations of drugs are able to control the release of drugs and reduce absorption variability. The oral administration of lipid nanoparticles is possible as aqueous dispersion or alternatively transformed into a traditional dosage forms such as tablets, pellets, capsules, or powders in sachets. The ability to incorporate drugs into lipid nanocarriers offers a new prototype in drug delivery that could be used for passive and active drug targeting. Lipid nanoparticles for topical application could be formulated with high content of lipid matrix or dispersed in creams or gels to give it 'body'. With the development and interest in lipid particulate drug delivery systems shown by pharmaceutical formulation scientists, a future full of lipid nanoparticle products in the market is envisaged.

Author details

Anthony A. Attama* and Mumuni A. Momoh
Department of Pharmaceutics, Faculty of Pharmaceutical Sciences, University of Nigeria, Nsukka, Enugu State, Nigeria

---

* Corresponding Author

Philip F. Builders
Department of Pharmaceutical Technology and Raw Material Development, National Institute for Pharmaceutical Research and Development, Idu, Abuja, Nigeria

6. References

[1] Northern Lipids Inc. (2008) Lipid Based Drug Formulation. http://www.northernlipids.com/ourfacilities.htm. (accessed 17 April 2012).

[2] Muller RH, Radtke M, Wissing SA. Solid Lipid Nanoparticles (SLN) and Nanostructured Lipid Carriers (NLC) in Cosmetic and Dermatological Preparations. Adv. Drug Deliv. Rev. 2002; 54(Suppl. 1): S131–S155.

[3] Muller RH. Medicament Vehicle for the Controlled Administration of an Active Agent, Produced from Lipid Matrix-Medicament Conjugates. 2000; WO0067800.

[4] Jain KK. Drug Delivery Systems - An Overview. In: Jain KK. (ed.) Drug Delivery Systems. Totowa: Humana Press; 2008. p1-50.

[5] Lipids-Chemistry Encyclopaedia- structure, water, proteins, number, name, molecule. http://www.chemistryexplained.com/Kr-Ma/Lipids.html#ixzz1sJCOSV00. (accessed 17 April 2012).

[6] Stuchlík M, Žák S. Lipid-based Vehicle for Oral Drug Delivery. Biomed. Papers 2001; 145(2): 17–26.

[7] Attama AA, Nkemnele MO. *In Vitro* Evaluation of Drug Release from Self Micro-Emulsifying Drug Delivery Systems Using a Novel Biodegradable Homolipid from *Capra hircus*. Int. J. Pharm. 2005; 304 4-10.

[8] Müller RH, Mehnert W, Lucks JS, Schwarz C, Mühlen A, Weyhers H, Freitas C, Riihl D. Solid Lipid Nanoparticles (SLN)- An Alternative Colloidal Carrier System for Controlled Drug Delivery. Eur. J. Pharm. Biopharm. 1995;41: 62-69.

[9] Attama AA, Müller-Goymann CC. Effect of Beeswax Modification on the Lipid Matrix and Solid Lipid Nanoparticle Crystallinity. Colloids Surf. A: Physicochem. Eng. Aspects. 2008;315: 189-195.

[10] Müller RH, Souto EB, Radtke M. PCT application PCT/EP00/04111. 2000.

[11] Schwarz C, Mehnert W, Lucks JS, Muller RH. Solid Lipid Nanoparticles (SLN) for Controlled Drug Delivery: I. Production, Characterization and Sterilization. J. Control. Rel. 1994;30: 83–96.

[12] Olbrich C, Geßner A, Kayser O, Muller RH. Lipid-Drug Conjugate (LDC) Nanoparticles as Novel Carrier System for the Hydrophilic Antitrypanosomal Drug Diminazene diaceturate. J. Drug Target. 2002;10(5): 387–396.

[13] Onuigbo EB, Okore VC, Ngene AA, Esimone CO, Attama AA. Preliminary Studies of a Stearylamine-based Cationic Liposome. J. Pharm. Res. 2011;10(1): 25-29.

[14] Onuigbo EB, Okore VC, Esimone CO, Ngene A, Attama AA. Preliminary Evaluation of the Immunoenhancement Potential of Newcastle Disease Vaccine Formulated as a Cationic Liposome. Avian Pathology 2012. DOI: 10.1080/03079457.2012.691154.

[15] Cevc G, Gebauer D, Stieber J, Schatzlein A, Blume G. Ultraflexible Vesicles Transfersomes, have an Extremely Low Pore Penetration Resistance and Transport

Therapeutic Amounts of Insulin Across the Intact Mammalian Skin. Biochim. Biophys. Acta 1998;1368: 201–215.

[16] Cevc G, Schaltzlein A, Richardsen H. Ultradeformable Lipid Vesicles can Penetrate the Skin and Other Semi-Permeable Barriers Unfragmented. Evidence from Double Label CLSM Experiments and Direct Size Measurements. Biochim. Biophys. Acta 2002;1564: 21–30.

[17] Uchegbu IF, Vyas SP. Non-ionic Surfactant Based Vesicles (Niosomes) in Drug Delivery. Int. J. Pharm. 1998;172: 33-70.

[18] Conacher M, Alexander J, Brewer JM. Niosomes as Immunological Adjuvants. In: Uchegbu I. (ed.) Synthetic Surfactant Vesicles. Singapore: International Publishers Distributors; 2000. p185–205.

[19] Onuigbo EB. Evaluation of Cationic Liposome- or Noisome-Based Antigen Delivery Systems for Newcastle Disease Vaccine. Ph.D. thesis. University of Nigeria, Nsukka; 2011.

[20] Lakshmi PK, Devi GS, Bhaskaran S, Sacchidanand S. Niosomal Methotrexate Gel in the Treatment of Localized Psoriasis: Phase I and phase II Studies. Indian J. Dermatol. Venereal. Leprol. 2007;73(3): 157-161.

[21] Guo C, Wang J, Cao F, Lee RJ, Zhai G. Lyotropic Liquid Crystal Systems in Drug Delivery. Drug Discov. Today 2010;15: 1032-1040.

[22] Charles L, Attama AA. Current State of Nanoemulsions in Drug Delivery. J. Biomat. Nanobiotechnol. 2011;2: 626-639.

[23] Kotta S, KhanvAW, Pramod K, Ansari SH, Sharma RK, Ali J. Exploring Oral Nanoemulsions for Bioavailability Enhancement of Poorly Water-soluble Drugs. Expert Opin. Drug Deliv. 2012;9(5): 585-598.

[24] Hagemann JW. Thermal Behaviour and Polymorphism of Acylglycerides. In: Garti N, Sato K. (eds.) Crystallization and Polymorphism of Fats and Fatty Acids. Surfactant Science Series, Vol. 31. New York: Marcel Dekker; 1988. p9-95.

[25] Westesen K, Siekmann B, Koch MHJ. Characterization of Submicron-sized Drug Carrier Systems Based on Solid Lipids by Synchrotron Radiation X-ray Diffraction. Prog. Colloid Polym. Sci. 1993;93: 356.

[26] Jenning V, Thünemann AF, Gohla SH. Characterisation of a Novel Solid Lipid Nanoparticle Carrier System Based on Binary Mixtures of Liquid and Solid Lipids. Int. J. Pharm. 2000;199(2): 167–177.

[27] Friedrich I, Reichl S, Müller-Goymann CC. Drug Release and Permeation Studies of Nanosuspensions Based on Solidified Reverse Micellar Solutions (SRMS). Int. J. Pharm. 2005;305(1-2): 167-175.

[28] Schubert MA, Harms M, Müller-Goymann CC. Structural Investigations on Lipid Nanoparticles Containing High Amounts of Lecithin. Eur. J. Pharm. Sci. 2006;27(2-3): 226-236.

[29] Attama AA, Schicke BC, Müller-Goymann CC. Further Characterization of Theobroma Oil-Beeswax Admixtures as Lipid Matrices for Improved Drug Delivery Systems. Eur. J. Pharm. Biopharm. 2006;64: 294-306.

[30] Attama AA, Müller-Goymann CC. A Critical Study of Novel Physically Structured Lipid Matrices Composed of a Homolipid from *Capra hircus* and Theobroma Oil. Int. J. Pharm. 2006;322: 67-78.

[31] Attama AA, Reichl S, Müller-Goymann CC. Diclofenac Sodium Delivery to the Eye: *In Vitro* Evaluation of Novel Solid Lipid Nanoparticle Formulation Using Human Cornea Construct. Int. J. Pharm. 2008;355: 307-313.

[32] Attama AA, Weber C, Müller-Goymann CC. Assessment of drug permeation from SLN formulated with a novel structured lipid matrix through artificial skin construct bio-engineered from HDF and HaCaT cell lines. J. Drug Deliv. Sci. Technol. 2008;18(3) 181-188.

[33] Severino P, Andreani T, Sofia-Macedo A, Fangueiro JF, Santana M-H A, Silva AM, Souto EB. Current State-of-Art and New Trends on Lipid Nanoparticles (SLN and NLC) for Oral Drug Delivery. J. Drug Deliv. 2012; doi:10.1155/2012/750891.

[34] Kalam MA, Sultana Y, Ali A, Aqil M, Mishra AK, Chuttani K. Preparation, Characterization and Evaluation of Gatifloxacin Loaded Solid Lipid Nanoparticles as Colloidal Ocular Drug Delivery System. J. Drug Target. 2010; 18(3): 191–204.

[35] Göppert TM, Müller RH. Adsorption Kinetics of Plasma Proteins on Solid Lipid Nanoparticles for Drug Targeting. Int. J. Pharm. 2005; 302(1-2): 172–186.

[36] Varshosaz J, Tabbakhian M, Mohammadi MY. Formulation and Optimization of Solid Lipid Nanoparticles of Buspirone HCl for Enhancement of its Oral Bioavailability. J. Liposome Res. 2010; 20(4): 286–296.

[37] Pandita D, Ahuja A, Velpandian T, Lather V, Dutta T, Khar RK. Characterization and *In Vitro* Assessment of Paclitaxel Loaded Lipid Nanoparticles Formulated using Modified Solvent Injection Technique. Pharmazie 2009; 64(5): 301–310.

[38] Lipids - Chemistry Encyclopedia - structure, water, proteins, number, name, molecule http://www.chemistryexplained.com/Kr-Ma/Lipids.html#ixzz1sJC5I4CP (accessed 17 April 2012).

[39] http://www.web-books.com/MoBio/Free/Ch1B2.htm (accessed 3 June 2012).

[40] Attama AA, Reichl S, Müller-Goymann CC. Sustained Release and Permeation of Timolol from Surface Modified Solid Lipid Nanoparticles through Bio-engineered Human Cornea. Current Eye Res. 2009;34(8): 698-705.

[41] Xie S, Zhu L, Dong Z, Wang Y, Wang X, Zhou W. Preparation and Evaluation of Ofloxacin-loaded Palmitic Acid Solid Lipid Nanoparticles. Int. J. Nanomed. 2011; 6: 547-555.

[42] Battaglia L, Gallarate M, Cavalli R, Trotta M. Solid Lipid Nanoparticles Produced Through a Coacervation Method. J. Microencapsul. 2010; 27(1): 78–85.

[43] Severino P, Pinho SC, Souto EB, Santana MHA. Crystallinity of Dynasan114 and Dynasan118 Matrices for the Production of Stable Miglyol-loaded Nanoparticles. J. Thermal Analysis Calorimetry 2012; 108:101–108.

[44] Başaran E, Demirel M, Sirmagül B, Yazan Y. Cyclosporine A Incorporated Cationic Solid Lipid Nanoparticles for Ocular Delivery. J. Microencapsul. 2010; 27(1): 37–47.

[45] Attama AA, Müller-Goymann CC. Investigation of Surface-modified Solid Lipid Nanocontainers Formulated with a Heterolipid-templated Homolipid. Int. J. Pharm. 2007; 334: 179-189.

[46] Montenegro L, Campisi A, Sarpietro M G et al. *In Vitro* Evaluation of Idebenone-loaded Solid Lipid Nanoparticles for Drug Delivery to the Brain. Drug Dev. Ind. Pharm. 2011; 37(6): 737–746.

[47] Vivek K, Reddy H, Murthy RSR. Investigations of the Effect of the Lipid Matrix on Drug Entrapment, *In Vitro* Release, and Physical Stability of Olanzapine-loaded Solid Lipid Nanoparticles. AAPS PharmSciTech. 2007; 8(4) Article no. 83.

[48] Rawat MK, Jain A, Singh S. *In Vivo* and Cytotoxicity Evaluation of Repaglinide-loaded Binary Solid Lipid Nanoparticles after Oral Administration to Rats. J. Pharm. Sci. 2011; 100(6): 2406–2417.

[49] Shah M, Chuttani K, Mishra AK, Pathak K. Oral Solid Compritol 888 ATO Nanosuspension of Simvastatin: Optimization and Biodistribution Studies. Drug Dev. Ind. Pharm. 2011; 37(5): 526–537.

[50] del Pozo-Rodríguez A, Delgado D, Solinís M A et al. Solid Lipid Nanoparticles as Potential Tools for Gene Therapy: *In Vivo* Protein Expression after Intravenous Administration. Int. J. Pharm. 2010; 385(1-2): 157–162.

[51] Nnamani PO, Adikwu MU, Attama AA, Ibezim EC (2010). SRMS142 Based Solid Lipid Microparticles: Application in Oral Delivery of Glibenclamide to Diabetic Rats. Eur. J. Pharm. Biopharm. 76(1) 68 - 74.

[52] Attama AA, Schicke BC, Müller-Goymann CC. Novel Physically Structured Lipid Matrices of Beeswax and a Homolipid from *Capra hircus* (Goat Fat): A Physicochemical Characterization. J. Drug Deliv. Sci. Technol. 2007;17(2): 103-112.

[53] Attama AA, Schicke BC, Paepenmüller T, Müller-Goymann CC. Solid Lipid Nanodispersions Containing Mixed Lipid Core and a Polar Heterolipid: Characterization. Eur. J. Pharm. Biopharm. 2007; 67: 48-57.

[54] Mozafari MR. Liposomes: an Overview of Manufacturing Techniques. Cellular Mol. Biol. Letters 2005;10: 711–719.

[55] Cortesi R, Esposito E, Luca G, Nastruzzi C. Production of Lipospheres as Carriers for Bioactive Compounds. Biomaterials 2002;23: 2283– 2294.

[56] Lippacher A, Müller RH, Mäder K. Semisolid SLN Dispersions for Topical Application: Influence of Formulation and Production Parameters on Viscoelastic Properties. Eur. J. Pharm. Biopharm. 2002;53(2): 155-160.

[57] Gasco MR. Method for Producing Solid Lipid Microspheres having a Narrow Size Distribution, US Patent No. 5250236; 1993.

[58] Sjostrom B, Bergensthal B. Preparation of Submicron Drug Particles in Lecithin-stabilized o/w Emulsion I: Model Studies of the Precipitation of Cholesteryl acetate. Int. J. Pharm. 1992;88: 53-62.

[59] Siekmann B, Westesen K. Investigation on Solid Lipid Nanoparticle Prepared by Precipitation in o/w Emulsion. Eur. J. Pharm. Biopharm. 1996;43: 104-109.

[60] Attama AA. SLN, NLC, LDC: State of the Art in Drug and Active Delivery. Recent Patents Drug Deliv. Form. 2011;5(3): 178-187.

[61] Westesen K, Bunjes H, Koch MH. Physicochemical Characterization of Lipid Nanoparticles and Evaluation of their Drug Loading Capacity and Sustained Release. J. Control. Rel. 1997;48: 223-236.

[62] Müller RH, Mäder K, Gohla SH. Solid Lipid Nanoparticles (SLN) for Controlled Drug Delivery- A Review of the State of the Art. Eur. J. Pharm. Biopharm. 2000;50: 161-177.

[63] Abdel-Mottaleb MMA, Neumann D, Lamprecht A. In Vitro Drug Release Mechanism from Lipid Nanocapsules (LNC). Int. J. Pharm. 2010;390: 208–213.

[64] zur Mühlen A, Schwarz C, Mehnert W. Solid Lipid Nanoparticles (SLN) for Controlled Drug Delivery- Drug Release and Release Mechanism. Eur. J. Pharm. Biopharm. 1998;45: 149–155.

[65] Aggarwal P, Hall JB, McLeland CB, Dobrovolskaia MA, McNeil SE. Nanoparticle Interaction with Plasma Proteins as it Relates to Particle Biodistribution, Biocompatibility and Therapeutic Efficacy. Adv. Drug Deliv. Rev. 2009;61: 428–437.

[66] Westesen K, Siekmann B. Investigation of the Gel Formation of Phospholipid-stabilized Solid Lipid Nanoparticles. Int. J. Pharm. 1997;151: 35-45.

[67] Lippacher A, Müller RH, Mäder K. Investigation on the Viscoelastic Properties of Lipid Based Colloidal Drug Carriers. Int. J. Pharm. 2000;196(2): 227-230.

[68] Unruh T, Westesen K, Bösecke P, Lindner P, Koch MHJ. Self-assembly of Triglyceride Nanocrystals in Suspension. Langmuir 2002;18(5): 1796-1800.

[69] Illing A, Unruh T, Koch MHJ. Investigation on Particle Self Assembly in Solid Lipid-based Colloidal Drug Carrier Systems. Pharm. Res. 2004;21(4): 592-597.

[70] Mehnert W, Mäder K. Solid Lipid Nanoparticles: Production, Characterization and Applications. Adv. Drug Deliv. Rev. 2001;47(2-3): 165–196.

[71] Westesen K, Wehler T. Physicochemical Characterization of a Model Intravenous Oil-in-water Emulsion. J. Pharm. Sci. 1992;81: 777-786.

[72] Heiati H, Phillips NC, Tawashi R. Evidence for Phospholipid Bilayer Formation in Solid Lipid Nanoparticles Formulated with Phospholipid and Triglyceride. Pharm. Res. 1996;13: 1406-1410.

[73] Schubert MA, Harms M, Müller-Goymann CC. Structural Investigations on Lipid Nanoparticles Containing High Amounts of Lecithin. Eur. J. Pharm. Sci. 2006;27(2-3): 226-236.

[74] Westesen K, Bunjes H. Do Nanoparticles Prepared from Lipids Solid at Room Temperature Always Possess a Solid Lipid Matrix. Int. J. Pharm. 1995;115: 129-131.

[75] Zimmermann E, Müller RH. Electrolyte-and pH-stabilities of Aqueous Solid Lipid Nanoparticle (SLN) Dispersions in Artificial Gastrointestinal Media. Eur. J. Pharm. Biopharm. 2001;52(2): 203-210.

[76] Olbrich C, Müller RH. Enzymatic Degradation of SLN- Effect of Surfactant and Surfactant Mixtures. Int. J. Pharm. 1991;180(1): 31-39.

[77] des Rieux A, Fievez V, Garinot M, Schneider YJ, Preat V. Nanoparticles as Potential Oral Delivery Systems of Proteins and Vaccines: A Mechanistic Approach. J. Control. Rel. 2006;116(1): 1-27.

[78] Bargoni A, Cavalli R, Caputo O, Fundaro A, Gasco MR, Zara GP. Solid Lipid Nanoparticles in Lymph and Plasma after Duodenal Administration to Rats. Pharm. Res. 1998;15(5): 745-750.

[79] Souto EB, Doktorovova S. Solid Lipid Nanoparticle Formulations, Pharmacokinetic and Biopharmaceutical Aspects in Drug Delivery. Methods Enzymol. 2009;464(C): 105-129.

[80] Pandey R, Sharma S, Khuller GK. Oral Solid Lipid Nanoparticle-based Antitubercular Chemotherapy. Tuberculosis 2005;85(5-6): 415-420.

[81] Harms M, Müller-Goymann CC. Solid Lipid Nanoparticles for Drug Delivery. J. Drug Del. Sci. Tech. 2011;21(1): 89-99.

[82] Almeida AJ, Souto EB. Solid Lipid Nanoparticles as a Drug Delivery System for Peptides and Proteins. Adv. Drug Deliv. Rev. 2007;59: 478-490.

[83] del Pozo-Rodriguez A, Delgado D, Solinís MA, Gascón AR. Lipid Nanoparticles as Vehicles for Macromolecules: Nucleic Acids and Peptides. Recent Pat. Drug Deliv. Formul. 2011;5: 214-226.

[84] Hussein R. Charakterisierung von Hartfettmatrices und Lipidnanosuspensionen mit Phospholipon 90H. Ph.D. thesis. TU Braunschweig, Braunschweig. 2009.

[85] Müller RH, Petersen RD, Hommoss A, Pardeike J. Nanostructured Lipid Carriers (NLC) in Cosmetic Dermal Products. Adv. Drug Del. Rev. 2007;59(6): 522-530.

[86] Pardeike J, Hommoss A, Müller RH. Lipid Nanoparticles (SLN, NLC) in Cosmetic and Pharmaceutical Dermal Products. Int. J. Pharm. 2009;366(1-2): 170-184.

[87] Wissing SA, Müller RH. The Influence of the Crystallinity of Lipid Nanoparticles on their Occlusive Properties. Int. J. Pharm. 2002;242(1-2): 377-379.

[88] Wissing SA, Müller RH. Cosmetic Applications for Solid Lipid Nanoparticles (SLN). Int. J. Pharm. 2003;254(1): 65-68.

[89] Villalobos-Hernandez JR, Müller-Goymann CC. Sun Protection Enhancement of Titanium Dioxide Crystals by the Use of Carnauba Wax Nanoparticles: The Synergistic Interaction Between Organic and Inorganic Sunscreens at Nanoscale. Int. J. Pharm. 2006;322(1-2): 161-170.

[90] Villalobos-Hernandez JR, Müller-Goymann CC. In vitro Erythemal UV-A Protection Factors of Inorganic Sunscreens Distributed in Aqueous Media Using Carnauba Wax-Decyl Oleate Nanoparticles. Eur. J. Pharm. Biopharm. 2007;65(1): 122-125.

[91] Cavalli R, Gasco MR, Chetoni P, Burgalassi S, Saettone MF. Solid Lipid Nanoparticles (SLN) as Ocular Delivery System for Tobramycin. Int. J. Pharm. 2002;238(1-2): 241-245.

[92] Bur M, Henning A, Hein S, Schneider M, Lehr CM. Inhalative Nanomedicine-Opportunities and Challenges. Inhalation Toxicol. 2009;21(Suppl. 1): 137-143.

[93] Nassimi M, Schleh C, Lauenstein HD, Hussein R, Hoymann HG, Koch W, Pohlmann G, Krug N, Sewald K, Rittinghausen S, Braun A, Müller-Goymann CC. A Toxicological Evaluation of Inhaled Solid Lipid Nanoparticles Used as a Potential Drug Delivery System for the Lung. Eur. J. Pharm. Biopharm. 2010;75(2): 107-116.

[94] Pandey R, Khuller GK. Solid Lipid Particle-based Inhalable Sustained Drug Delivery System Against Experimental Tuberculosis. Tuberculosis 2005;85(4): 227-234.

[95] Innovative Nanoscale Therapeutics. Camurus. http://www.camurus.com/ (accessed 17 April 2012).

[96] Yasukawa T, Tabata Y, Kimura H, Ogura Y. Recent Advances in Intraocular Drug Delivery Systems. Recent Patents Drug Deliv. Formul. 2011;5: 1-10.

[97] Battaglia L, Gallarate M. Lipid Nanoparticles: State of the Art, New Preparation Methods and Challenges in Drug Delivery. Expert Opin. Drug Deliv. 2012;9(5): 497-508.

[98] Hommoss A. Nanostructured Lipid Carriers (NLC) in Dermal and Personal Care Formulations. Ph.D. thesis. Freie Universität Berlin, Berlin. 2008.

[99] Puri D, Bhandari A, Sharma P, Choudhary D. Lipid Nanoparticles (SLN, NLC): A Novel Approach for Cosmetic and Dermal Pharmaceutical. J. Global Pharma. Technol. 2010; 2(5):1-15.

Chapter 7

Nanocarrier Systems
for Transdermal Drug Delivery

José Juan Escobar-Chávez, Isabel Marlen Rodríguez-Cruz,
Clara Luisa Domínguez-Delgado, Roberto Díaz-Torres,
Alma Luisa Revilla-Vázquez, Norma Casas Aléncaster

Additional information is available at the end of the chapter

1. Introduction

The nanomedicine which is the application of technologies on the scale of 1 to 500 nm to diagnose and treat diseases, it has become a very relevant topic nowadays. During the last century, there has been a lot of new research and patents regarding nanomedicine in health sciences [1]. The objective of nanomedicine is to diagnose and preserve the health without side effects with noninvasive treatments. To reach these goals, nanomedicine offers a lot of new tools and capabilities. The manipulation that nanomedicine provides to the drugs and other materials in the nanometer scale can change the basic properties and bioactivity of materials. The solubility, increment in surface area, control release and site-targeted delivery are some characteristics that nanotechnology can manipulate on drug delivery systems.

Nanotechnology applied to health sciences contains new devices used in surgery, new chips for better diagnostics, new materials for substituting body structures and some structures capable to carry drugs through the body for treatment of a lot of diseases. These structures can be made of a lot of different materials and they are very different in structure and chemical nature. All these nanostructures are called nanocarriers and they can be administrated into the organisms by topical and transdermal routes [2]. Nanocarriers are a powerful weapon against a lot of illnesses since they are so small to be detected by immune system and they can deliver the drug in the target organ. For that reason, drug doses using nanocarriers and side effects decrease a lot.

The idea for using these tiny systems is not as new as we think but the use of nanocarriers in pharmaceutical products is not frequent, since the technology is expensive for certain types of nanoparticles and because nanocarriers need to be evaluated for demonstrating they do not have toxic effects. Nowadays the controversy of biological effects due to nanostructures is an open discussion, in one hand, the nanotechnologist continue making new and more sophisticated nanocarriers and in the other hand, toxicologist continue evaluating possible damaging effects.

Whatever it happens, nanotechnology is the new era and nanomedicine cannot be taking off. New nanocarriers will be created and the entire scientist working in nanomedicine bet for it to be the cure of diseases that in this moment are difficult to deal with [3]

The application of preparations to the skin for medical purposes is as old as the history of medicine itself, with references to the use of ointments and salves found in the records of Babylonian and Egyptian medicine. The historical development of permeation research is well described by Hadgraft & Lane [4]. Over time, the skin has become an important route for drug delivery in which topical, regional or systemic effects are desired. Nevertheless, skin constitutes an excellent barrier and presents difficulties for the transdermal delivery of therapeutic agents, since few drugs possess the characteristics required to permeate across the stratum corneum in sufficient quantities to reach a therapeutic concentration in the blood. In order to enhance drug transdermal absorption different methodologies have been investigated developed and patented [5,6]. Improvement in physical permeation-enhancement technologies has led to renewed interest in transdermal drug delivery. Some of these novel advanced transdermal permeation enhancement technologies include: iontophoresis, electroporation, ultrasound, microneedles to open up the skin and more recently the use of transdermal nanocarriers [3,7-10].

A number of excellent reviews that have been published contain detailed discussions concerning many aspects of transdermal nanocarriers [11-17]. The present chapter shows an updated overview of the use of submicron particles and other nanostructures in the pharmaceutical field, specifically in the area of topical and transdermal drugs. This focus is justified due to the magnitude of the experimental data available with the use of these nanocarriers. The development of submicron particles and other nanostructures in the pharmaceutical and cosmetic fields has been emerged in the last decades for designing best formulations for application through the skin [18-21].

2. The skin

The skin is the largest organ of the body [22-24], accounting for more than 10% of body mass, and the one that enables the body to interact more intimately with its environment. Essentially, the skin consists of four layers: The SC, that is the outer layer of the skin (non-viable epidermis), and forms the rate-controlling barrier for diffusion for almost all compounds. It is composed of dead flattened, keratin-rich cells, the corneocytes. These dense cells are surrounded by a complex mixture of intercellular lipids, namely, ceramides, free fatty acids, cholesterol, and cholesterol sulphate. Their most important feature is that they are structured as ordered bilayer arrays [25-28]. The other layers are: the remaining layers of the epidermis (viable epidermis), the dermis, and the subcutaneous tissue (**Figure 1**). There are also several associated appendages: hair follicles sweat ducts, glands and nails [29,30].

Many agents are applied to the skin either deliberately or accidentally, with either beneficial or deleterious outcomes. The main interest in dermal absorption assessment is related to: a) Local effects in dermatology (e.g., corticosteroids for dermatitis); b) transport through the skin seeking a systemic effect (e.g., nicotine patches, hormonal drug patches, etc.) [31]; c) surface effects (e.g., sunscreens, cosmetics, and anti-infectives) [32,33]; d) targeting of deeper tissues (e.g., nonsteroidal anti-inflammatory agents) [34-37]; and e) unwanted absorption (e.g., solvents in the workplace, pesticides or allergens) [38,39].

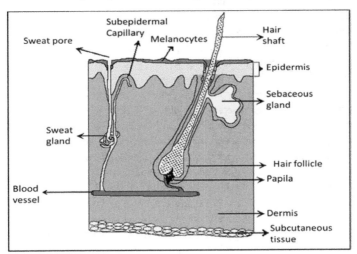

Figure 1. Schematic representation of skin layer.

2.1. Epidermis

2.1.1. Stratum corneum

The stratum corneum is the heterogeneous outermost layer of the epidermis and is approximately 10-20 μm thick. The stratum corneum consists of about 15 to 25 layers of flattened, stacked, hexagonal, and cornified cells embedded in an intercellular matrix of lipids. These lipid domains form a continuous structure so they are considered to play a crucial role in the maintenance of the skin barrier that helps avoid transepidermal water loss. Each cell is approximately 40 μm in diameter and 0.5 μm thick [40].

The stratum corneum barrier properties may be partly related to its very high density (1.4 g/cm³ in the dry state) and its low hydration of 15–20 %, compared with the usual 70 % for the body. Each stratum corneum cell is composed mainly of insoluble bundled keratins (70 %) and lipid (20 %) encased in a cell envelope, accounting for about 5% of the stratum corneum weight. The permeability barrier is located within the lipid bilayers in the intercellular spaces of the stratum corneum [6-8] and consists of ceramides (40–50%), fatty acids (15–25%), cholesterol (20–25%) and cholesterol sulphate (5–10 %) [41-45].

The barrier function is further facilitated by the continuous desquamation of this horny layer with a total turnover of the stratum corneum occurring once every 2–3 weeks. The stratum corneum functions as a barrier are to prevent the loss of internal body components, particularly water, to the external environment. The cells of the stratum corneum originate in the viable epidermis and undergo many morphological changes before desquamation. Thus, the epidermis consists of several cell strata at varying levels of differentiation.

The origins of the cells of the epidermis lie in the basal lamina between the dermis and viable epidermis. In this layer there are melanocytes, Langerhans cells, Merkel cells, and two major keratinic cell types: the first functioning as stem cells having the capacity to divide and produce new cells; the second serving to anchor the epidermis to the basement membrane [46]. The basement membrane is 50–70 nm thick and consists of two layers, the lamina densa and lamina lucida, which comprise mainly proteins, such as type IV collagen, aminin, nidogen and fibronectin. Type IV collagen is responsible for the mechanical stability of the basement membrane, whereas laminin and fibronectin are involved with the attachment between the basement membrane and the basal keratinocytes. The cells of the basal lamina are attached to the basement membrane by hemidesmosomes, which are found on the ventral surface of basal keratinocytes [47]. Hemidesmosomes appear to comprise three distinct protein groups: two of which are bullous pemphigoid antigens (BPAG1 and BPAG2), and the other epithelial cellspecific integrins [48-50]. BPAG1 is associated with the organization of the cytoskeletal structure and forms a link between the hemidesmosome structure and the keratin intermediate filaments. The integrins are transmembrane receptors that mediate attachment between the cell and the extracellular matrix. Human epidermal basal cells contain integrins $\alpha_2\beta_1$, $\alpha_3\beta_1$ and $\alpha_6\beta_4$. Integrin $\alpha_6\beta_4$ and BPAG2 appear to be the major hemidesmosomal protein contributors to the anchoring of the keratinocyte, spanning from the keratin intermediate filament, through the lamina lucida, to the lamina densa of the basement membrane [51]. In the lamina densa, these membrane-spanning proteins interact with the protein laminin-5 which, in turn, is linked to collagen VII, the major constituent of the anchoring fibrils within the dermal matrix. It has also been suggested that both BPAG2 and integrin $\alpha_6\beta_4$ mediate in the signal transductions required for hemidesmosome formation and cell differentiation and proliferation. Integrin $\alpha_3\beta_1$ is associated with actin and may be linked with laminin-5. Epidermal wounding results in an up-regulation of these proteins that appears to be involved with cell motility and spreading. The importance of maintaining a secure link between the basal lamina cells and the basement membrane is obvious, and the absence of this connection results in chronic blistering diseases such as pemphigus and epidermolysis bullosa.

2.2. Dermis

The dermis is about 0.1–0.5 cm thick and consists of collagenous (70 %) and elastin fibres. In the dermis, glycosaminoglycans or acid mucopolysaccharides, are covalently linked to peptide chains to form proteoglycans, the ground substance that promotes the elasticity of the skin. The main cells present are the fibroblasts, which produce the connective tissue components of collagen, laminin, fibronectin and vitronectin; mast cells, which are involved in the immune and inflammatory responses; and melanocytes involved in the production of the pigment melanin [51]. Nerves, blood vessels and lymphatic vessels are also present in the dermis.

Contained within the dermis is an extensive vascular network providing for the skin nutrition, repair, and immune responses for the rest of the body, heat exchange, immune response, and thermal regulation. Skin blood vessels derive from those in the subcutaneous tissues (hypodermis), with an arterial network supplying the papillary layer, the hair follicles, the sweat and apocrine glands, the subcutaneous area, as well as the dermis itself. These arteries feed into arterioles, capillaries, venules, and, thence, into veins. Of particular importance in this vascular network is the presence of arteriovenous anastomoses at all levels in the skin. These arteriovenous anastomoses, which allow a direct shunting of up to 60% of the skin blood flow between the arteries and veins, thereby avoiding the fine capillary network, are critical to the skin's functions of heat regulation and blood vessel control. Blood flow changes are most evident in the skin in relation to various physiological responses and include psychological effects, such as shock ("draining of color from the skin") and embarrassment ("blushing"), temperature effects, and physiological responses to exercise, hemorrhage, and alcohol consumption.

The lymphatic system is an important component of the skin in regulating its interstitial pressure, mobilization of defense mechanisms, and in waste removal. It exists as a dense, flat meshwork in the papillary layers of the dermis and extends into the deeper regions of the dermis. Also present in the dermis are a number of different types of nerve fibers supplying the skin, including those for pressure, pain, and temperature [52]. Epidermal appendages such as hair follicles and sweat glands are embedded in the dermis [53].

2.3. Hypodermis

The deepest layer of the skin is the subcutaneous tissue or hypodermis. The hypodermis acts as a heat insulator, a shock absorber, and an energy storage region. This layer is a network of fat cells arranged in lobules and linked to the dermis by interconnecting collagen and elastin fibers. As well as fat cells (possibly 50% of the body's fat); the other main cells in the hypodermis are fibroblasts and macrophages. One of the major roles of the hypodermis is to carry the vascular and neural systems for the skin. It also anchors the skin to underlying muscle. Fibroblasts and adipocytes can be stimulated by the accumulation of interstitial and lymphatic fluid within the skin and subcutaneous tissue [54]. The total thickness of skin is about 2–3 mm, but the thickness of the stratum corneum is only about 10–15 μm.

2.4. Skin appendages

There are four skin appendages: the hair follicles with their associated sebaceous glands, eccrine and apocrine sweat glands, and the nails, but these occupy only about 0.1 % of the total human skin surface.

The pilosebaceous follicles have about 10 to 20 % of the resident flora and cannot be decontaminated by scrubbing. The hair follicles are distributed across the entire skin surface with the exception of the soles of the feet, the palms of the hand and the lips. A smooth muscle, the erector pilorum, attaches the follicle to the dermal tissue and enables hair to stand up in response to fear. Each follicle is associated with a sebaceous gland that varies in size from 200 to 2000 µm in diameter. The sebum secreted by this gland consisting of triglycerides, free fatty acids, and waxes, protects and lubricates the skin as well as maintaining a pH of about 5. Sebaceous glands are absent on the palms, soles and nail beds. Sweat glands or eccrine glands respond to temperature via parasympathetic nerves, except on palms, soles and axillae, where they respond to emotional stimuli via sympathetic nerves [51]. The eccrine glands are epidermal structures that are simple, coiled tubes arising from a coiled ball, of approximately 100 µm in diameter, located in the lower dermis. It secretes a dilute salt solution with a pH of about 5, this secretion being stimulated by temperature-controlling determinants, such as exercise and high environmental temperature, as well as emotional stress through the autonomic (sympathetic) nervous system. These glands have a total surface area of about 1/10,000 of the total body surface. The apocrine glands are limited to specific body regions and are also coiled tubes. These glands are about ten times the size of the eccrine ducts, extend as low as the subcutaneous tissues and are paired with hair follicles.

Nail function is considered as protection. Nail plate consists of layers of flattened keratinized cells fused into a dense but elastic mass. The cells of the nail plate originate in the nail matrix and grow distally at a rate of about 0.1 mm/day. In the keratinization process the cells undergo shape and other changes, similar to those experienced by the epidermal cells forming the stratum corneum. This is not surprising because the nail matrix basement membrane shows many biochemical similarities to the epidermal basement membrane [55,56]. Thus, the major components are highly folded keratin proteins with small amounts of lipid (0.1–1.0%). The principal plasticizer of the nail plate is water, which is normally present at a concentration of 7–12 %.

3. Skin functions

Many of the functions of the skin can be classified as essential to survival of the body bulk of mammals and humans in a relatively hostile environment. In a general context, these functions can be classified as a protective, maintaining homeostasis or sensing. The importance of the protective and homeostatic role allows the survival of humans in an environment of variable temperature; water content (humidity and bathing); and the presence of environmental dangers, such as chemicals, bacteria, allergens, fungi and radiation. In a second context, the skin is a major organ for maintaining the homeostasis of the body, especially in terms of its composition, heat regulation, blood pressure control, and excretory roles. It has been argued that the basal metabolic rate of animals differing in size should be scaled to the surface area of the body to maintain a constant temperature through the skin's thermoregulatory control [57]. Third, the skin is a major sensory organ in terms of sensing environmental influences, such as heat, pressure, pain, allergen, and microorganism entry. Finally, the skin is an organ that is in a continual state of regeneration and repair. To fulfill each of these functions, the skin must be tough, robust, and flexible, with effective communication between each of its intrinsic components mentioned above.

The stratum corneum also functions as a barrier to prevent the loss of internal body components, particularly water, to the external environment. The epidermis plays a role in temperature, pressure, and pain regulation.

Appendage functions are following: hair follicle and sebaceous gland fulfill with protect (hair) and lubricate (sebum), eccrine and apocrine glands have the functions of cooling and vestigial secondary sex gland, respectively; and nails has the function of to protect.The hypodermis acts as a heat insulator, a shock absorber and an energy storage region. One of the major roles of the hypodermis is to carry the vascular and neural systems for the skin.

4. Routes of drug penetration through the skin

The determination of penetration pathways of topically applied substances into the skin is the subject of several investigations. The permeation of drugs through the skin includes the diffusion through the intact epidermis y through the skin appendages. These skin appendages are hair follicles and sweat glands which form shunt pathways through the intact epidermis, occupying only 0.1% of the total human skin [58]. It is known drug permeation through the skin is usually limited by the stratum corneum. Two pathways through the intact barrier may be identified, the intercellular and transcellular route (**Figure 2**):

a.   The intercellular lipid route is between the corneocytes.

Interlamellar regions in the stratum corneum, including linker regions, contain less ordered lipids and more flexible hydrophobic chains. This is the reason of the non-planar spaces between crystalline lipid lamellae and their adjacent cells outer membrane. Fluid lipids in skin barrier are crucially important for transepidermal diffusion of the lipidic and amphiphilic molecules, occupying those spaces for the insertion and migration through intercellular lipid layers of such molecules [59,60]. The hydrophilic molecules diffuse predominantly "laterally" along surfaces of the less abundant, water filled inter-lamellar spaces or through such volumes; polar molecules can also use the free space between a lamella and a corneocyte outer membrane to the same end [61].

b.   The transcellular route contemplates the crossing through the corneocytes and the intervening lipids [24].

Intracellular macromolecular matrix within the stratum corneum abounds in keratin, which does not contribute directly to the skin diffusive barrier but supports mechanical stability and thus intactness of the stratum corneum. Transcellular diffusion is practically unimportant for transdermal drug transport [62]. The narrow aqueous transepidermal pathways have been observed using confocal laser scanning microscopy (CLSM). Here regions of poor cellular and intercellular lipid packing coincide with wrinkles on skin surface and are simultaneously the sites of lowest skin resistance to the transport of hydrophilic entities. This lowest resistance pathway leads between clusters of corneocytes at the locations where such cellular groups show no lateral overlap.

The better sealed and more transport resistant is the intra-cluster/inter-corneocyte pathway [63]. Hydrophilic conduits have openings between ≥5 μm (skin appendages) and ≤10 nm (narrow inter-corneocyte pores). So sweat ducts (≥50 μm), pilosebaceous units (5–70 μm), and sebaceous glands (5–15 μm) represent the largest width/lowest resistance end of the range. Junctions of corneocytes-clusters and cluster boundaries fall within the range [64]. It was determined that the maximally open hydrophilic conduits across skin are approximately 20–30 nm wide, including pore penetrant/opener thickness [63]. Another studies revealed the width of the negatively charged hydrophilic transepidermal pores expanded by electroosmosis to be around of 22–48 nm [65]. Lipophilic cutaneous barrier is governed by molecular weight and distribution coefficient rather than molecular size [66]. The relative height of cutaneous lipophilic barrier consequently decreases with lipophilicity of permeant, but molecules heavier than 400–500 Da are so large permeants to find sufficiently wide defects in the intercellular lipidic matrix to start diffusing through the lipidic parts of cutaneous barrier [64, 66,67].

The contribution to transdermal drug transport can increases with the pathways widening or multiplication, for example such that is caused by exposing the stratum corneum to a strong electrical (electroporation/iontophoresis), mechanical (sonoporation/sonophoresis), thermal stimulus, or suitable skin penetrants [59].

Recently, follicular penetration has become a major focus of interest due to the drug targeting to the hair follicle is of great interest in the treatment of skin diseases. However due to follicular orifices only occupying 0.1% of the total skin surface area, it was assumed as a non important route. But a variety of studies shown the hair follicles as could be a way to trough the skin [68- 73]. Such follicular pathway also has been proposed for topical administration of nanoparticles and microparticles and it has been investigated in porcine skin, because in recent studies the results have confirmed the *in vitro* penetration into the porcine hair follicles might be considered similar to those on humans *in vivo*. After topical application of dye sodium fluorescein onto porcine skin mounted in Franz diffusion cells with the acceptor compartment beneath the dermis, the fluorescence was detected on the surface, within the horny layer, and in most of the follicles confirming the similarity in the penetration between porcine and human skin [72]. So nanoparticles have been studied in porcine skin revealing in the surface images that polystyrene nanoparticles accumulated preferentially in the follicular openings, this distribution was increased in a time-dependent manner, and the follicular localization was favored by the smaller particle size [74]. In other investigations, it has been shown by differential stripping the influence of size microparticles in the skin penetration. It can act as efficient drug carriers or can be utilized as follicle blockers to stop the penetration of topically applied substances [73].

It has already been postulated that certain molecules can hydrogen bond to groups present on the surfaces of follicular pores [75]. However, more studies have to be made in order to identify all the molecular properties that influence drug penetration into hair follicles.

Nowadays, there are currently a number of methods available for quantifying drugs localized within the skin or various layers of the skin. To date, a direct, non-invasive quantification of the amount of topically applied substance penetrated into the follicles had not been possible. Therefore, stripping techniques, tape stripping and cyanoacrylate skin surface biopsy have been used to remove the part of the stratum corneum containing dye topically applied [76]. Thus, the "differential stripping" has been shown as a new method that can be used to study the penetration of topically applied substances into the follicular infundibula non-invasively and selectively [20,26,30,76,77].

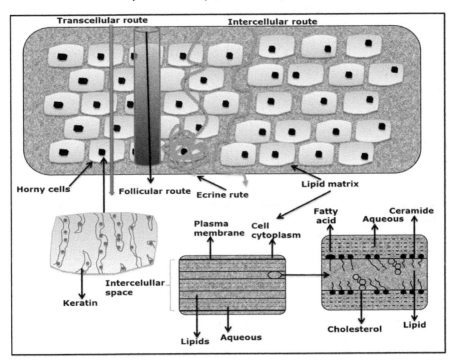

Figure 2. Schematic representation of penetration routes of drugs throughout the skin.

5. Advantages and disadvantages of transdermal drug delivery

Transdermal drug delivery systems offer several important advantages over more traditional approaches, in addition to the benefits of avoiding the hepatic first-pass effect, and higher patient compliance, the additional advantages and the disadvantages [78-80] that transdermal drug delivery offers can be summarized as follows in Table 1.

Advantages of transdermal drug delivery	Disadvantages of transdermal drug delivery
Longer duration of action	Possibility of local irritation at the site of application
Reduction in dosing frequency	Erythema, itching, and local edema can be caused by the drug, the adhesive, or other excipients in the patch formulation
More uniform plasma levels	The skin's low permeability limits the number of drugs that can be delivered in this manner
Useful for drugs that require relatively consistent plasma levels	
It is an alternative route of administration to accommodate patients who cannot tolerate oral dosage forms (specially for nauseated or unconscious patients)	
Improved bioavailability	
Reduction of side effects	
Flexibility of terminating the drug administration by simply removing the patch from the skin	

Table 1. Main advantages and disadvantages of transdermal drug delivery

6. Nanocarrier systems

Nanocarriers have demonstrated increased drug absorption, penetration, half-life, bioavailability, stability, etc. Nanocarriers are so small to be detected by immune system and they can deliver the drug in the target organ using lower drug doses in order to reduce side effects. Nanocarriers can be administrated into the organisms by all the routes; one of them is the dermal route. The nanocarriers most used and investigated for topical/transdermal drug delivery in the pharmaceutical field are shown in **Figure 3** and **Table 2**.

6.1. Nanoparticles

Nanoparticles are smaller than 1,000 nm. Nowadays, it is possible to insert many types of materials such as drugs, proteins, peptides, DNA, etc. into the nanoparticles. They are constructed from materials designed to resist pH, temperature, enzymatic attack, or other problems [81]. Nanoparticles can be classified as nanospheres or nanocapsules (See **Figure**

4). Nanospheres are solid-core structures and nanocapsules are hollow-core structures. Nanoparticles can be composed of polymers, lipids, polysaccharides and proteins [82,83]. Nanoparticles preparation techniques are based on their physicochemical properties. They are made by emulsification-diffusion by solvent displacement, emulsification-polymerization, in situ-polymerization, gelation, nanoprecipitation, solvent evaporation/extraction, inverse salting out, dispersion polymerization and other derived from these one.

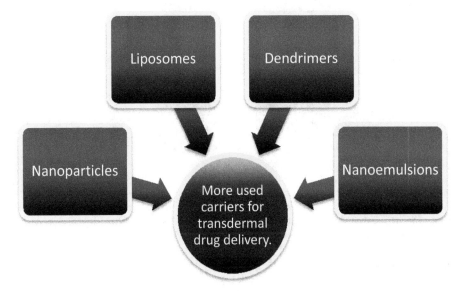

Figure 3. More used transdermal nanocarriers

6.2. Nanoemulsions

Nanoemulsions are isotropic dispersed systems of two non miscible liquids, normally consisting of an oily system dispersed in an aqueous system (o/w nanoemulsion), or an aqueous system dispersed in an oily system but forming droplets or other oily phases of nanometric sizes (100 nm). They can be stable (methastable) for long times due to the extremely small sizes and the use of adequate surfactants. Nanoemulsions can use hydrophobic and hydrophilic drugs because it is possible to make both w/o or o/w nanoemulsions [84]. They are non-toxic and non-irritant systems and they can be used for skin or mucous membranes, parenteral and non parenteral administration in general and they have been used in the cosmetic field. Nanoemulsions can be prepared by three methods mainly: high-pressure homogenization, microfluidization and phase inversion temperature. Transdermal delivery using nanoemulsions has been reduced due to the stability problems inherent to this dosage form.

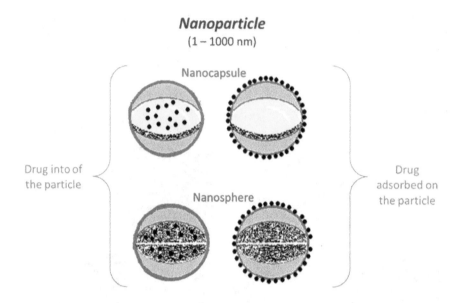

Figure 4. Nanospheres and nanocapsules are small vesicles used to transport drugs. Nanospheres are typically solid polymers with drugs embedded in the polymer matrix. Nanocapsules are a shell with an inner space loaded with the drug of interest. Both systems are useful for controlling the release of a drug and protecting it from the surrounding environment.

6.3. Liposomes

Liposomes are hollow lipid bilayer structures (**Figure 5**) that can transport hydrophilic drugs inside the core and hydrophobic drugs between the bilayer [85]. They are structures made of cholesterol and phospholipids. They can have different properties depending on the excipients included and the process of their elaboration. The nature of liposomes makes them one of the best alternatives for drug delivery because they are non-toxic and remain inside the bloodstream for a long time. Liposomes can be surface-charged as neutral, negative or positive, depending on the functional groups and pH medium. Liposomes can encapsulate both lipophilic and hydrophilic drugs in a stable manner, depending on the polymer added to the surface [86]. There are small unilamellar vesicles (25 nm to 100nm), medium-sized unilamellar vesicles (100 nm and 500nm), large unilamellar vesicles, giant unilamellar vesicles, oligolamellar vesicles, large multilamellar vesicles and multivesicular vesicles (500 nm to microns). The thickness of the membrane measures approximately 5 to 6 nm. These shapes and sizes depend of the preparation technique, the lipids used and process variables. Depending on these parameters, the behavior both in vivo and in vitro can change and opsonization processes, leakage profiles, disposition in the body and shelf life are different due to the type of liposome [86].

Liposomes preparation techniques follow three basic steps with particular features depending on safety, potential scale up and simplicity: 1) Lipid must be hydrated, 2) Liposomes have to be sized and 3) Nonencapsulated drug has to be removed. The degree of transdermal drug penetration is affected by the lamellarity, lipid composition, charge on the liposomal surface, mode of application and the total lipid concentrations [87].

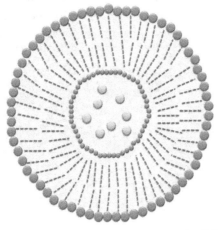

Figure 5. Liposomes are spherical vesicles that comprise one or more lipid bilayer structures enclosing an aqueous core. They protect encapsulated drugs from degradation. Liposomes can also be functionalized to improve cell targeting and solubility

6.4. Dendrimers

Dendrimers are monodisperse populations that are structurally and chemically uniform (**Figure 6**). They allow conjugation with numerous functional groups due to the nature of their branches. The amount of branches increases exponentially and dendrimers growth is typically about 1 nm per generation [88]. The dendrimers classification is based on the number of generations. After the creation of a core, the stepwise synthesis is called first generation; after that, every stepwise addition of monomers creates the next generation. This approach allows an iterative synthesis, providing the ability to control both molecular weight and architecture.

The kind of polymer chosen to construct the dendrimer by polimerization is very important with regard to the final architecture and features. In addition, the use of branched monomers has the peculiarity of providing tailored loci for site-specific molecular recognition and encapsulation. Notably, 3D and fractal architecture, as well as the peripheral functional groups, provide dendrimers with important characteristic physical and chemical properties. In comparison with linear polymers, dendritic structures have "dendritic voids" that give these molecules important and useful features. These spaces inside dendrimers can mimic the molecular recognition performed by natural proteins.

Furthermore, dendrimers have a high surface-charge density due to ionizable groups that help them to attach drugs by electrostatic forces, regardless of the stoichimetry. This dendrimer-drug association provides drugs with better solubility, increasing their transport through biological membranes and sometimes increasing drug stability. The number of molecules that can be incorporated into dendrimers is related to the number of surface functional groups; therefore, later-generation dendrimers are more easily incorporated into dendritic structure. However, not all the functional groups are available for interaction due to steric volume, molecule rotation or stereochemistry effects. Dendrimers can have positive and negative charges, which allows them to complex different types of drugs [89].

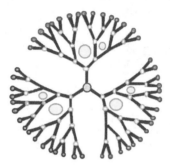

Figure 6. Dendrimers are highly branched polymers with a controlled three-dimensional structure around a central core. They can accommodate more than 100 terminal groups.

6.5. Advantages and limitations of using nanocarriers for transdermal drug delivery

As it is has been mentioned before, the search for new strategies able to enhance the topical and transdermal penetration of drugs has become essential [61]. Different carrier systems have been proposed in an attempt to favour the transport of drugs through the skin, enabling drug retention and in some cases allowing a controlled release. Skin penetration is essential to a number of current concerns, for example, contamination by microorganisms and chemicals, drug delivery to skin (dermatological treatments) and through skin (transdermal treatments), and skin care and protection (cosmetics) [103-106].

Follicular penetration has become a major focus of interest due to the drug targeting to the hair follicle is of great interest in the topical treatment of skin diseases. However due to follicular orifices only occupying ~0.1% of the total skin surface area, it was assumed as a non important route. But recently, a variety of studies have shown that the hair follicles represent a important way to trough the skin and some techniques have been used to test the penetration of drugs loaded nanoparticles/microsparticles [70,72,73,107-109]. Confocal laser scanning microscopy which permits optical sectioning of thick tissues and cells and their subsequent computerized three-dimensional reconstruction, has been used to study the entry of drugs through the skin [110]. It was visualized in the fresh human scalp skin on-line the diffusion processes of a model fluorophore into the hair follicle at different depths [72]. Such follicular pathway also has been proposed for topical administration of nanoparticles and microparticles using porcine skin. Recent studies have confirmed that the *in vitro* penetration into the porcine hair follicles might be considered similar to those on humans *in vivo* [73]. Studies in porcine skin revealed in the surface images that polystyrene nanoparticles accumulated preferentially in the follicular openings, this distribution was increased in a time-dependent manner, and the follicular localization was favored by the smaller particle size [76]. In other investigations, it has been shown by differential stripping the influence of size microparticles in the skin penetration. It can act as efficient drug carriers or can be utilized as follicle blockers to stop the penetration of topically applied substances [75]. An alternative technique is multiphoton microscopy (MPM) especially two-photon excitation microscopy has been widely used in imaging biological specimens treated with nanoparticles [111-114]. The near-infrared light used in the two-photon microscope can penetrate deeper in highly scattering tissues such as *in vivo* human skin than confocal microscopes operated with ultraviolet excitation [115]. Futhermore, this technique provides both cellular and extracellular structural information, with subcellular resolution helpful for clinical dermatological diagnosis, both *ex vivo* and *in vivo*. In addition, it can be used to characterize stratum corneum structures, visualize and quantify transcutaneous drug delivery, detect skin cancers, explore collagen structural transitions, and watch laser–skin interactions [116,117]. A common method used for quantifying drugs localized within the skin or various layers of the skin are the tape stripping and cyanoacrylate skin surface biopsy techniques, which have been used to remove the part of the stratum corneum containing dye topically applied. Thus, the "differential stripping" has been shown as a new method that can be used to study the penetration of topically applied substances into the follicular infundibula non-invasively and selectively [118]. It has been reported in a previous *in vitro* permeation studies using tape stripping, that triclosan-loaded nanoparticles penetrated into the skin and their retention favoured a local effect. Moreover, polymeric nanoparticles are expected to be able to form a depot in the hair follicles, providing a targeted controlled drug delivery [33,119].

In general, the principal advantages of microparticles and nanoparticles over conventional formulations such as creams, solutions, ointments, lotions, gels, and foams, is that the second ones have different absorption characteristics and aesthetic properties, and they also have some major limitations, such as poor penetration and uncontrolled drug release. Furthermore, tolerability and safety end points, such as irritation, dryness, erythema, itching, stinging and burning will be key factors in determining its usefulness. It happens because using a traditional system, drug delivery is sometimes rapid and topical or plasmatic concentrations can result in toxic effects. However, for the case of nanoparticles a smaller amount of the drug is necessary and due to the targeted nature of delivery [120]. Topical or transdermal drug deliveries have many advantages over the other routes: fewer side effects, increased patient compliance, controlled release, and the lack of a hepatic first pass [121].

Nanocarrier	Size range	Preparation methods	Characteristics	References
Polymeric nanoparticles	10-1000 nm	-In situ polymerization -Emulsification-evaporation, -Emulsification-diffusion, -Emulsification-diffusion by solvent displacement.	Solid or hollow particles wich have entraped, binded or encapsulated drugs.	[33]
Solid lipid nanoparticles	50-1000 nm	-High-pressure homogenization.	Similar to polymeric nanoparticles but made of solid lipids.	[90]
Inorganic Nanoparticles	<50nm	-Sol-gel technique	Nanometric particles, made up of inorganic compounds such as silica, titania and alumina.	[91]
Liposomes	25 nm-100 μm	-Sonication -Extrusion, -Mozafari method	Vesicles composed of one or more concentric lipid bilayers, separated by water or aqueous buffer compartments.	[92]
Dendrimers	3–10 nm	-Polymerization	Macromolecular high branched structures.	[93]
Quantum dots	2-10nm	-Colloidal assembly, viral assembly, -Electrochemical assembly.	Made up of organic surfactants, precursors and solvents.	[94]
Lipid globules	1-100 nm	-Emulsification espontaneous systems.	Multicomponent fluid made of water, a hydrophobic liquid, and one or several surfactants resulting in a stable system.	[95]
Lipid microcylinders	<1 μm	-Self emulsification	Self organizing system in which surfactants crystallize into tightly packed bilayers that spontaneously form cylinders.	[96]

Ethosomes	<400 nm	-Cold method -Hot method	Non invasive delivery carriers that enable drugs to reach the deep skin layers and/or the systemic circulation.	[97]
Aquasomes	60-300 nm	-Self-assembling of hydroxyapatite by coprecipitation method	The particle core is composed of noncrystalline calcium phosphate or ceramic diamond, and it is covered by a polyhydroxyl oligomeric film.	[98]
Pharmacosomes	<200 nm	-Hand-shaking method -Ether-injection method	Pure drug vesicles formed by amphiphilic drugs.	[99]
Colloidosomes	200nm – 1.5 μm	-Self-assembly of colloidal particles at the interface of emulsion droplets	Hollow capsules with elastic shells.	[100]
Niosomes	10-1000 nm	-Self-assembly of nonionic Surfactant	Bilayered structures made of non-ionic surfactant vesicles.	[101]
Nanoemulsions	20-200nm	-High-pressure homogenization. -Microfluidization. -Phase Inversion temperature	Submicron emulsions o/w or w/o.	[102]

Table 2. Examples of nanocarriers used for drug delivery.

It has been reported that nanoencapsulation of drugs (nano-medicines) increases their efficacy, specificity, tolerability and therapeutic index [122-124]. These nano-formulations are reported to be superior to traditional medicine with respect to controlled release, targeted delivery and therapeutic impact. The targeting capabilities of nanomedicines are influenced by particle size, surface charge, surface modification, and hydrophobicity. Of these, nanoparticle size distribution is an important factor in determining the interaction with the cell membrane and their penetration across physiological barriers, being dependent on the tissue, target site and circulation [125]. Example of this are the nanostructured lipid carriers (NLC) by their structure (lipid nanoparticles with solid matrix) increase in loading capacity, physical and chemical long-term stability, triggered release and potentially supersaturated topical formulations with respect to solid lipid nanoparticles (SLN). Other advantages of NLC include improvement in stabilisation of incorporated compounds, controlled release, occlusivity, film formation on skin including in vivo effects on the skin. Lipid nanoparticles have been observed as a good option for transdermal delivery because they can be prepared in different sizes and it is possible to modify surface polarity in order to improve skin penetration [126,127]. From the upper skin, nanoparticles can reach deeper skin regions because they exhibit mechanical flexion [128].

Additionaly, transdermal nanocarriers are able to reach target organs because they can be attached to antibodies, antigens, vitamins and other molecules to be more specific. Nanoparticles can travel largely undetected by the immune system depending of the nanocarriers size of the antigen added as well as its composition. So, by hiding functional groups or protecting these groups with other molecules, drugs can be released specifically in the target organ. Consecuently, nanoparticles can even travel from the skin to lymph nodes, representing a promising tool for immunomodulation [129]. One of the first strategies for transdermal delivery were the liposomes. The nature of liposomes makes them one of the best alternatives for drug delivery because they are non-toxic and remain inside the bloodstream for a long time [130-133]. Nevertheless, some factors affect the degree of transdermal drug penetration such as the lamellarity, the lipid composition, the charge on the liposomal surface, the mode of application and the total lipid concentrations [89,134]. For that reason, flexible vesicles called transfersomes or transformable liposomes have been compared with those rigid vesicles to enhance penetration [135-142]. The lipids present in the liposome bilayer can interact with lipids present in the stratum corneum changing the structure of the upper skin. This change is beneficial for the penetration of lipophilic drugs into the stratum corneum [143]. Some liposomes may have a deformable structure and pass through the stratum or may accumulate in the channel-like regions in the stratum corneum, depending upon their composition [144,145]. In order to obtain transformable liposomes more flexible, they are prepared using surfactants or alcohol (ethosomes) in the lipid bilayer, to be able to deform them when a pressure is applied in the transdermal route.

Some limitations for nanocarriers are the important tests and regulations that should be carried out to ensure an adequate characterization, analytical evaluation, toxicological and pharmacological assessment, which is necessary to determine the efficacy of using these nanostructures in therapies and diagnosis because of their tiny size, their high surface energy, their composition, their architecture, their attached molecules, etc. Those things are frequently reviewed for the dendrimers. One of the main advantages is that they have multivalency and it is possible to get control of the functional groups on the surface [146,147]. Due to their form and size (1–10 nm), these molecules can carry drugs, imaging agents, and can interact with lipids present in membranes, because it was reported a better permeation in cell cultures and intestinal membranes. They also increased the permeation of lipophilic drugs instead of hydrophilic drugs. The main problems with this kind of transdermal carrier are poor biodegradation and inherent cytotoxicity [148]. To obtain dendrimers less toxic, dendrimers have been linked to peptides. Dendrimers-peptides are formed from amino acids linked via peptide-amide bonds to the branches of dendrimers in the core or on the surface to get down the toxicity. Then, they are bio-transformed to produce amino-acid derivatives. Besides, the synthesis of these structures is less expensive and purification does not present any difficulty [149,150].

It is suggested in future research to elucidate the interactions between nanocarriers and other molecules as well as interactions between nanocarriers and biological entities. The toxicology of nanostructures is also a current concern. Materials behave very differently when they are diminished to nanosizes. Traditional laws do not work at this "meso-scale" in the same way as they function at the macro-scale. On the macro scale, bulk properties in a material predominate over surface properties. At the micro-scale, surface properties tend to dominate. At the meso-scale, both types of properties play significant roles [151,152]. Furthermore, the effects of metabolized/altered nanostructures on the biological system are difficult to predict. Regulatory agencies are taking action to assess new Nanotechnology-based products.

In addition, the fabrication of nanocarriers scaling up from the lab at the industrial production is difficult and the materials used to prepare nanocarriers are very expensive in the majority of the cases.

7. Applications of nanocarrier systems in topical/transdermal delivery

Nanocarriers as drug delivery systems were first intended for use in parenteral or oral routes of administration and as such still continue to be the focus of many studies [153]. However skin application of these nanocarriers, and especially for liposomes, polymeric and lipidic nanoparticles, also makes sense when considering surface effects (film formation and occlusive effects), local effects in the skin (drug delivery in the epidermis and dermis) and systemic effects (deeper drug permeation and transdermal delivery). In potential uses apart from those concerned with surface effects the nanocarrier has to overcome the SC barrier in order to deliver the drug more or less deeply into skin layers. Recent advances in the study of penetration mechanisms deal with the control of the intercellular penetration route by the crystalline state of lipids, and the penetration through skin appendages (the follicular pathway) that appears to contribute much more than was previously thought. Applications dependent on skin penetration that have received special attention include transdermal delivery of nano- and microparticles by hair follicles, especially for nanoparticles which penetrate hair follicles very efficiently targeting the skin immune system in order to develop new vaccination strategies, and problems relating to skin diseases [154,155].

Options for topical and transdermal delivery are the solid lipid nanoparticles (SLNs) and nanostructured lipid carriers (NLCs) [156]. Some drugs such as triptolide, triamcinolone acetonide acetate, cyclosporin A have been used to be entrapped in SLN [157-159]. SLN can be admixed to an already commercially available and established topical formulation, e.g. a cosmetic day cream. Admixing the SLN leads to an increase in occlusivity while still maintaining the 'light character' of the day cream and avoiding the glossiness of more occlusive night creams. This phenomena is explained in **Figure 7**. However, having a highly occlusive night cream already, addition of SLN will have little or no effect [156].

Lipid nanoparticles are other options to load arthemeter and econazole nitrate [160,161]. Celecoxib [162]. It was compared the permeability of coenzima Q 10 incorporated in NLC and in an emulsion with the same lipid contain. The occlusion effect of the cream was also investigated. The result showed a higher permeability of the molecule and a higher occlusive effect for the NLC than for the emulsion as it could be observed in **Figures 8 and 9** [163].

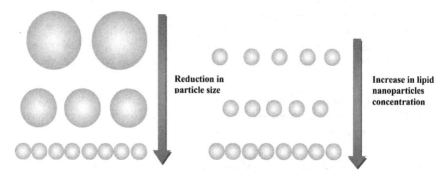

Figure 7. The occlusion factor of lipid nanoparticles depends on various factors: at identical lipid content, reducing the particle size leads to an increase in particle number, the film becomes denser (left) and therefore the occlusion factor increases. At a given particle size, increasing the lipid concentration increases particle number and density of the film (right) which also leads to a higher occlusion factor.

Different studies shown lipid nanoparticles were able to enhance the chemical stability of compounds sensitive to light, oxidation and hydrolysis. Enhancement of chemical stability after incorporation into lipid nanocarriers was proven for many cosmetic actives, e.g. coenzyme Q10 [164-166], ascorbyl palmitate [164,167], tocopherol (vitamin E) [165] and retinol (vitamin A) [168-170].

Three vitamin derivatives including vitamin C (ascorbyl tetraisoplamitate), vitamin E (tocopherol acetate) and vitamin A (retinyl palmitate) were also loaded in PLGA nanospheres, for skin whitening and anti-wrinkles/aging applications due vitamin C suppresses the blemishes because it limits the activity of tyrosinase, which promotes melanin production. Furthermore, it increases collagen formation to reduce wrinkles, and prevents cell oxidation by eliminating active oxygen. As to vitamin E and A, they also act as antioxidant and collagen promoter, respectively. They were able to reach the target areas in a stable form, sustain the pharmacological effect for a long time and be effective to reduce the wrinkles and produce a whitening effect [171]. In a sense, the idea of nanoparticle design for drug delivery systems in cosmetics applications is important.

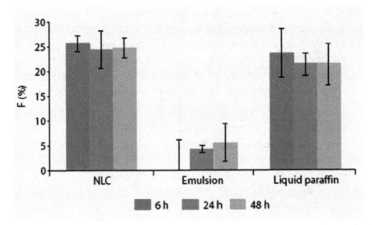

Figure 8. Occlusion factor (F) of NLC, emulsion and liquid paraffin (with permission from authors) [163].

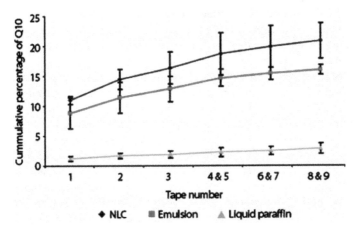

Figure 9. Tape stripping test: summation of coenzyme Q10 found in the tapes related to the applied amount (with permission from authors) [163].

As it was described before, the follicles are deep invaginations inside skin where the SC is thinner, the vascularisation is denser, and there are several targets of interest along a follicle structure from both cosmetic and pharmaceutical viewpoints [172]. Here, minoxidil which is an antihypertensive has been introduced in a block of copolymer poly (ε-caprolactone)-block-poly(ethyleneglycol) to treat the alopecia areata disorder , by widening blood vessels and opening potassium channels, it allows more oxygen, blood, and nutrients to the follicle. This disorder is an inflammatory condition, often reversible hair loss affecting mainly children and young adults. Clinically, round hairless patches appear on the scalp while hair follicles remain intact. This skin disorder is related with the distal part of the human hair follicle immune system, especially with the interacting intraepithelial T cells. The cause of this condition is diverse and seems to involve T cell–mediated immunologic changes, neuropeptides, genetic disposition to autoimmunity, and distress [30,173,174]. As the infundibulum of the hair follicle is surrounded by an extensive capillary network and the permeability of its epithelium allows the transport of molecules or particles to the blood circulatory system. There is a high density of immune cells in and around the infundibulum epithelium which could be targets also for hair follicle immune system and topical vaccination.

The sebaceous glands associated with hair follicles provide another potential target for delivering drugs against acne, androgenetic alopecia and other sebaceous gland dysfunctions. Different nanoparticles formulations have been prepared in order to treat acne vulgaris, which is an inflammatory disease of the pilosebaceous units, most densely concentrated on the face and torso [175]. Pathogenesis is multifactorial, but *Propionibacterium acnes* a Gram-positive bacterium plays a central role in the promotion of inflammation in acne. The most commonly formulations are prepared with different topical antimicrobials, either alone or in combination with other drugs. It is expected that an agent able to inhibit *P. acnes* growth and to suppress the inflammatory response will provide significant benefits to patients with acne vulgaris [30,176,177]. For that reason triclosan has been used in several systems. It was reported the characterization of triclosan loaded polymeric nanoparticles. They showed a good encapsulation efficiency and also a good physical stability representing an alternative as a treatment of acne [33]. Triclosan loaded nanoparticles made of chitosan and cyclodextrins were prepared using a very simple ionic gelation technique. This new approach permits to enhance the entrapment of hydrophobic drugs by forming molecular inclusion complexes with cyclodextrins in aqueous media. Such a device could be of interest for conferring protection to some specific drug molecules through the complexation followed by entrapment in the polymer matrix [109]. Another drug used to treat this disorder is tretinoin (all-*trans*-retinoic acid) which is the active form of a metabolic product of Vitamin A, also called retinoic acid. Tretinoin-loaded nanocapsules improved tretinoin photostability, independently on the type of oily phase used (capric/caprylic triglycerides and sunflower seed oil) in this study, and represent a potential system to be incorporated in novel topical or systemic dosage forms containing tretinoin [178].

Formulations of nanoparticles are often used in combination with penetration chemical and physical enhancers to modify the physical state of the stratum corneum, affecting the degree of transdermal drug penetration. DNA has been entrapped in nanoparticle of polysaccharide such as chitosan/poly-γ-glutamic acid and in a multifunctional core-shell polymeric nanoparticle of PLGA core and a positively-charged glycol chitosan (GC) shell. Another drugs used in the preparation of nanoparticles made of propyl-starch derivatives are flufenamic acid, testosterone and caffeine [179,180]. Insulin is a protein which has also been introduced in chitosan nanoparticles [83]. Poly (lactide-co-glycolide) polymer has been used to prepare biodegradables nanoparticles containing dexamethasone phosphate and 5-Fluorouracil [181,182]. Chlorhexidine loaded polymeric nanoparticle are used to treat cutaneous infections [183].

Inflammatory skin diseases account for a large proportion of all skin disorders and constitute a major health problem worldwide. Psoriasis, atopic dermatitis, poison ivy, and eczema are another skin disorders. Contact dermatitis, atopic dermatitis, and psoriasis represent the most prevalent inflammatory skin disorders and share a common efferent T-lymphocyte mediated response. Oxidative stress and inflammation have recently been linked to cutaneous damage in T-lymphocyte mediated skin diseases, particularly in contact dermatitis [184]. Poison ivy and atopic dermatitis may also present with bullous and vesicular changes [185]. Lipid nanoparticles have been investigated to improve the treatments of skin diseases such as atopic eczema, psoriasis, skin mycosis and inflammations. Apart from the treatment of skin diseases by topical application, e.g. gastrointestinal side effects of non-steroidal anti-inflammatory drugs can be decreased by topical antirheumatic therapy. Drugs under investigations for dermal application using lipid nanoparticles at the present are for instance glucocorticoids, retinoids, non-steroidal anti-inflammatory drugs, COX-2 inhibitors and antimycotics. It was showed that it is possible to enhance the percutaneous absorption with lipid nanoparticles. These carriers may even allow drug targeting to the skin or even to its substructures. Thus they might have the potential to improve the benefit/risk ratio of topical drug therapy [186].

Perioral dermatitis is commonly seen in women aged 20–35 years. It presents as red papules that form superficial plaques around the perioral area, nasolabial folds and/or lower eyelids. It is minimally itchy [187,188]. Topical corticosteroids are the first-line therapy of acute exacerbations of atopic dermatitis and contact dermatitis. Prednicarbate is superior to the halogenated glucocorticoids because of an improved benefit/risk ratio. However, at the present the separation of desired anti-inflammatory effects and undesired antiproliferative effects is still not satisfying. Therefore, lipid nanoparticles were investigated as a delivery system for prednicarbate. The report show an improved extent of prednicarbate uptake by human skin *in vitro*, if applied as SLN dispersion or cream containing prednicarbate-loaded SLN. The authors found that a prednicarbate targeting to the epidermis [189]. This is particular relevant because prednicarbate in the dermis is responsible for the induction of irreversible skin atrophy while the inflammatory process is most pronounced within the epidermis [186]. Therefore, a better benefit/risk ratio is expected for the application of pretnicarbate in SLN containing topical formulations.

Tretinoin, a metabolite of vitamin A is used for topical treatment of various proliferateive and inflammatory skin diseases such as psoriasis, acne (as mentioned before), photo aging, epidermotropic T-cell lymphomas and epithelial skin cancer. One of the major disadvantages associated with the topical application of tretinoin is local skin irritation such as erythrema, peeling and burning as well as increased sensitivity to sunlight. To overcome these problems tretinoin was incorporated into SLN [190]. *In vitro* permeation studies through rat skin indicated that SLN-based tretinoin gel has a permeation profile comparable to that of the market tretinoin cream. Furthermore, Draize patch test showed that SLN-based tretinoin gel resulted in remarkably less erythremic episodes compared to the currently marketed tretinoin cream (**Figure 10**). Therefore, also for formulations containing tretinoin-loaded SLN a better benefit/risk ratio is expected.

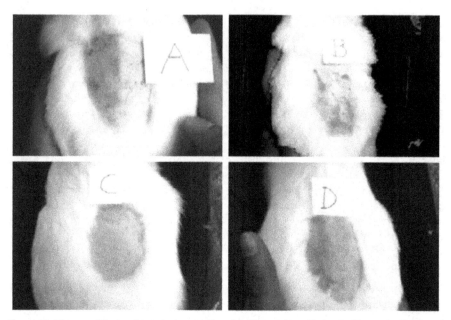

Figure 10. Pictures of Draize skin irritation studies carried out on New Zealand rabbits 24 h after application of (A) control (no application); (B) marketed formulation (Retino-A® cream); (C) SLN-based gel without tretinoin; (D) SLN-based gel containing tretinoin (0.05%, w/w). The Marketed tretinoin cream clearly shows erythemal lesions, which are not visible in SLN based tretinoin gel [190]. "Reprinted from International Journal of Pharmaceutics, 345/1-2, Kumar A. Shah, Abhijit A. Date,Medha D. Joshi,Vandana B. Patravale, Solid lipid nanoparticles (SLN) of tretinoin: Potential in topical delivery, 163-171., Copyright (2007), with permission from Elsevier"

Liposomes which were one of the first strategies for transdermal delivery are being successfully used in cancer therapy [139,141]. However to date, many liquid-type nanocosmetics carriers, such as liposomes, are structurally unstable. Specifically, when passing through the skin, they adhere to the inside walls of the skin cells causing the collapse of phospholipid association bodies and the leak of their encapsulated ingredients. As a result, their ability to transport active ingredients to deep skin is not likely good. Some authors report the use of flexible vesicles called transfersomes or transformable liposomes in comparison with rigid vesicles to enhance penetration [148,191]. The application of transformable liposomes more flexible, which are prepared using surfactants or alcohol (ethosomes) in the lipid bilayer, to be able to deform them when a pressure is applied in the transdermal route has been increased.

In some researches, dendrimers are used for transdermal drug delivery. They show promising results in the delivery of drugs such as tamsulosin [192], indomethacin [193], ketoprofen and diflunisal [194] and 5-fluorouracil [195]. The main problems with this kind of transdermal carrier are poor biodegradation and inherent cytotoxicity [158]. In order to get down the toxicity dendrimers have been linked to peptides (dendrimers-peptides) from amino acids linked via peptide-amide bonds to the branches of dendrimers in the core or on the surface [159,160].

For 5-fluorouracil (5FU) (log P = −0.89) which is one hydrophilic model drug used to treat skin diseases, has been reporte to have very poor penetration in skin [196-198]. Many strategies to increase skin permeation of this drug have been tested: prodrugs, terpenes, fatty acids, iontophoresis, sonophoresis, laser ablation and dendrimers which increased 5FU permeation across the skin by altering the skin structure [198-203].

Nowadays transdermal delivery using nanoemulsions it is not so used as nanoparticles or liposomes delivery due to the stability problems inherent to this dosage form. Nevertheless, Gamma Tocopherol, Caffeine, Plasmid DNA, Aspirin, Methyl Salicylate, Insulin, Nimesulide have been included in nanoemulsion. The use of these nanocarriers to deliver analgesics, corticosteroids, anti cancer agents, etc. is very important since these drugs are able to act immediately because they do not need to cross extra barriers. The drug is bioavailable easily and faster [204-210].

8. Conclusions

Nanocarriers have shown many advantages for topical and trasdermal delivery of drugs. It could be shown already for various drugs that topical/trandermal formulations containing nanoparticles can enhance the penetration into the skin increasing treatment efficiency, target the epidermis or follicles, reducing side effects. Furthermore, an increased activities as well as prolonged activities have been reported. These delivery systems can deliver both hydrophilic and lipophilic molecules. Advances with regard to materials, fabrication methods and techniques facilitate the development of new and better nanocarriers. Nonetheless, future researches must ensure the benefit and evaluate the risk ratio for many drugs included in nanocarriers.

Author details

José Juan Escobar-Chávez
Unidad de Investigación Multidisciplinaria, Laboratorio 12: Sistemas Transdérmicos y Materiales Nanoestructurados, Facultad de Estudios Superiores Cuautitlán-Universidad Nacional Autónoma de México, Estado de México

Isabel Marlen Rodríguez-Cruz
Departamento de Enseñanza e Investigación, Hospital Regional de Alta Especialidad de Zumpango. Zumpango, Estado de México

Clara Luisa Domínguez-Delgado
Departamento de Ingeniería y Tecnología. Sección de Tecnología Farmacéutica, Facultad de Estudios Superiores Cuautitlán-Universidad Nacional Autónoma de México, Estado de México

Roberto Díaz- Torres

Unidad de Investigación Multidisciplinari,. Laboratorio 9: Toxicología y genética, Facultad de Estudios Superiores Cuautitlán-Universidad Nacional Autónoma de México, Estado de México

Alma Luisa Revilla-Vázquez

Laboratorio de Desarrollo de Métodos Analíticos, Facultad de Estudios Superiores Cuautitlán-Universidad Nacional Autónoma de México, Cuautitlán Izcalli, Estado de México

Norma Casas Aléncaster

Laboratorio de Propiedades Reológicas de Alimentos, Facultad de Estudios Superiores Cuautitlán-Universidad Nacional Autónoma de México, Cuautitlán Izcalli, Estado de México

Acknowledgement

Dr. José Juan Escobar-Chávez wishes to acknowledge PAPIIT TA200-312, Cátedra PACIVE NCONS-17 and PAPIME 203612. We are also grateful with Dr. Müller and Dr. Pardeike for permission of their figures. The authors report no conflict of interests.

9. References

[1] Brower V. Is nanotechnology ready for primetime? Journal of National Cancer Institute 2006; 98:9-11.

[2] Escobar-Chávez JJ, Rodriguez Cruz IM, Dominguez-Delgado CL. Chemical and Physical enhancers for transdermal drug delivery. In: Gallelli L (ed.) Pharmacology. Rijeka: InTech; 2012. p397-433.

[3] Díaz-Torres R. Transdermal nanocarriers. In: José Juan Escobar-Chávez/Virginia Merino (Eds.) Current Technologies to Increase the Transdermal Delivery of Drugs. The Netherlands: Bentham Science Publishers; 2010. p120-40.

[4] Hadgraft J, Lane ME. Skin permeation: The years of enlightenment. International Journal of Pharmaceutics 2005, 305 (1-2):2-12.

[5] Barry BW. Novel mechanisms and devices to enable successful transdermal drug delivery. European Journal of Pharmaceutical Sciences 2001; 14(2):101–4.

[6] Rizwan M, Aqil M, Talegaonkar S, Azeem A, Sultana Y, Ali A. Enhanced transdermal drug delivery techniques: an extensive review of patents. Recent Patents on Drug Delivery & Formulations 2009; 3:(2), pp. 105-24,

[7] Escobar-Chávez JJ & Merino V eds. Current Technologies to increase the Transdermal Delivery of Drugs. The Netherlands: Bentham Science Publishers; 2010.

[8] Escobar-Chávez JJ, Bonilla-Martínez D, Villegas-González A, Rodríguez-Cruz IM, Domínguez-Delgado CL. The use of sonophoresis in the administration of drugs through the skin. Journal of Pharmacy and Pharmaceutical Sciences 2009; 12(1): 88-115.

[9] Escobar-Chávez JJ, Merino V, López-Cervantes M, Rodríguez-Cruz IM, *et al*. The use of iontophoresis in the administration of nicotine and new non-nicotine drugs through the skin for smoking cessation. Current Drug Discovery Technologies 2009; 6(3):171-185.

[10] Escobar-Chávez JJ, Bonilla-Martínez D, Villegas-González A, Revilla-Vazquez AL. The electroporation as an efficient physical enhancer for transdermal drug delivery. Journal of Clinical Pharmacology 2009; 49(11):1262-83.

[11] Papakostas D, Rancan F, Sterry W, Blume-Peytavi U, Vogt A. Nanoparticles in dermatology. Archives of Dermatology Research 2011; 303(8):533-50.

[12] Kristl J, Teskac K, Grabnar PA. Current view on nanosized solid lipid carriers for drug delivery to the skin. Journal of Biomedical Nanotechnology 2010; 6(5):529-42.

[13] Schroeter A, Engelbrecht T, Neubert RH, Goebel AS. New nanosized technologies for dermal and transdermal drug delivery: A review. Journal of Biomedical Nanotechnology 2010; 6(5):511-28.

[14] Neubert RH. Potentials of new nanocarriers for dermal and transdermal drug delivery. European Journal of Pharmaceutics and Biopharmaceutics 2011; 77(1):1-2.

[15] Desai P, Patlolla RR, Singh M. Interaction of nanoparticles and cell-penetrating peptides with skin for transdermal drug delivery. Molecular Membrane Biology 2010; 27(7):247-59.

[16] Chourasia R Jain SK. Drug targeting through pilosebaceous route. Current Drug Targets 2009; 10(10):950-67.

[17] Gasco MR, Gasco P. Nanovector. Nanomedicine (London) 2007; 2(6):955-60.

[18] Magdassi S. Delivery systems in cosmetics. Colloids and Surfaces A 1997; 123-124:671-679.

[19] Luppi B, Cerchiara T, Bigucci F, Basile R, Zecchi V. Polymeric nanoparticles composed of fatty acids and polyvinylalcohol for topical application of sunscreens. Journal of Pharmacy and Pharmacology 2004;56:407-411.

[20] Kaur IP, Agrawal R. Nanotechnology: a new paradigm in cosmeceuticals. Recent Patents in Drug Delivery Formulations 2007;1:171-182.

[21] Alvarez-Roman R, Barre G, Guy RH, Fessi H. Biodegradable polymer nanocapsules containing a sunscreen agent: preparation and photoprotection. European Journal of Pharmaceutics and Biopharmaceutics 2001;52:191-195.

[22] Escobar Chávez JJ, Merino-Sanjuan V, López-Cervantes M, et al. The tape stripping technique as a method for drug quantification in skin. Journal of Pharmacy and Pharmaceutical Sciences 2008; 11(1):104-130.

[23] Potts RO, Francoeur ML. The influence of stratum corneum morphology on water permeability. Journal of Investigative Dermatology 1991; 96, 495-499.

[24] Potts RO, Guy RH. Predicting skin permeability. Pharmaceutical Research 1992; 9(5):663-669.

[25] Ellias PM. Epidermal barrier function: intercellular lamellar lipid structures, origin, composition and metabolism. Journal of Controlled Release 1991;15,199-208.

[26] Escobar-Chávez JJ, Melgoza-Contreras LM, López-Cervantes M, et al. The tape stripping technique as a valuable tool for evaluating topical applied compounds. In: Gary W. Caldwell /Atta-ur-Rahman / Z.Yan / M. Iqbal Choudhary (Eds.) Frontiers in

Drug Design & Discovery, The Netherlands: Bentham Science Publishers; 2009. Vol. 4, p189-227.

[27] Hadgraft J. Skin, the final frontier. International Journal of Pharmaceutics 2001; 224 (1-2):1-18.

[28] Guy RH and Hadgraft J. Transdermal drug delivery. New York: Marcel Dekker, Inc., p. 1-23, (2003).

[29] Nevill AM. The need to scale for differences in body size and mass: and explanation of Klieber's 0.75 mass exponent. Journal of Applied Physiology 1994; 2870-2873.

[30] Domínguez-Delgado CL, Rodríguez-Cruz IM. & López-Cervantes M. The skin a valuable route for administration of drugs. In: José Juan Escobar-Chávez/Virginia Merino (Eds). Current Technologies To Increase The Transdermal Delivery Of Drugs. The Netherlands: Bentham Science Publishers Ltd; 2010. p1-22.

[31] Escobar-Chávez JJ, Merino V, Díez-Sales O, Nácher-Alonso A, Ganem-Quintanar A, Herráez M, Merino-Sanjuán M. Transdermal nortriptyline hydrochloride patch formulated within a chitosan matrix intended to be used for smoking cessation. Pharmaceutical Development Technology 2011, 16 (2):162-9.

[32] Escobar-Chávez JJ, López-Cervantes M, Naïk A, Kalia YN, Quintanar-Guerrero D, Ganem Quintanar A. Applications of the thermoreversible Pluronic F-127 gels in pharmaceutical formulations, Journal of Pharmacy and Pharmaceutical Sciences 2006; 9(3):339-358.

[33] Domínguez-Delgado CL, Rodríguez-Cruz IM, Escobar-Chávez JJ, Calderón-Lojero IO, Quintanar-Guerrero D, Ganem A. Preparation and characterization of triclosan nanoparticles intended to be used for the treatment of acne. European Journal of Pharmaceutics and Biopharmaceutics 2011,79(1):102-7.

[34] Fang JY, Leu YL, Wang YY, and Tsai YH. *In vitro* topical application and *in vivo* phramacodynamic evaluation of nonivamide hydrogels using Wistar rat as an animal model, European Journal of Pharmaceutical Sciences 2002;15(5):417-423.

[35] Shin SC, Cho CW,Oh IJ. Effects of non ionic surfactants as permeation enhancers towards piroxicam from the poloxamer gel through rat skins, International Journal of Pharmaceutics 2001; 222(2), 199-203.

[36] Liaw J, Lin Y-Ch. Evaluation of poly(ethylene oxide)-poly(propylene oxide)-poly(ethylene oxide) (PEO-PPO-PEO) gels as a release vehicle for percutaneous fentanyl. Journal of Controlled Release 2000; 68:273-282.

[37] Wang YY, Hong CT, Chiu WT, Fang JY. *In vitro* and *in vivo* evaluations of topically applied capsaicin and nonivamide from hydrogels, International Journal of Pharmaceutics 2000; 224,1-2.

[38] Mattorano DA, Kupper LL, Nylander-French LA. Estimating dermal exposure to jet fuel (naphthalene) using adhesive tape strip samples. The Annals of Occupational Hygiene 2004; 48(2): 139–146.

[39] Chao Y-Ch, Nylander-French LA. Determination of Keratin Protein in a Tape stripped Skin Sample from Jet Fuel Exposed Skin. The Annals of Occupational Hygiene 2004; 48(1):65–73.

[40] Kenneth AW. Dermatological and transdermal formulations, New York, USA: Marcel Dekker Inc; 2002.

[41] Gray GM, White RJ, Williams RH, Yardley HJ. Lipid composition of the superficial stratum corneum cells of the epidermis. British of Journal Dermatology 1982; 106:59–63.

[42] Wertz PW, Downing DT. Ceramides of pig epidermis: structure determination. Journal of Lipid Research 1983; 24: 759-65.

[43] Long SA, Wertz PW, Strauss SJ, Downing DT. Human stratum corneum polar lipids and desquamation. Archives in Dermatology Research 1985; 277: 284-87.

[44] Wertz PW, Miethke MC, Long SA, Strauss JS, Downing DT. The composition of ceramides from human stratum corneum and from comedones. Journal of Investigative Dermatology 1985; 84: 410–12.

[45] Melnik BC, Hollmann J, Erler E, Verhoeven B, Plewig G. Microanalytical screening of all major stratum corneum lipids by sequential high-performance thin-layer chromatography. Journal of Investigative Dermatology 1989; 92: 231-34.

[46] Lavker RM, Sun T. Heterogeneity in epidermal basal keratinocytes: morphological and functional correlations. Science 1982; 215: 1239-41.

[47] Borradori L, Sonnenberg A. Structure and function of hemidesmosomes: more than simple adhesion complexes. Journal of Investigative Dermatology 1999; 112:411-18.

[48] Sawamura D, Li K, Chu M–L, Uitto J. Human bullous pemphigoid antigen (BPAG1): amino acid sequences deduced from cloned cDNAs predict biologically important peptide segments and protein domains. Journal of Biological Chemistry 1991; 266: 17784-90.

[49] Li K, Tamai K, Tan EML, Uitto J. Cloning of type XVII collagen. Complementary and genomic DNA sequences of mouse 180-kDa bullous pemphigoid antigen (BPAG2) predict an interrupted collagenous domain, a transmembrane segment, and unusual features in the 5'-end of the gene and the 3'-untranslated region of mRNA. Journal of Biological Chemistry 1993; 268: 8825-34.

[50] Stepp MA, Spurr–Michaud S, Tisdale A, Elwell J, Gipson IK. α6β4 Integrin heterodimer is a component of hemidesmosomes. Proceedings of the National Academy of Sciences 1990; 87: 8970-74.

[51] Burgeson RE, Christiano AM. The dermal–epidermal junction. Current Opinion in Cell Biology 1997; 9:651–58.

[52] Cross SE, Roberts MS. Subcutaneous absorption kinetics of interferon and other solutes. Journal of Pharmacy and Pharmacology 1993; 45: 606-09.

[53] Melski JW. The anatomy and physiology of the skin. In:Principles and Practice of Skin Excisions. Amsterdam: IEJEMEC & GBEJEMEC (eds), 1996; pp. 1–14.

[54] Steinstrasser I, Merkle HP. Dermal metabolism of topically applied drugs: Pathways and models reconsidered. Pharmaceutica Acta Helvetiae 1995; 70:3–24.

[55] Szuba A, Rockson SG. Lymphedema: anatomy, physiology and pathogenesis. Vascular Medicine 1997; 2: 321-26.

[56] Cameli N, Picardo M, Perrin C. Expression of integrins in human nail matrix. British Journal of Dermatology 1994; 130: 583–88.

[57] Philpott MP. Defensins and acne. Molecular Immunology 2003; 40: 457-462.

[58] Illel B. Formulation for transfollicular drug administration: some recent advances. Critical Reviews in Therapeutic Drug Carrier Systems 1997;14: 207-19.

[59] Xiang TX, Anderson BD. Influence of chain ordering on the selectivity of dipalmitoylphosphatidylcholine bilayer membranes for permeant size and shape. Biophysical Journal 1998; 75: 2658–71.

[60] Geinoz S, Guy RH, Testa B, Carrupt PA. Quantitative structure–permeation relationships (QSPeRs) to predict skin permeation: a critical evaluation. Pharmaceutical Research 2004; 21: 83–92.

[61] Cevc G. Drug delivery across the skin. Expert Opinion on Investigational Drugs 1997; 6: 1887–37.

[62] Cevc G, Vierl U. Nanotechnology and the transdermal route. A state of the art review and critical appraisal. Journal of Controlled Release 2010; 141(3):277-99.

[63] Schätzlein A, Cevc G. Non-uniform cellular packing of the stratum corneum and permeability barrier function of intact skin: a high-resolution confocal laser scanning microscopy study using highly deformable vesicles (Transfersomes). British Journal of Dermatology 1998; 138: 583–92.

[64] Mitragotri S. Modeling skin permeability to hydrophilic and hydrophobic solutes based on four permeation pathways. Journal of Controlled Release 2003; 86: 69–92.

[65] Aguilella V, Kontturi K, Murtomäki L, Ramírez P. Estimation of the pore size and charge density in human cadaver skin. Journal of Controlled Release 1994; 32: 249–57.

[66] Johnson ME, Blankschtein D, Langer R. Evaluation of solute permeation through the stratumcorneum: lateral bilayer diffusion as the primary transport mechanism. Journal of Pharmaceutical Science 1997; 86:1162–72.

[67] Guy R. Transdermal drug delivery. 2a ed; Marcel Dekker. New York, USA, 2003.

[68] Meidan VM, Docker M, Walmsley AD, Irwin WJ. Low intensity ultrasound as a probe to elucidate the relative follicular contribution to total transdermal absorption. Pharmeceutical Research 1998; 15: 85–92.

[69] Ogiso T, Shiraki T, Okajima K, et al. Transfollicular drug delivery: penetration of drugs through human scalp skin and comparison of penetration between scalp and abdominal skins in vitro. Journal of Drug Targeting 2002; 10:369–78.

[70] Dokka S, Cooper SR, Kelly S, Hardee GE, Karras JG. Dermal delivery of topically applied oligonucleotides via follicular transport in mouse skin. Journal of Investigative Dermatology 2005; 124: 971–75.

[71] Grams YY, Whitehead L, Lamers G, Sturman N, Bouwstra JA. Online diffusion profile of a lipophilic dye in different depths of a hair follicle in human scalp skin. Journal of Investigative Dermatology 2005; 125:775–82.

[72] Jacobi U, Toll R, Sterry W, Lademann J. Follicles play a role as penetration pathways in *in vitro* studies on porcine skin? An optical study. Laser Physics 2005; 15: 1594–98.

[73] Teichmann A, Ossadnik M, Richter H, Sterry W, Lademann J. Semiquantitative determination of the penetration of a fluorescent hydrogel formulation into the hair follicle with and without follicular closure by microparticles by means of differential stripping. Skin Pharmacology and Physiology 2006; 19: 101–5.

[74] Alvarez-Román R, Naik A, Kalia YN, Guy RH, Fessi H. Skin penetration and distribution of polymeric nanoparticles. Journal of Controlled Release 2004; 99:53–62.

[75] Essa EA, Bonner MC, Barry BW. Human skin sandwich for assessing shunt route penetration during passive and iontophoretic drug and liposome delivery. Journal of Pharmacy and Pharmacology 2002; 54: 1481–90.

[76] Escobar-Chávez JJ, López-Cervantes M, Ganem Rondero A. Conventional Methods for Cutaneous Drug Sampling. In: Narasimha Murthy (Ed.). Dermatokinetics of therapeutic agents. Boca Raton: CRC Press Taylor and Francis Group; 2011, p81-130.

[77] Teichmann A, Jacobi U, Ossadnik M, *et al.* Differential stripping: determination of the amount of topically applied substances penetrated into the hair follicles. Journal of Investigative Dermatology 2005; 125: 264–69.

[78] Prochazka AV. New developments in smoking cessation. Chest 2000;117(4) Suppl 1:169S-175S.

[79] Wilkosz MF, Bogner RH. Trandermal drug delivery. Part 1: Current status. US pharmacist 2003; 28(4).

[80] http://www.ezinearticles.com/?Transdermal-Drug-Delivery,-Transdermal-Patches&id=155961 (accessed: 1May 2012).

[81] Huang X, Du Y, Yuan H & Hu F. Preparation and pharmacodynamics of low-molecular-weight chitosan nanoparticles containing insulin. Carbohydrate Polymers 2009; 76:368-373.

[82] Goswami S, Bajpai J & Bajpai AK. Designing Gelatin Nanocarriers as a Swellable System for Controlled Release of Insulin: An In-Vitro Kinetic Study. Journal of Macromolecular Science 2010; 47:119-130.

[83] Rodríguez-Cruz IM, Domínguez-Delgado CL, Escobar-Chávez JJ, Leyva-Gómez G, Ganem-Quintanar A, Quintanar-Guerrero D. Nanoparticle infiltration to prepare solvent-free controlled drug delivery system. International Journal of Pharmaceutics 2009; 371:177-181.

[84] Sonneville-Aubrun O, Simonnet JT & Alloret FL. Nanoemulsions: a new vehicle for skincare products. Advances in Colloid and Interface Science 2004; 108-109:145-149.

[85] Bangham AD. Liposomes: the Babraham connection. Chemistry and Physics of Lipids 1993; 64:275-285.

[86] Rodriguez-Justo O & Moraes ÂM. Analysis of process parameters on the characteristics of liposomes prepared by ethanol injection with a view to process scale-up: Effect of temperature and batch volume. Chemical Engineering Research and Design 2011;89(6):785-792.

[87] Cevc G, Blume G. Lipid vesicles penetrate into intact skin owing to the transdermal osmotic gradients and hydration force. Biochimica et Biophysica Acta 1992; 1104:226-232.

[88] Svenson S, Tomalia DA. Dendrimers in biomedical applications – reflections on the field. Advanced Drug Delivery Reviews 2005; 57:2106-2129.

[89] Kabanov VA, Zezin AB, Rogacheva VB, Gulyaeva ZG, Zansochova MF, Joosten JGH & Brackman J. Polyelectrolyte behavior of astramol poly(propyleneimine) dendrimers. Macromolecules 1998; 31:142-5144.

[90] Almeida AJ, Souto E. Solid lipid nanoparticles as a drug delivery system for peptides and proteins. Advanced Drug Delivery Reviews 2007; 59:478-490.

[91] García-González CA, Sampaio da Sousa AR, Argemí A, López Periago A, Saurina J, Duarte CM & Domingo C. Production of hybrid lipid-based particles loaded with inorganic nanoparticles and active compounds for prolonged topical release. International Journal of Pharmaceutics 2009; 382(1-2): pp.296-304.

[92] El Maghraby GM, Barry BW & Williams AC. Liposomes and skin: From drug delivery to model membranes. European Journal of Pharmaceutical Sciences 2008; 34:203-222.

[93] Menjoge AR, Kannan RM & Tomalia DA. Dendrimer-based drug and imaging conjugates: design considerations for nanomedical applications. Drug Discovery Today 2010;15:171-185.

[94] Rzigalinski BA, Strobl JS. Cadmium-containing nanoparticles: Perspectives on pharmacology and toxicology of quantum dots. Toxicology and Applied Pharmacology 2009; 238:280-288.

[95] Dan Y, Liu H, Gao W & Chen S. Activities of essential oils from Asarum heterotropoides var. mandshuricum against five phytopathogens. Crop Protection 2010; Vol. 29, No. 295-299.

[96] Dodla MC, Bellamkonda RV. Differences between the effect of anisotropic and isotropic laminin and nerve growth factor presenting scaffolds on nerve regeneration across long peripheral nerve gaps. Biomaterials 2008; 29:33-46.

[97] Elsayed MMA, Abdallah OY, Naggar VF & Khalafallah NM. Deformable liposomes and ethosomes: Mechanism of enhanced skin delivery. International Journal of Pharmaceutics 2006; 322:60-66.

[98] Rojas-Oviedo I, Salazar-López RA, Reyes-Gasga J & Quirino-Barreda CT. Elaboration and structural analysis of aquasomes loaded with Indomethacin. European Journal of Pharmaceutical Sciences 2007; 32:223-230.

[99] Jin Y, Tong L, Ai P, Li M & Hou X. Self-assembled drug delivery systems: 1. Properties and *in vitro/in vivo* behavior of acyclovir self-assembled nanoparticles (SAN). International Journal of Pharmaceutics 2006; 309:199-207.

[100] Rossier-Miranda FJ, Schroën CGPH & Boom RM. Colloidosomes: Versatile microcapsules in perspective. Colloids and Surfaces A: Physicochemical and Engineering Aspects 2009; 343:43-49.

[101] Hong M, Zhu S, Jiang Y, Tang G & Pei Y. Efficient tumor targeting of hydroxycamptothecin loaded PEGylated niosomes modified with transferrin. Journal of Controlled Release 2009; 133:96-102.

[102] Elnaggar YSR, El-Massik MA & Abdallah OY. Self-nanoemulsifying drug delivery systems of tamoxifen citrate: Design and optimization. International Journal of Pharmaceutics 2009; 380(1-2):133-141.

[103] Kim JC, Song ME, Kim MJ, Lee EJ, Park SK, Rang MJ, Ahn HJ. Preparation and characterization of triclosan-containing vesicles. Colloids and Surfaces B 2002; 26 235–241.

[104] Pardeike J, Hommoss A, Müller RH. Lipid nanoparticles (SLN, NLC) in cosmetic and pharmaceutical dermal products. International Journal of Pharmaceutics 2009; 366 170–184.

[105] Cevc G. Lipid vesicles and other colloids as drug carriers on the skin, Advanced Drug Delivery Reviews 2004; 56 675– 711.

[106] Maestrelli F, Garcia-Fuentes M, Mura P, Alonso MJ. A new drug nanocarrier consisting of chitosan and hydoxypropylcyclodextrin, European Journal of Pharmaceuitics and Biopharmaceutics 2006; 63 79–86.

[107] Alvarez-Román R, Naik A, Kalia YN, Fessi H, Guy RH. Visualization of skin penetration using confocal laser scanning microscopy. European Journal of Pharmaceutics and Biopharmaceutics 2004; 58 301–316.

[108] Ogiso T, Shiraki T, Okajima K, Tanino TT, Iwaki MM. and Wada TT. Transfollicular drug delivery: penetration of drugs through human scalp skin and comparison of penetration between scalp and abdominal skins in vitro. Journal of Drug Targeting 2002; 10:369–78.

[109] Jacobi U, Toll R, Sterry W, Lademann J. Follicles play a role as penetration pathways in in vitro studies on porcine skin?. An optical study. Laser Physics Letters 2005; 15: 1594–98.

[110] Wilson T., (1990). Confocal Microscopy. Academic Press, London.

[111] Gerritsen HC, and De Grauw CJ. Imaging of optically thick specimen using two-photon excitation microscopy. Microscopy Research andTechnique 1999; 47, 206–209.

[112] Denk W, Delaney KR, Gelperin A, Kleinfeld D, Strowbridge BW, Tank DW, and Yuste R. Anatomical and functional imaging of neurons using 2-photon laser scanning microscopy. Journal of Neuroscience Methods 1994; 54, 151–162.

[113] Svoboda K, Denk W, Kleinfeld D, and Tank DW. In vivo dendritic calcium dynamics in neocortical pyramidal neurons. Nature 1997; 385, 161–165.

[114] Xu C, and Webb WW. Nonlinear and two-photon induced fluorescence. In:Topics in Fluorescence Spectroscopy. New York, USA: J. R. Lakowicz, editor, 1997.

[115] Denk WJ, Strickler JH, and Webb WW. Two-photon laser scanning fluorescence microscopy. Science 1990; 248, 73-76.

[116] Tsai TH, Jee SH, Dong CY, Lin SJ. Multiphoton microscopy in dermatological imaging. Journal Dermatological Science 2009; 56, 1-8.

[117] Paoli J, Smedh M, Ericson MB. Multiphoton laser scanning microscopy—a novel diagnostic method for superficial skin cancers. Seminars in Cutaneous Medicine and Surgery 2009; 28, 190-195.

[118] Chen T., Langer R., Weaver J. C. (1998) Skin electroporation causes molecular transport across the stratum corneum through localized transport regions. Journal of Investigative Dermatology Symposium Proceedings 1998; 3(2):159-65.

[119] Domínguez- Delgado CL. Estudio sobre el transporte a través de piel *in vitro* de triclosán, formulado en una dispersión de nanopartículas poliméricas, como alternativa para el tratamiento del acné. Efecto del laureato de sacarosa como promotor de absorción. Informe de investigación de Maestría. Posgrado en Ciencias Químicas, UNAM, 2008.

[120] Thiboutot D, Zaenglein A, Weiss J, Webster G, Calvarese B, Chen D. An aqueous gel fixed combination of clindamycin phosphate 1.2% and benzoyl peroxide 2.5% for the once-daily treatment of moderate to severe acne vulgaris: assessment of efficacy and safety in 2813 patients. Journal of American Academy of Dermatology 2008; 59: 792-800.

[121] Chien YW. (1987). Transdermal therapeutic systems. In: Controlled Drug Delivery Fundamentals and Applications. Robinson J. R., Lee V. H. L, editors. New York, USA: Marcel Dekker, Inc. p. 523-549.

[122] Schroeder U, Sommerfeld P, Ulrich S, Sabel BA. Nanoparticle technology for delivery of drugs across the blood–brain barrier. Journal of Pharmaceutical Science 1998; 87, 1305–1307.

[123] Raghuvanshi RS, Katare YK, Lalwani K, Ali MM, Singh O and Panda AK. Improved immune response from biodegradable polymer particles entrapping tetanus toxoid by use of different immunization protocol and adjuvants. International Journal of Pharmaceutics 2002; 245: 109–121.

[124] Leroux JC, Allemann E, De Jaeghere F, Doelker E, Gurny R. Biodegradable nanoparticles—from sustained release formulations to improved site specific drug delivery. Journal of Controlled Release 1996; 39, 339.

[125] Brannon-Peppas L, Blanchette JO. Nanoparticle and targeted systems for cancer therapy, Advanced Drug Delivery Reviews 2004; 56: 1649–1659.

[126] Haag R. Supramolecular drug-delivery systems based on polymeric core-shell architectures. Angewandte Chemie International Edition 2004; 43:278-282.

[127] Radowski MR, Shukla A, von Berlepsch H, Bottcher C, Pickaert G, Rehage H, Haag R. Supramolecular aggregates of dendritic multishell architectures as universal nanocarriers. Angewandte Chemie International Edition 2007; 46:1265-1269.

[128] Tinkle SS, Antonini JM, Rich BA, Roberts JR, Salmen R, DePree K, Adkins EJ. Skin as a route of exposure and sensitization in chronic beryllium disease. Environmental Health Perspectives 2003; 111:1202-1208.

[129] Kim S, Lim YT, Soltesz EG, De Grand AM, Lee J, Nakayama A. Near-infrared fluorescent type II quantum dots for sentinel lymph node mapping. Nature Biotechnology 2004; 22:93-97.

[130] Symon Z, Peyser A, Tzemach D, Lyass O, Sucher E, Shezen E, Gabizon A. Selective delivery of doxorubicin to patients with breast carcinoma metastases by stealth liposomes. Cancer 1999; 86:72-78.

[131] Gonçalves A, Braud AC, Viret F, Genre D, Gravis G, Tarpin C. Phase I study of pegylated liposomal doxorubicin (Caelyx) in combination with carboplatin in patients with advanced solid tumors. Anticancer Research 2003; 23:3543-3548.

[132] Seiden M. V, Muggia F, Astrow A, Matulonis U, Campos S, Roche M. A phase II study of liposomal lurtotecan (OSI-211) in patients with topotecan resistant ovarian cancer. Gynecologic Oncology 2004; 93:229-232.

[133] El Maghraby GMM, Williams AC, Barry BW. Can drug-bearing liposomes penetrate intact skin? Journal of Pharmacy and Pharmacology 2006; 58:415-429.

[134] Weiner N, Williams N, Birch G, Ramachandran C, Shipman C, Flynn G. Topical delivery of liposomally encapsulated interferon evaluated in a cutaneous herpes guinea pig model. Antimicrobial Agents and Chemotherapy 1989; 33:1217-1221.

[135] Planas ME, Gonzalez P, Rodriguez L, Sanchez S, Cevc G. Noninvasive percutaneous induction of topical analgesia by a new type of drug carrier, and prolongation of local pain insensitivity by anesthetic liposomes. Anesthesia and Analgesia 1992; 75:615-621.

[136] Sentjurc M, Gabrijelcic V. Transport of liposome-entrapped molecules into the skin as studied by electron paramagnetic resonance imaging methods. In: Non-Medical Application of liposomes. Lasic B, editor. New York, USA; CRC Press.1995, pp 91-114.

[137] Cevc G., Gebauer D., Stieber J., Schatzlein A., Blume G., (1998) Ultraflexible vesicles, Transfersomes, have an extremely low pore penetration resistance and transport therapeutic amounts of insulin across the intact mammalian skin. Biochimica et Biophysica Acta 1998; 1368:201-215.

[138] Paul A, Cevc G, Bachhawat BK. Transdermal immunisation with an integral membrane component, gap junction protein, by means of ultradeformable drug carriers, transfersomes. Vaccine 1998; 16:188-195.

[139] Van den Bergh BA, Bouwstra JA, Junginger HE, Wertz PW. Elasticity of vesicles affects hairless mouse skin structure and permeability. Journal of Controlled Release 1999; 62:367-379.

[140] Guo J, Ping Q, Sun G, Jiao C. Lecithin vesicular carriers for transdermal delivery of cyclosporin A. International Journal of Pharmaceutics 2000; 194:201-207.

[141] Guo J, Ping Q, Zhang L. Transdermal delivery of insulin in mice by using lecithin vesicles as a carrier. Drug Delivery 2000; 7:113-116.

[142] Vrhovnik K, Kristl J, Sentjurc M, Smid-Korbar J. Influence of liposome bilayer fluidity on the transport of encapsulated substances into the skin, studied by EPR. Pharmaceutical Research 1998; 15:525-530.

[143] Egbaria K, Ramachandran C, Weiner N. Topical application of liposomally entrapped cyclosporin evaluated by *in vitro* diffusion studies with human skin. Skin Pharmacology 1991; 4:21-28.

[144] Cevc G, Schatzlein A, Richardsen H. Ultradeformable lipid vesicles can penetrate the skin and other semi-permeable barriers unfragmented. Evidence from double label CLSM experiments and direct size measurements. Biochimica et Biophysica Acta 2002; 1564:21-30.

[145] Honeywell-Nguyen PL, de Graaff A, Junginger HE, Bouwstra JA. Interaction between elastic and rigid vesicles with human skin *in vivo*. Proceedings International Symposium of Controlled Release Bioactive Materials 2000; 27:237-238.

[146] Esfand R, Tomalia DA. Poly(amidoamine) (PAMAM) dendrimer: from biomimicry to drug delivery and biomedical applications. Drug Discovery Today 2001; 6:427-436.

[147] D'Emanuele A, Attwood D. Dendrimerdrug interactions. Advanced Drug Delivery Reviews 2005; 57:2147-2162.

[148] Parekh HS. The Advance of Dendrimers - A Versatile Targeting Platform for Gene/Drug Delivery. Current Pharmaceutical Design 2007; 13:2837-2850.

[149] Niederhafner P, Šebestík J, Ježek J. Peptide dendrimers. Journal of Peptide Science 2005; 11:757-788.

[150] Cloninger MJ. Biological applications of dendrimers. Current Opinion in Chemical Biology 2002; 6:742-748.

[151] Medintz IL, Uyeda HT, Goldman ER, Mattoussi H. Quantum dot bioconjugates for imaging, labeling and sensing. Nature Materials 2005; 4:435-446.

[152] Caruthers SD, Wickline SA, Lanza GM. Nanotechnological applications in medicine. Current Opinion in Biotechnology 2007; 18:26-30.

[153] Arshady R. (1999).Microspheres, microcapsules, & liposomes. London: Citus books.

[154] Lademann J, Richter H, Teichmann A, Otberg N, Blume-Peytavi U, Luengo J, Weiss B, Schaefer UF, Lehr CM, Wepf R, Sterry W. Nanoparticles-an efficient carrier for drug delivery into the hair follicles. European Journal of Pharmaceutics and Biopharmaceutics 2007; 66:159–64.

[155] Bolzinger MA, Briançon S, Pelletier J, Chevalier Y. Penetration of drugs through skin, a complex rate-controlling membrane. Current Opinion in Colloid and Interface Science 2012; doi:10.1016/j.cocis.2012.02.001

[156] Müller RH, Radtke M, Wissing SA. Solid lipid nanoparticles (SLN) and nanostructured lipid carriers (NLC) in cosmetic and dermatological preparations. Advance Drug Delivery Reviews 2002; 54:S131-S155.

[157] Mei Z, Chen H, Weng T, Yang Y, Yang X. Solid lipid nanoparticle and microemulsion for topical delivery of triptolide. European Journal of Pharmaceutics and Biopharmaceutics 2003; 56:189-196.

[158] Liu W., Hu M., Liu W., Xue C., Xu H., Yang X. Investigation of the carbopol gel of solid lipid nanoparticles for the transdermal iontophoretic delivery of triamcinolone acetonide acetate. International Journal of Pharmaceutics 2008; 364:135-141.

[159] Ugazio E, Cavalli R, Gasco MR. Incorporation of cyclosporin A in solid lipid nanoparticles (SLN). International Journal of Pharmaceutics 2002; 241:341-344.

[160] Aditya NP, Patankar S, Madhusudhan B, Murthy RSR, Souto EB. Arthemeter-loaded lipid nanoparticles produced by modified thin-film hydration: Pharmacokinetics, toxicological and *in vivo* anti-malarial activity. European Journal of Pharmaceutical Science 2010; 40:448-455.

[161] Sanna V, Caria G, Mariani A. Effect of lipid nanoparticles containing fatty alcohols having different chain length on the ex vivo skin permeability of Econazole nitrate. Powder Technology 2010; 201:32-36.

[162] Joshi M, Patravale V. Nanostructured lipid carrier (NLC) based gel of celecoxib. International Journal of Pharmaceutics 2008; 346:124-132.

[163] Pardeike J, Müller RH. Coenzyme Q10 loaded NLCs: preparation, occlusion properties and penetration enhancement *(Cutanova Cream NanoRepair Q10)*. Pharmaceutical Technology Europe 2007; 19: 46–49.

[164] Teeranachaideekul V, Souto EB, Junyaprasert V B, Müller RH. Cetyl palmitate-based NLC for topical delivery of Coenzyme Q10-Development, physicochemical characterization and *in vitro* release studies. European Journal of Pharmaceutical Science 2007; 67:141-148.

[165] Dingler A. Feste Lipid-Nanopartikel als kolloidale Wirstoffträgersysteme zur dermalen Applikation. Institut für Pharmazie. Freie Universität, Berlin, 1998.

[166] Puglia C, Filosa R, Peduto A, de Caprariis P, Rizza L, Bonina F, Blasi P. Evaluation of alternative strategies to optimize ketorolac transdermal delivery. AAPS Pharmaceutical Science Technology 2006; 7, 1–9 (Article 64).

[167] Teeranachaideekul V, Mülle, RH, Junyaprasert VB. Encapsulation of ascorbyl palmitate in nanostructured lipid carriers (NLC)-effects of formulation parameters on physicochemical stability. International Journal of Pharmaceutics 2007; 340, 198–206.

[168] Jenning V.Solid Lipid Nanoparticles (SLN) as a Carrier System for the Dermal Application of Retinol. Free University of Berlin, Berlin, 1999.

[169] Jenning V, Gohla SH. Encapsulation of retinoids in solid lipid nanoparticles (SLN). Journal of Microencapsulation 2001; 18, 149–158.

[170] Jee JP, Lim SJ, Park JS, Kim CK. Stabilization of all-trans retinol by loading lipophilic antioxidants in solid lipid nanoparticles. European Journal of Pharmaceutics and Biopharmaceutics 2006; 63, 134–139.

[171] Tsujimoto H and Hara K. Application 21-Development of functional skincare cosmetics using biodegradable PLGA nanospheres. Nanoparticle Technology Handbook (Second Edition), 2012, pp 501-506.

[172] Patzelt A, Richter H, Knorr F, Schäfer U, Lehr CM, Dähne L, Sterry W, Lademann J. Selective folicular targeting by modification of the particle sizes. Journal of Controlled Release 2011; 150:45–8.

[173] Shim J, Seok KH, Park W, Han S, Kim J, Chang I. Transdermal delivery of mixnoxidil with block copolymer nanoparticles. Journal of Controlled Release 2004; 97:477-484.

[174] Cetin ED, Savk E, Uslu M, Eskin M, Karul A. Investigation of the inflammatory mechanisms in alopecia areata. The American Journal of Dermatopathology 2009; 31: 53-60.

[175] Zaenglein AL, Graber EM, Thiboutot DM, Strauss JS, Wolff K, Goldsmith LA, Katz SI, Gilchrest B, Paller AS, Leffell D. J., editors., Chapter 78. Acne vulgaris and acneiform eruptions. 2009. Fitzpatrick's Dermatology in General Medicine. 7e: http://www.accessmedicine.com/content.aspx?aID=2963025

[176] Gollnick H, Cunliffe W, Berson D, Dreno B, Finlay A, Leyden JJ, Shalita AR, Thiboutot D. Management of acne: a report from the global alliance to improve outcomes in acne. Journal of the American Academy of Dermatology 2003; 49, S1-S37.

[177] Bojar RA, Holland KT. Acne and Propionibacterium acnes. Clinical Dermatology 2004; 22, 375–9.

[178] Ourique AF, Pohlmann AR, Guterres SS, Beck RCR. Tretinoin-loaded nanocapsules: Preparation, physicochemical characterization, and photostability study. International Journal of Pharmaceutics 2008; 352: 1–4.

[179] Lee P, Peng S, Su C, Mi F, Chen H, Wei M, Lin HJ, Sung HW. The use of biodegradable polymeric nanoparticles in combination with a low-pressure gene gun for transdermal DNA delivery. Biomaterials 2008; 29:742-751.

[180] Santander-Ortega MJ, Stauner T, Loretz B, Ortega-Vinuesa JL, Bastos-González D, Wenz G, Schaefer UF, Lehr CM. Nanoparticles made from novel starch derivatives for transdermal drug delivery. Journal of Controlled Release 2010;141:85-92.

[181] Thote AJ, Gupta RB. Formation of nanoparticles of a hydrophilic drug using supercritical carbon dioxide and microencapsulation for sustained release. Nanomedicine:Nanotechnology 2005; 1:85-90.

[182] McCarron PA, Hall M. Incorporation of novel 1-alkylcarbonyloxymethyl prodrugs of 5-fluorouracil into poly(lactide-co-glycolide) nanoparticles. International Journal of Pharmaceutics 2008; 348:115-124.

[183] Lboutounne H, Chaulet J, Ploton C, Falson F, Pirot F. Sustained ex vivo skin antiseptic activity of chlorhexidine in poly(ε-caprolactone) nanocapsule encapsulated form and as a digluconate. Journal of Controlled Release 2002; 82:319-334.

[184] Fuchs J, Zollner TM, Kaufmann R, Podda M. Redox-modulated pathways in inflammatory skin diseases. Free Radical Bioogy and Medicine 2001; 30: 337–53.

[185] Sanfilippo AM, Barrio V, Kulp-Shorten C, Callen JP. Common pediatric and adolescent skin conditions. Journal of Pediatric and Adolescent Gynecology 2003; 16: 269-83.

[186] Schäfer-Korting M, Mehnert W, Korting HC. Lipid nanoparticles for improved topical application of drugs for skin diseases. Advanced Drug Delivery Reviews 2007; 59, 427–443.

[187] Layton AM. Acne vulgaris and similar eruptions. Medicine 2005; 33: 44-48.

[188] Zouboulis ChC. Sebaceous glands, acne and related disorders: basic and clinical research, clinical entities and treatment. Journal of Investigative Dermatology 1997; 108: 371–98.

[189] Santos MC, Mehnert W, Schaller M, Korting HC, Gysler A, Haberland A, Schafer-Korting M. Drug targeting by solid lipid nanoparticles for dermal use. Journal of Drug Targeting 2002; 10, 489–495.

[190] Shah KA, Date AA, Joshi MD, Patravale VB. Solid lipid nanoparticles (SLN) of tretinoin: potential in topical delivery. International Journal of Pharmaceutics 2007; 345, 163–171.

[191] Cevc G, Gebauer D, Stieber J, Schatzlein A, Blume G.Ultraflexible vesicles, Transfersomes, have an extremely low pore penetration resistance and transport therapeutic amounts of insulin across the intact mammalian skin. Biochimica et Biophysica Acta 1998; 1368:201-215.

[192] Wang Z, Itoh Z, Hosaka Y, Kobayashi I, Nakano Y, Maeda I, Umeda F, Yamakawa J, Kawase M, Yag K. Novel Transdermal Drug Delivery System with Polyhydroxyalkanoate and Starburst Polyamidoamine Dendrimer. Journal of Bioscience and Bioengineering 2003; 95:541-543.

[193] Chauhan AS, Sridevi S, Chalasani KB, Jain AK, Jain SK, Jain NK, Diwan PV. Dendrimer-mediated transdermal delivery: Enhanced bioavailability of indomethacin. Journal of Controlled Release 2003; 90:335-343.

[194] Yiyun C, Na M, Tongwen X, Rongqiang F, Xueyuan W, Xiaomin W, Longping W. Transdermal delivery of nonsteroidal anti-inflammatory drugs mediated by polyamidoamine (PAMAM) dendrimer. Journal of Pharmaceutical Sciences 2007; 96:595-602.

[195] Venuganti VVK, Perumal OP. Effect of poly(amidoamine) (PAMAM) dendrimer on skin permeation of 5-fluorouracil. International Journal of Pharmaceutics 2008; 361:230-238.

[196] Cornwell PA, Barry BW. The routes of penetration of ions and 5-fluorouracil across human skin and the mechanisms of action of terpene skin penetration enhancers. International Journal of Pharmaceutics 1993; 94:189-194.

[197] Tsuji T, Sugai T. Topically administered fluorouracil in psoriasis. Archives in Dermatology 1975;105:208-212.

[198] Goette DK. Topical chemotherapy with 5-fluorouracil. A review. Journal of American Academy of Dermatology 1981; 4:633-649.

[199] Beall HD, Sloan KB. Topical delivery of 5-fluorouracil (5-FU) by 1, 3-bisalkylcarbonyl-5-FU prodrugs. International Journal of Pharmaceutics 2002; 231:43-49.

[200] Gao S, Singh J. Effect of oleic acid/ethanol and oleic acid/propylene glycol on the *in vitro* percutaneous absorption of 5-fluorouracil and tamoxifen and the macroscopic barrier property of porcine epidermis. International Journal of Pharmaceutics 1998; 165:45-55.

[201] Meidan VM, Walmsley AD, Docker MF, Irwin WJ. Ultrasound-enhanced diffusion into coupling gel during phonophoresis of 5-fluorouracil. International Journal of Pharmaceutics1999; 185:205-213.

[202] Merino V, Lopez A, Kalia YN, Guy RH. Electrorepulsion versus electroosmosis: effect of pH on the iontophoretic flux of 5-fluorouracil. Pharmaceutical Research 1999; 16:758-761.

[203] Lee WR., Shen SC, Wang KH, Hu CH, Fang JY. The effect of laser treatment on skin to enhance and control transdermal delivery of 5-fluorouracil. Journal of Pharmaceutical Science 2002; 91:1613-1626.

[204] Kuo F, Subramanian B, Kotyla T, Wilson TA, Yoganathan S, Nicolosi RJ. Nanoemulsions of an anti-oxidant synergy formulation containing gamma tocopherol have enhanced bioavailability and anti-inflammatory properties. International Journal of Pharmaceutics 2008; 363:206-213.

[205] Shakeel F, Ramadan W. Transdermal delivery of anticancer drug caffeine from water-in-oil nanoemulsions. Colloid Surface B 2010; 75:356-362.

[206] Wu H, Ramachandran C, Bielinska AU, Kingzett K, Sun R, Weiner ND, Roessler BJ. Topical transfection using plasmid DNA in a water-in-oil nanoemulsion. International Journal of Pharmaceutics 2001; 221:23-34.

[207] Subramanian B, Kuo F, Ada E, Kotyla T, Wilson T, Yoganathan S, Nicolosi R. Enhancement of anti-inflammatory property of aspirin in mice by a nano-emulsion preparation. International Immunopharmacology 2008; 8:1533-1539.

[208] Mou D, Chen H, Du D, Mao C, Wan J, Xu H, Yang J. Hydrogel-thickened nanoemulsion system for topical delivery of lipophilic drugs. International Journal of Pharmaceutics 2008; 353:270-276.

[209] Wu H., Ramachandran C, Weiner ND, Roessler BJ. Topical transport of hydrophilic compounds using water-in-oil nanoemulsions. International Journal of Pharmaceutics 2001; 220:63-75.

[210] Alves MP, Scarrone AL, Santos M, Pohlmann AR, Guterres SS. Human skin penetration and distribution of nimesulide from hydrophilic gels containing nanocarriers. International Journal of Pharmaceutics 2007; 341:215-220.

Chapter 8

Magnetic Nanoparticles: Synthesis, Surface Modifications and Application in Drug Delivery

Seyda Bucak, Banu Yavuztürk and Ali Demir Sezer

Additional information is available at the end of the chapter

1. Introduction

Magnetic nanoparticles (MNP) have gained a lot of attention in biomedical and industrial applications due to their biocompatibility, easy of surface modification and magnetic properties. Magnetic nanoparticles can be utilized in versatile ways, very similar to those of nanoparticles in general. However, the magnetic properties of these particles add a new dimension where they can be manipulated upon application of an external magnetic field. This property opens up new applications where drugs that are attached to a magnetic particle to be targeted in the body using a magnetic field. Often, targeting is achieved by attaching a molecule that recognizes another molecule that is specific to the desired target area. This often requires a chemical recognition mechanism and does not succeed as designed. Therefore, magnetic nanoparticles can offer a solution to carry drugs to the desired areas in the body.

Magnetic nanoparticles, although may contain other elements, are often iron oxides. Most common iron oxides are magnetite (Fe_3O_4), maghemite (γ-Fe_2O_3), hematite (α-Fe_2O_3) and geotite. Depending on the experimental conditions, one or more of the iron oxide phases may form. It is very important to carefully control the experimental conditions to ensure the presence of a single-phase.

Frequently encountered iron oxide nanoparticles in applications are superparamagnetic. Superparamagnetism is a form of magnetism, which is observed with small ferromagnetic or ferrimagnetic nanoparticles. In small enough nanoparticles, magnetization can randomly flip direction of nanoparticle under the influence of temperature. However, the magnetic susceptibility of superparamagnetic nanoparticles is much larger than the paramagnetic ones. Superparamagnetism occurs in nanoparticles that have single-domain, i.e. composed of a single magnetic domain. In this condition, it is considered that the magnetization of the nanoparticles is a single-giant magnetic moment, the sum of all the individual magnetic moments carried by the atoms of the nanoparticle. When an external magnetic field is applied to the superparamagnetic nanoparticles, they tend to align along the magnetic field, leading to a net magnetization. In the absence of an external magnetic field, however, the dipoles are randomly oriented and there is no net magnetization. The size dependence of magnetic properties of Fe_3O_4 nanoparticles synthesized from non-aqueous homogeneous solutions of polyols has been recently investigated (Caruntu et al., 2007). Out of the previously mentioned iron oxides, magnetite and maghemite are superparamagnetic and studies where these are used as magnetic nanoparticles will predominantly be focused in this summary.

Recent toxicity studies on magnetic nanoparticles are summarized to show the biocompatibility of these particles. Research on targeting drugs using MNPs show to be very promising and some examples are given. Hyperthermia, which is a complementary treatment for tumors that uses magnetic field to increase temperature and cause cell death, can be achieved using MNPs and some recent advances in this field are presented. At the end, a table summaries different types of MNP matrixes used for drug delivery applications.

2. Toxicity

One of the main reasons that made magnetic nanoparticles interesting for biomedical applications is their biocompatibility. As these particles are being used as drug delivery vehicles, their cytotoxicity should be investigated in detail. These particles have been shown to have low toxicity in human body by several *in vitro* and *in vivo* studies.

Ferric iron is normally transported by means of transferrin, which can bind the cell-surface localized transferrin receptor. Within the cell cytoplasm, the majority of the cytoplasmic iron pool is stored in specialized proteins called ferritin. Due to the physiological relevance of iron, MNPs were initially considered to be non-cytotoxic. MNPs can naturally be broken down resulting in the release of ferric iron which can then participate in the normal iron metabolism. It has, however, been recognized that the small size of MNPs might pose an additional hazard as the particles can reach high local concentrations within the cells and are generally more difficult to be efficiently cleared from the body (Rivera et al., 2010; Chan et al., 2002). Furthermore, free iron has been associated with the formation of free radicals, which would be particularly harmful to neural tissues already weakened by pathological processes (Winer et al., 2011).

It is important to note that in almost all the studies, the toxicity is shown to increase significantly above a certain administration level. Although high loadings (>100 µg/mL) of MNPs cause cytotoxicity, the concentrations needed for drug delivery applications are often below the toxic level for suitably coated MNPs (Karlsson et al., 2008).

Toxicity is often a result of serum proteins binding to the surface of the MNPs, altering the composition of the cell medium to which the cells are exposed (Mahmoudi et al., 2009). Coated nanoparticles induce lower toxicity not only due to the presence of the biocompatible coating, but also due to the lower adsorption sites for proteins, ions and other components in the medium (Mahmoudi et al., 2010).

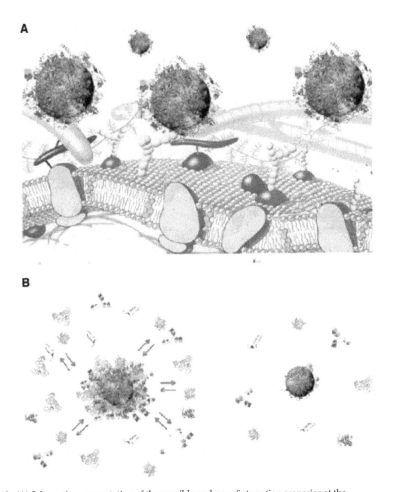

Figure 1. (A) Schematic representation of the possible exchange/interaction scenarios at the bionanointerface at the cellular level. (B) Schematic drawing of the structure of protein–nanoparticle in blood plasma confirming the existence of various protein binding (e.g. an outerweakly interacting layer of protein (full red arrows) and a hard slowly exchanging corona of proteins (right) (Mahmoudi et al., 2011)

Magnetite (Fe_3O_4) and maghemite (γ-Fe_2O_3) can show different cellular responses because of their ability to undergo oxidation/reduction reactions. In fact, magnetite has been shown to cause higher levels of oxidative DNA lesions (using comet assay) in A549 human lung epithelial cell line in the absence of decreased cell viability as compared to maghemite owing to its potential to undergo oxidation (Karlsson et al., 2009; Karlsson et al., 2008).

One of the most sensitive parameters in toxicity is the surface coating of the nanoparticles. The degree of surface coverage has been postulated to be the main parameter in cellular uptake as incomplete surface coverage was shown to promote opsonization and rapid endocytosis whereas fully coated MNPs escaped opsonization which, as a result, prolonged plasma half-life (Jung et al., 1995). The negatively charged uncoated MNPs have been shown to exhibit cytotoxicity above a certain threshold amount. Uncoated MNPs also have low solubilities which result in their precipitation in aqueous media impeding blood vessels in *in vivo* studies. In order to reduce the toxicity of MNPs, different coatings have been used. Häfeli at al. (Häfeli et al., 2009) have coated MNPs with polyethylene oxide (PEO) triblock copolymers (PEO-COOH-PEO) and found that the PEO tail block length inversely correlates with toxicity. PEO tail lengths above 2 kDa were suggested to be suitable for *in vivo* applications. Mahmoudi et al. (Mahmoudi et al., 2009) showed that uncoated particles induce greater toxicity than polyvinyl alcohol (PVA) coated magnetite particles. They also have shown that the toxicity of uncoated particles may significantly be reduced by substitution with surface-saturated uncoated particles. Coating maghemite particles with dimercaptosuccinic acid (DMSA) were shown to almost eliminate the toxicity of these particles (Auffan et al., 2006) by preventing direct contact between the particle and human dermal fibroblasts. However, in a different study using DMSA coated maghemite particles, a quantifiable model cell system is developed and showed that intercellular delivery of even moderate levels of MNPs may adversely affect cell function (Pisanic et al., 2007). Maghemite particles were coated with polyethylene imine (PEI)-g-polyethylene glycol (PEG) and their toxicity was compared with branched PEI coatings (Schweiger et al., 2011). Introduction of PEG was shown to have a shielding effect and resulted in lower toxicity Lee et al. (Lee et al., 2011) used ethylene glycol double layer stabilized maghemite nanoparticles and showed these to be non-toxic. PEG coating of magnetite particles also were shown to reduce the toxicity (Zhou et al., 2011).

When MNPs are embedded in chitosan to obtain magnetic chitosan particles, they have shown to exhibit relatively low cytotoxicity (Park et al., 2005) due to complete coverage of MNPs with chitosan.

Although dextran is a complex branched glucose that is often used in medical applications, dextran coated magnetite particles caused cell death as much as uncoated magnetite particles (Berry et al., 2003). Conversely, in a comparative study, uncoated magnetite, uncoated maghemite, dextran coated magnetite and dextran coated maghemite were investigated for cytotoxicity and neither of the samples exhibited cytotoxicity below 100 mg/mL and the only samples that demonstrated genotoxicity was the dextran coated maghemite (Singh et al., 2012). In a more extensive study, Ding et al. (Ding et al., 2010) showed that the cytotoxicity of dextran hybridized magnetite nanoparticles is cell-specific. This result suggests that the related cells should be concerned for the cytotoxicity evaluation.

A range of secondary surfactants around magnetic particles have been tested for toxicity *in vivo*. Citric and alginic acid surfactants were found to be significantly less toxic than starch, decanoic acid and PEG. This study shows the importance of optimizing surface coating to minimize toxicity (Kuznetsov et al., 1999).

In an *in vivo* study, albumin coated magnetite microspheres were shown to be well tolerated (Kuznetsov et al., 1999) Magnetite albumin microspheres bearing adriamycin (an anti-cancer drug) showed reduced toxicity to animal organs or cells compared to a single dose of adriamycin which reduces the side effects remarkably (Ma et al.,2000). However, in another study, albumin derivatized MNPs were found to cause membrane disruption, possibly due to the interaction of the protein with membrane fatty acids and phospholipids (Berry et al., 2003).

Low cytotoxicity compared to uncoated magnetite particles was evaluated of Fe_3O_4–PLLA– PEG–PLLA (PLLA: poly L-lactic acid) particles at the cellular level. They also create low genotoxic and immuntoxic at the molecular level. Acute toxicity tests showed quite a low toxicity which makes them have great potential for use in biomedical applications (Chen et al., 2012). Magnetite encapsulated in micelles of MPEG-PLGA (PLGA: poly (lactic-co-glycolic acid) exhibited no cytotoxicity (Ding et al., 2012).

More recently, particle size as opposed to coating degree has been suggested to exert chief influence on the rates of uptake by macrophages (Raynal et al., 2004). In *in vivo* studies, MNPs of 50 nm (dextran coated) and 4 μm (polystyrene coated) were used and shown to be safe for intraocular applications (Raju et al., 2011). Oral, intravenous and intraperitoneal administration of MNPs of about 20 nm did not exhibit toxicity (Zefeng et al., 2005). MNPs with 1,6 hexanediamine were shown to be safe after being administered by intracerebral or intraarterial inoculation to rats (Muldoon et al., 2005). MNPs of 40 nm were shown to be non-toxic to mES cells (Shundo et al., 2012).

Under the application of magnetic field, MNPs were shown to exhibit higher toxicities which lead to cell death (Simioni et al., 2007; Bae et al., 2011). This is the basis of a tumor treatment, hyperthermia, which will be summarized in detail in the later sections.

Despite such routine use of MNPs, the long-term effects and potential neurotoxicity have, as yet, not been evaluated extensively (Yildirimer et al., 2011).

The ability to use magnetic nanoparticles in biomedical applications due to their low cytotoxicity, stirred a big interest in the scientific community to use these particles as drug carriers. In drug delivery, there are mainly two goals; first is the targeting of the drug to the desired area in the body to reduce the side effects to other organs and second is the controlled release of the drug to avoid the classical overdosing/underdosing cycle. Magnetic nanoparticles may provide a solution to both these goals. The coating around the magnetic nanoparticle is optimized to carry and release the drug in the desired fashion, like in the case of most nanoparticles. However, the unique property of these particles is that they are magnetic, allowing being manipulated using an external magnetic field. This forms the basis of magnetic targeting where the drug-carrying magnetic particle is directed to a specific area upon application of a magnetic field.

3. Magnetic targeting

In order to investigate the magnetic targeting *in vitro*, an experimental setup that models a branched artery supplying a tumor region with parameters close to the real system has been constructed. The targeting of the particles was achieved and found to be dependent on the magnetic volume force in the branch point (Gitter et al., 2011). Using the same set-up, a novel quantitative targeting map that combines magnetic volume forces at characteristic points, the magnet position and quantitative data was constructed. Up to 97% of the nanoparticles were successfully targeted into the chosen branch (Gitter et al., 2011).

A device for magnetically targeted drug delivery system (MT-DDS), which can allow to navigate and to accumulate the drug at the local diseased part inside the body by controlling to magnetic field strength and/or gradient generated by the superconducting magnets was developed. Mn-Zn ferrite particles are injected to an experimental apparatus as a vein model of the Y-shaped glass tubes using multiple bulk superconductor magnets. This is a basic technology for magnetically targeted drug delivery system that provides the drug navigation in the blood vessel of the circulatory organs system, which shows the usefulness of the medicine transportation methodology for MT-DDS (Mishima et al., 2007).

To test seeding MNP in blood vessels and targeting the injected ones to these specific sites, experimental and computational models are constructed. To create strong and localized field gradients, microfluidic channels embedded with magnetic anchors were constructed using modified soft lithographic techniques to analyze the trapping process. Qualitative results from experimental investigations confirmed the legitimacy of the approach. It is demonstrated that capturing and aggregating magnetic microspheres at specified points in the vascular system is possible (Forbes et al., 2003).

Locally targeted drug delivery using two magnetic sources was theoretically modeled and experimentally demonstrated as a new method for optimizing the delivery of magnetic carriers in high concentration to specific sites in the human body. Experimental results have demonstrated that capturing superparamagnetic beads of both micrometer and sub-micrometer diameter at reasonably high concentrations is possible in flow conditions consistent with the dimensions and flow velocity occurring in the coronary artery in the human body. The same experiments performed with non-magnetic mesh resulted in no significant capture, indicating that the implant is responsible for providing the necessary magnetic field gradients and forces to capture the injected beads (Yellen et al., 2005).

There are several *in vivo* studies on magnetic targeting. Magnetic chitosan nanoparticles, were successfully targeted to tumor tissue for photodynamic therapy, resulting in low accumulation in skin and hepatic tissue (Sun et al., 2009).

Magnetic carbon nanotubes (MNT) with a layer of magnetite nanoparticles on their inner surface were prepared where the chemotherapeutic agents were incorporated into the pores. By using an externally placed magnet to guide the drug matrix to the regional lymph nodes, the MNTs are shown to be retained in the draining targeted lymph node for several days and continuously release chemotherapeutic drugs (Yang et al., 2008).

In an *in vitro* study, magnetic poly(ethyl-2-cyanoacrylate) (PECA) nanoparticles containing anti-cancer drugs were shown to release drug and have magnetic mobility under external magnetic field (Yang et al., 2006).

Intra-caroid administration of polyethyleneimine (PEI) modified magnetic nanoparticles in conjunction with magnetic targeting resulted in 30 fold increase in tumor entrapment of particles compared to that seen with intravenous administration (Chertok et al., 2010).

Magnetite-dextan composite particles were employed to deliver mitoxantrone *in vivo*. Mitoxantrone concentration in tumor tissue was found to be always significantly higher with magnetic targeting and the plasma iron concentrations fell after the application of the magnet, indicating the effectiveness of magnetic targeting (Krukemeyer et al., 2012).

In another study, mitoxantrone was bound to superparamagnetic Fe_3O_4-nanoparticles and the drug loaded nanoparticles were given through the femoral artery close to the tumor. The magnetic nanoparticles were attracted to the tumors by a focused external magnetic field during the application. Results from HPLC-biodistribution experiments showed that magnetic drug targeting allows to enrich the therapeutic agent up to 50 times higher in the desired body compartment (i.e. the tumor region) compared to the commonly used systemic application (Alexiou et al., 2011).

Magnetic nanoparticle seeds composed of magnetite carboxyl modified polydivinylbenzene and containing magnetite were studied *in vitro* for use as an implant in implant assisted-magnetic drug targeting (IA-MDT). In the presence of a 70mT external magnetic field, the MNP seeds were captured first from a fluid stream passing through a 70% porous polymer scaff old that was designed to mimic capillary tissue. This is then used to capture magnetic drug carrier particles (MDCPs) with the same magnetic field (Mangual et al., 2011).

Poly-[aniline-co-N-(1-one-butyric acid) aniline] (SPAnH) coated Fe_3O_4 particles with 1,3-bis(2-chloroethyl)-1-nitrosourea (BCNU). Bound-BCNU-3 could be concentrated at targeted sites *in vitro* and *in vivo* using an externally applied magnet. When applied to brain tumors, magnetic targeting was found to increase the concentration and retention of bound-BCNU-3 (Hua et al., 2011).

The accumulation of superparamagnetic nanoparticles with starch coating in gliosarcomas were enhanced by magnetic targeting and quantified by MR imaging (Chertok et al., 2008).

PEG-modified cross linked starch coated magnetite particles for magnetic targeting studies *in vivo*. Selective, enhanced brain tumor targeting of intravenously administered PEG-MNPs was confirmed in a 9L-glioma rat model. Tumor targeting results, were promising and warranted both the further development of drug-loaded PEG-MNPs and concurrent optimization of the magnetic targeting strategy utilized (Cole et al., 2011).

Super high-magnetization nanocarriers (SHMNCs) comprising of a magnetic Fe_3O_4 (SHMNPs) core and a shell of aqueous stable self-doped poly[N-(1-onebutyric acid))aniline (SPAnH), which have a high drug loading capacity (27.1 wt%) of doxorubicin (DOX) were prepared. These nanocarriers enhanced the drug's thermal stability and maximized the efficiency with which it is delivered by magnetic targeting therapy to MGH-U1 bladder cancer cells, in part by avoiding the effects of p-glycoprotein (P-gp) pumps to enhance the intracellular concentration of DOX (Hua et al., 2011).

Magnetic particles are also targeted to tumor area so tumors can be imaged. Iron oxides particles are often used as contrast agents for MRI. In fact, magnetite is an FDA approved contrast agent. In this summary, magnetic particles used for MRI will not be covered as the focus of this study is to make a comprehensive summary on magnetic drug delivery.

As seen in the abovementioned studies, magnetic targeting is an efficient way to target drugs to the desired area, commonly to tumors. However, in some studies along with magnetic targeting, targeting ligands are also used. In the absence of magnetic targeting, targeting is achieved using ligands on drug carriers that specifically bind to receptors in the targeted area. A common ligand used for this purpose is folate (or folic acid). Folate has a high affinity for the folate receptor protein which is commonly expressed on the surface of many human cancers. If folate is tagged to a drug carrying nanoparticle, the folate binds to the folate receptor on the surface of cancer cell and the conjugate is uptaken via endocytosis, completing the targeted drug delivery. A schematic representation of a magnetic particle with targeting ligands is shown in Figure 2.

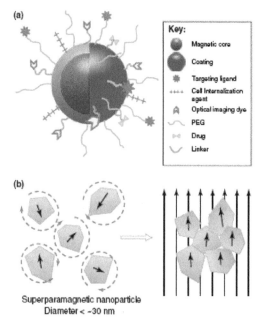

Figure 2. (a) Schematic representation of the "core–shell" structure of MNPs and multi-functional surface decoration. MNPs consist of a magnetic iron oxide core coated with a biocompatible material (e.g. polysaccharide, lipid, protein, small silane linkers, etc.). Functional groups on the surface of coatings are often used to link ligands for molecular targeting, cellular internalization, optical imaging, enhanced plasma residence and/or therapy. The variety of moieties that decorate the MNP surface imparts the nanoparticle with its multi-functional, theranostic character. (b) Illustration of superparamagnetic MNP response to applied magnetic fields. MNPs comprise rotating crystals that align with the direction of an applied magnetic field. Crystal reorientation provides the high magnetic

susceptibility and saturation magnetization observed for this material. The circular dashed lines around the superparamagnetic nanoparticles on the left illustrate the randomization of their orientation, due to temperature effects, in the absence of a magnetic field. (Cole et al.2011).

Magnetic nanocarriers were synthesized based on superparamagnetic iron oxide particles with biocompatible Pluronic F127 and poly(dl-lactic acid) (F127-PLA) copolymer chemically conjugated with folic acid (FA), carrying DOX. Magnetic particles were guided to targeted site by the aid of external magnetic field, and correspondingly the therapeutic efficacy of anti-tumor drug can be improved. These qualitative results were carried out with simply statistical analysis, which suggested that the dual targeting mechanisms can lead to better therapeutic results (Huang et al., 2012).

Superparamagnetic iron oxide nanocrystals and DOX are co-encapsulated into PLGA/polymeric liposome core–shell nanocarriers withcholesterol with or without folate. The folate-targeting DOX loaded magnetic core–shell nanocarriers were shown to have better targeting effect to the Hela cells *in vitro* than their non-folate targeting counterparts (Wang et al., 2012).

Thermosensitive magnetic liposomes with DPPC:cholesterol:DSPE-PEG2000:DSPE-PEG2000-Folate (DPPC: Dipalmitoylphosphatidylcholine; DSPE: 1,2-distearoyl-sn-glycero-3-phosphoethanolamine) at 80:20:4.5:0.5 molar ratio were prepared containing DOX. This carrier, when physically targeted to tumor cells in culture by a permanent magnetic field yielded a substantial increase in cellular uptake of DOX as compared to Caelyx® (a commercially available liposomal doxorubicin preparation), non-magnetic folate-targeted liposomes (FolDox) and free DOX in folate receptor expressing tumor cell lines (KB and HeLa cells) (Pradhan et al., 2010).

Magnetic nanoparticles with mesoporous core-shell structure of silica were prepared and successfully modified with a fluorescent polymer chain as a labeling segment and folic acid as the cancer targeting moiety and loaded with a drug for directional release. The drug carrier was shown to be able to drill into the cell membranes and obtain a sustained release of the anticancer drug into the cytoplasm. The *in vitro* cellular uptake of the drug demonstrated that the drug-loaded nanocomposites could effectively target the tumor cells (Chen et al., 2010).

Nanoparticles of Fe_3O_4 core with fluorescent SiO_2 shell were synthesized and grafted with hyperbranched polyglycerol (HPG-grafted $Fe_3O_4@SiO_2$ nanoparticles) conjugated with folic acid. Significant preferential uptake of the folic acid-conjugated nanoparticles by human ovarian carcinoma cells (SKOV-3) as compared to macrophages and fibroblasts were shown by *in vitro* studies (Wang et al., 2011).

Magnetite nanoparticles are decorated through the adsorption of a polymeric layer (carboxymethly chitosan) around the particle surface and are conjugated with fluorescent dye, targeting ligand, and drug molecules for improvement of target specific diagnostic and possible therapeutics applications. Acrylic acid, folic acid, particles (Fe_3O_4-CMC-AA-FA) and DOX was loaded into the shell of the MNPs and release study was carried out at different pH. The Fe_3O_4-CMC-AA-FA-DOX NPs showed a significant growth inhibition for HeLa cells in a dose dependent manner in comparison to NIH3T3 cells. This study indicates that Fe_3O_4-CMC-AA-FA is able to provide a single nanoscale construct, which is capable of tumor cell-targeting, imaging, and drug delivery functions. This is the first description of a chitosan based MNPs system possessing all of the above mentioned capabilities (Sahu et al., 2012).

Other ligands than folate have also been used for active targeting of nanoparticles. DOX on 5-carboxylfluorescein (FAM) labeled AGKGTPSLETTP peptide (A54) coupled starch-coated iron oxide nanoparticles demonstrated the specificity of DOX-loaded A54-SIONs (SION: superparamagnetic iron oxide) to BEL-7402 cells *in vitro*. The microscopy images proved that DOX-loaded A54-SIONs were successfully targeted to tumor tissue of nude mice with an external magnetic field *in vivo* (Yang et al., 2009).

Ligand-modified CPT-SAIO@SiO_2 nanocarriers were used for the delivery of an anticancer agent (encapsulated camptothecin (CPT)). It was found that the modified nanocarriers showed reasonably high drug load efficiency for CPT and a high uptake rate by cancer cells overexpressing EGFR through clathrin-mediated endocytosis. The intracellular release of the CPT molecules via an external magnetic stimulus proved to be technically successful and ensured much higher therapeutic efficacy than that obtained with the free drug (Tung et al., 2011).

Cetuximab-immuno micelles in which the anti-EGFR (Epidermal growth factor receptor) (EGFR), monoclonal antibody was linked to poly(ethylene glycol)-block-poly(ε-caprolactone) (PEG–PCL) These micelles were loaded with DOX and Fe_3O_4 superparamagnetic iron oxide. It was demonstrated that the immunomicelles inhibited cell proliferation more effectively than their nontargeting counterparts. Cetuximab-immunomicelles bind more efficiently to the cancer cells that overexpress epidermal growth factor receptor, leading to a higher quantity of superparamagnetic iron oxide and DOX being transported into these cells (Liao et al., 2011).

An anticancer drug was conjugated onto the PEGylated SPIO (SPIO: superparamagnetic iron oxide) nanocarriers via pH-sensitive bonds. Tumor-targeting ligands, cyclo(Arg-Gly-Asp-D-Phe-Cys) (c(RGDfC)) peptides, and PET 64Cu chelators, macrocyclic 1,4,7-triazacyclononane-N, N0, N00-triacetic acid (NOTA), were conjugated onto the distal ends of the PEG arms. cRGD-conjugated SPIO nanocarriers exhibited a higher level of cellular uptake than cRGD-free ones *in vitro*. These nanocarriers demonstrated promising properties for combined targeted anticancer drug delivery and PET/MRI dual-modality imaging of tumors (Yang et al., 2011).

Polymeric liposomes (PEG/RGD-MPLs); composed of amphiphilic polymer octadecyl-quaternized modified poly (γ-glutamic acid) (OQPGA), PEGylated OQPGA, RGD peptide grafted OQPGA and magnetic nanoparticles. It provided a possibility to responded to external permanent magnet with superparamagnetic characteristics, when was used for magnetic tissue targeting *in vivo*. The cell uptake results suggested that the PEG/RGDMPLs (with RGD and magnetic particles) exhibited more drug cellular uptake than non RGD and non magnetism carriers in MCF-7 cells (Su et al., 2012).

All these studies show that magnetic targeting is an efficient way to target drugs to tumor area. Coupled with active targeting using appropriate ligands, ligand-modified drug loaded magnetic nanoparticles, upon application of an external magnetic field provide excellent systems for effective drug targeting. Once targeting of magnetic particles to the desired area takes place, one of the most frequently used tumor treatments is hyperthermia. When magnetic nanoparticles are in the vicinity of the tumor and are subjected to an alternating magnetic field, dissipate heat and raise the temperature of the tumor, resulting in tumor cell death.

4. Hyperthermia treatment

Temperatures between 40°C and 45°C are generally being referred to as hyperthermia. Temperatures up to 42°C can render cancer cells more susceptible to the effect of irradiation and cause a certain degree of apoptosis, whereas temperatures >45°C are termed thermoablation and cause direct cell killing (necrosis) (Elsherbini et al., 2011).

In clinical applications of magnetic nanoparticle hyperthermia for cancer treatment it is very important to ensure a maximum damage to the tumor while protecting the normal tissue (Salloum et al., 2009). Although magnetic nanoparticle hyperthermia in cancer treatment holds great potential, it is severely limited by the fact that the anticipated heating distribution is difficult to control, and it leads to uneven and inadequate temperature elevation in tumor tissue. Transport of particles in tissue involves processes including extracellular transport of the carrier solution, transport of particles in the carrier solutions, and interaction between the particles and cell surface. The extracellular transport of nanoparticles in tumors is not well understood (Salloum et al., 2008).

Hyperthermia is almost always used with other forms of cancer therapy, such as radiation therapy and chemotherapy. Hyperthermia may make some cancer cells more sensitive to radiation or harm other cancer cells that radiation cannot damage. When hyperthermia and radiation therapy are combined, they are often given within an hour of each other. Hyperthermia can also enhance the effects of certain anticancer drugs (Van der Zee, 2002; Wust et al., 2002).

Numerous clinical trials have studied hyperthermia in combination with radiation therapy and/or chemotherapy. These studies have focused on the treatment of many types of cancer, including sarcoma, melanoma, and cancers of the head and neck, brain, lung, esophagus, breast, bladder, rectum, liver, appendix, cervix, and peritoneal lining (mesothelioma) (Falk et al., 2001; Feldman et al., 2003; Chang et al., 2001). Many of these studies, but not all, have shown a significant reduction in tumor size when hyperthermia is combined with other treatments. However, not all of these studies have shown increased survival in patients receiving the combined treatments (Van der Zee, 2002; Wust et al., 2002).Unique advantages of magnetic nanomaterials for hyperthermia based and combined therapies are schematically shown in Figure 3.

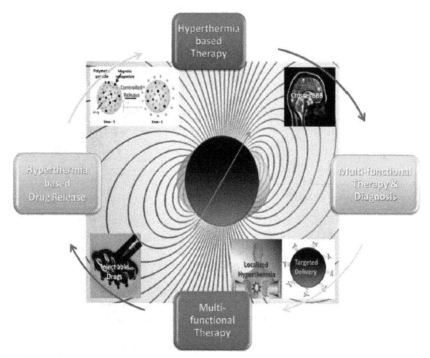

Figure 3. A schematic representation of some of the unique advantages of magnetic nanomaterials for hyperthermia-based therapy and controlled drug delivery (Kumar & Mohammad, 2011).

Magnetic losses in an alternating magnetic field to be utilized for heating arise due to different processes of magnetization reversal in the particle system: (1) hysteresis, (2) Néel or Brown relaxation, and (3) frictional losses in viscous suspensions (Hergt et al., 2006).

The magnetization of superparamagnetic nanoparticles can spontaneously change orientation under the influence of thermal energy. The magnetization oscillates between its two equilibrium positions. The typical time between two orientation changes is given by the Néel relaxation time $\tau_N = \tau_0 e^{\frac{KV}{k_B T}}$, where τ_0 is an attempt time with a value around 10^{-9}-10^{-10} seconds.

In the absence of a magnetic field, magnetic nanoparticles in solution move randomly, a movement called Brownian motion. When magnetic field is applied to magnetic nanoparticles in a fluid, magnetic nanoparticles rotate and progressively align with the magnetic field due to the torque generated by the interaction of the magnetic field with the magnetization. The time taken for a magnetic nanoparticle to align with a small external magnetic field is given by the Brown relaxation time: $\tau_B = \frac{3\eta V}{k_B T}$, where η is the solvent viscosity. The delay between the magnetic field rotation and the magnetization rotation leads to a hysteresis. The area of this hysteresis loop is dissipated in the environment as thermal energy, which used in magnetic hyperthermia.

When an alternating magnetic field (AMF) is applied to a magnetic material, due to magnetic hysteresis, an energy is dissipated called the Specific Absorption Rate (SAR) and is expressed in W/g of nanoparticles.

The SAR of a given material is given by $SAR = Af$, where A is the area of the hysteresis loop and f the alternation frequency of the magnetic field. A is expressed in J/g and is also called the "specific losses" of the material, hence SAR may also be referred to as Specific Loss Power (SLP) in some studies.

The value of SAR estimated for the same material by several research groups may vary because it depends on several parameters like the physical and chemical properties of the carrier fluid, coating materials, frequency and amplitude of applied field, size and shape of Fe_3O_4 nanoparticles (Elsherbini et al., 2011).

An optimized SAR distribution in terms of A is developed by optimizing an algorithm to inversely determine the optimum heating patterns induced by multiple nanoparticle injections (Salloum et al., 2009). For hyperthermia applications, high SAR values are required. One way to achieve this is to increase the magnetic field strength but the average magnetic field strength should be kept below 30 mT to avoid the formation of eddy currents, which can induce toxicity (Alphandéry et al., 2012).

The study of SPA as a function of particle size shows that the average size and size distribution of the nanoparticles constituting a heating agent are central parameters for the design of efficient heating nanoparticles (Goya et al., 2008).

Unfortunately a direct comparison of particle composition and size is very difficult to make. In one study multidomain ferrite particles were prepared and SAR data is compared with small magnetite particles with and without dextran coating. Large ferrite particles (200-400 nm) had considerably lower power absorption per mass than smaller particles of the same composition although both particle size distributions were relatively broad (Jordan et al., 1993). However particles with large sizes are shown not reach inner cell (Martín-Saavedra et al., 2010).

By performing calorimetry measurements with Pluronic F127 coated Fe_3O_4 monodisperse particles it was shown that at a given frequency, heating rates of superparamagnetic particles are dependent on particle size, in agreement with earlier theoretical predictions. Results also indicate a broadening of SLP with sample polydispersity as predicted (Gonzales-Weimuller et al., 2009).

Similarly, a mean particle diameter in the single domain size range (20–70 nm) combined with a small size distribution width are shown to enhance SLP (Hergt et al., 2007).

Previous studies have shown a linear relationship between tissue iron concentration and heating rate in targeted magnetic hyperthermia treatment (Pardoe et al., 2003). A critical component of arterial embolization hyperthermia (AEH) is shown to be the concentration and distribution of ferromagnetic particles in the normal hepatic parenchyma (NHP), as well as in the tumor tissue. If the distribution of particles in NHP is heterogeneous, with areas of high concentration, then unwanted areas of necrosis may result during AEH (Moroz et al., 2002).

In another study, several types of magnetic iron oxide nanoparticles representative for different preparation methods (wet chemical precipitation, grinding, bacterial synthesis, magnetic size fractionation) are used for a comparative study (Hergt et al., 2006). Commercially available very small superparamagnetic particles are claimed to be suboptimal for effective tumor heating. In contrast, superparamagnetic magnetite nanoparticles were shown to be appropriate for inducing hyperthermia with radiofrequency to Ehrlich tumors (Elsherbini et al., 2011).

No correlation was found between the magnetic moment of a single particle and SPA values for MNPs in the superparamagnetic regime. The optimum particle diameter is suggested to be near the critical size for the single- to multi-domain transition for Fe_3O_4 phase, although the relation between SPA mechanisms and incipient domain walls is still to be determined (Goya et al., 2008).

When using magnetic nanoparticles as a heating source for magnetic particle hyperthermia it is of particular interest to know if the particles are free to move in the interstitial fluid or are fixed to the tumor tissue. The immobilization state determines the relaxation behaviour of the administered particles and thus their specific heating power (Dutz et al., 2011). If the particles are not able to rotate and a temperature increase due to Brown relaxation can be neglected. An investigation showed that carboxymethyl dextran coated magnetic particles are fixed rather strongly to the tumor tissue after injection into a tumor (Dutz et al., 2011).

The effect of Néel relaxation on magnetic nanoparticles unable to move or rotate are studied and losses in linearly and circularly polarized fields are compared (De Châtel et al., 2009). In frequencies lower than the Larmor frequency, linear polarization is found to be the better source of heat power, at high frequencies (beyond the Larmor frequency) circular polarization is preferable. If Néel relaxation in isotropic sample is the dominant mechanism, the technical complications of generating a circularly polarized field in difficult geometry need not be considered.

In order to reach the required temperature with minimum particle concentration in tissue the specific heating power (SHP) of MNP should be as high as possible. The dependence of specific heating power of the size of superparamagnetic particles on the frequency and amplitude of the external alternating magnetic field is found to obey the predictions of relaxation theory. For small mean sizes (about 6 nm) the heating capability is negligibly small whereas larger particles deliver heating suitable for hyperthermia (Glöckl et al., 2006).

Data on SLP commonly reported in the literature show remarkable scattering of the orders of magnitude of 10–100W g^{-1} for a field amplitude of 10 kA m^{-1} and frequency of about 400 kHz (Hergt et al., 2006).

In summary:

1. The SLP of MNP must be considerably increased for achieving useful therapy temperatures in small tumors (at present smaller than 10mm diameter).

2.   The main practical problem with MPH is an inadequate MNP supply to the tumor. For IT injection inhomogeneity of MNP distribution in tissue may lead to local temperature differences which do not allow for differentiation of hyperthermia and thermoablation. As a result of insufficient temperature enhancement in parts of the tumor there is a risk of proliferation of surviving tumor cells.

3.   For systemic supply of MNP (e.g. antibody targeting) the target enrichment with MNP must be considerably enhanced for achieving therapy temperature. In particular, the therapy of small targets (metastases below presently diagnostic limit) seems to be a questionable hope (Hergt et al., 2007).

The specific loss power useful for hyperthermia is restricted by serious limitations of the alternating field amplitude and frequency. Large values of SLP of the order of some hundreds of W g^{-1} at 400 kHz and 10 kA m^{-1} are found for particles with mean size of about 18 nm provided that the size distribution is sufficiently narrow. A very large value of SLP of nearly 1 kW g^{-1} is found for bacterial magnetosomes having a mean diameter of the magnetite crystals of about 35 nm (Hergt et al., 2006).

MNPs modified with amino silane, which is commonly used in biomedicine, bacterial magnetosomes (BM) exhibit a better heating effect under AMF. Although both particles are found to enhance reduction in cell viability by hyperthermia using MNPs and magnetosomes of the same concentration, current of lower intensity is needed by BMs to produce a similar inhibitory effect in the tumor cell (Liu et al., 2012).

When chains of magnetosomes, which are bound to each other by a filament made of proteins, are incubated in the presence of cancer cells and exposed to an alternating magnetic field of frequency 198 kHz and average magnetic field strength of 20 or 30 mT, they produce efficient inhibition of cancer cell proliferation. This behavior is explained by a high cellular internalization, a good stability in solution and a homogenous distribution of the magnetosome chains, which enables efficient heating (Alphandéry et al., 2012).

When magnetosome chains are heated, the filament binding the magnetosomes together is denatured and individual magnetosomes are obtained which are prone to aggregation, are not stable in solution and do not produce efficient inhibition of cancer cell proliferation under application of an alternating magnetic field (Alphandéry et al., 2012).

Poly(ethylene glycol) methyl ether methacrylate and dimethacrylate with iron oxide as implantable biomaterials. It was demonstrated that the temperature of the hydrogels can be controlled by changing the AMF strength so that the gels either reached hyperthermic (42–45 °C) or thermoablative (60–63 °C) temperatures. The final temperature the hydrogel nanocomposites reach can be tailored to either one of these temperature ranges. The hydrogels were heated in an AMF, and the heating response was shown to be dependent on both iron oxide loading in the gels and the strength of the magnetic field (Meenach et al., 2010).

Cationic magnetoliposome containing both magnetic fluid and the photosensitizer-based complex (CB:ZnPc-ML) were prepared using the thin lipid film method. This result shows that the application of light and AC magnetic field together can be much more effective than the each of the two treatments applied separately (Bolfarini et al., 2012).

Combined effect of magnetic hyperthermia and chemotherapy was evaluated using drug loaded PCPG magnetoliposomes. Thermosensitive drug release took place under the influence of magnetic field and this combined therapy was shown to be more efficient than either treatment alone (Kulshrestha et al., 2012).

It was demonstrated that the temperature achieved with ferromagnetic MNPs was higher than that achieved with superparamagnetic MNPs, even with the same uptake amount into cells. This is due to heating efficiency differences between hysteresis loss and magnetic relaxation. Heat generation predominantly occurs by hysteresis loss rather than by magnetic relaxation. Heat produced by nanoparticles incorporated into cells and adsorbed on cell membranes should be critical for damaging cells, compared with heat produced from outside cells (Baba et al., 2012).

According to some, the well-known iron oxide ferro fluids become undesirable because their iron atoms are poorly distinguishable from those of hemoglobin. A suggested solution is to use mixed-ferrites (MFe_2O_4 where $M\frac{1}{4}Co$, Mn, Ni, Zn) to have a range of magnetic properties. These ferrites have attracted special attention because they save time, and because of their low inherent toxicity, ease of synthesis, physical and chemical stabilities and suitable magnetic properties (Sharifi et al., 2012).

Giri et al. studied citrate coated ferrite particles below 100 nm sizes. Saturation magnetization is found to decrease for coated materials as magnetization is proportional to the amount of weight for the same magnetic material. The coercivity is found to be sufficient for hysteresis loss heating in hyperthermia. The magnetic hysteresis data indicate that these samples (coated) exhibit sufficient hysteresis losses to obtain the temperature required for the destruction of the tumorous cells.

Ferrite particles were prepared in a chitosan matrix at varying ratios (Park et al., 2005). The time period needed for reaching hyperthermia shortened upon increase of chitosan ratio while the saturation magnetization decreases. Optimization of ferrite-chitosan ratio may be promising for hyperthermia applications.

Co-Ti ferrite nanoparticles of 6-12 nm were shown to be suitable for hyperthermia applications (Ichiyanagia et al., 2012). Zn-Gd ferrite particles are suitable but if you cap them with poly (ethylene glycol) PEG, they are not useful (Yao et al., 2009). Co ferrite particles of 7.5 nm copolymerized with poly(methacrylate) and poly(2-hydroxyethylmethacrylate) were shown to be suitable for hyperthermia (Hayashi et al., 2012). $CoFe_2O_4$ ferrite particles (ferromagnetic) were shown to be suitable for hyperthermia (Skumiel, 2006).

Examining the heating produced by nanoparticles of various materials, barium-ferrite and cobalt-ferrite are unable to produce sufficient MFH heating, that from iron-cobalt occurs at a far too rapid rate to be safe, while fcc iron-platinum, magnetite, and maghemite are all capable of producing stable controlled heating. Iron-cobalt MNPs induce temperature changes that are too large, whereas barium-ferrite and cobalt-ferrite MNPs do not provide enough heat to treat a tumor. Simulations showed that magnetite, fcc iron-platinum, and maghemite MNPs are well suited for MFH, making it possible to heat tumors above 41 °C while keeping the surrounding healthy tissue temperatures below this value (Kappiyoor et al., 2010).

The thermoreversible hydrogels (poloxamer, chitosan), which accommodated 20% w/v of the magnetic microparticles, proved to be inadequate. Alginate hydrogels, however, incorporated 10% w/v of the magnetic microparticles, and the external gelation led to strong implants localizing to the tumor periphery, whereas internal gelation failed in situ. The organogel formulations, which consisted of precipitating polymers dissolved in single organic solvents, displayed various microstructures. A 8% poly(ethylene-vinyl alcohol) in DMSO (DMSO: Dimethyl sulfoxide) containing 40% w/v of magnetic microparticles formed the most suitable implants in terms of tumor casting and heat delivery (Le Renard et al., 2010).

Cell culture experiments showed that, by adjusting the amount of magnetic microspheres MMS and the time of exposure to AMF, heat treatments of mild to very high intensities could be achieved using maghemite nanoparticles embedded in mesoporous silica matrix (Martín-Saavedra et al., 2010). The heating effect of iron containing multi walled carbon nanotubes of 10-40 nm were studied and shown to be suitable (Krupskaya et al., 2009).

Several magnetic fluids are shown to be suitable for hyperthermia application. In a comparative study, 16 commercial magnetic fluids are investigated and most suitable ones are distinguished (Kallumadil et al., 2009). Magnetite microcapsules of 20-30 μm embedded in agar phantom exhibited heat generation under an alternating magnetic field (Miyazaki et al., 2012). Magnetite nanoparticles of 10 nm in an aerogel matrix are potential hyperthermia agents where the aerogel matrix can be used for drug loading for combined therapy (Lee et al., 2012).

As can be seen from the aforementioned studies, although there is not a clear definition for an ideal magnetic material for hyperthermia, there are several materials that can be employed, depending on the particular situation. Combined therapies of drug delivery and hyperthermia are promising future outlooks in this field.

Magnetic Drug Carriers

Being potential candidates for drug delivery due to their low toxicity and ability to be targeted, magnetic particles are often coated to stabilize them against precipitation, ensure their low cytotoxicity and to carry the drug in a matrix.

In *in vivo* applications SPION particles should be coated to prevent the drug molecule conjugations and to limit interactions with non-targeted cell sides, to prevent particle agglomeration and for enhanced drug loading and release. Different approaches in SPION coating resulting different assembly of polymers are summarized in Figure 4. In polysaccharide coating and coating with copolymers, the resulted particles are found as uniformly encapsulated cores. In another coating approach, polymer molecules anchored to the magnetic particle surface resulting in a brush like structure. Liposome and micelle forming molecules results a core shell structure with magnetic particles in the core. These structures can be used in drug encapsulation with retaining hydrophobic regions. (Veiseh et al., 2010).

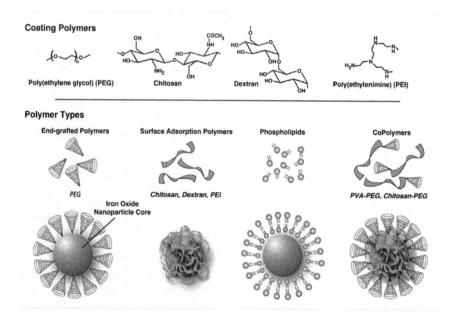

Figure 4. Illustration depicting the assembly of polymers onto the surface of magnetic nanoparticle cores (Veiseh et al., 2010).

Different particles are designed as drug delivery vehicles and a summary of these particles are given in Table 1.

Type of magnetic nanoparticle	Particle size	Coating agent	Drug	Design matrix	Drug release mechanism	Ref
Fe₃O₄	Core diameter of 10 - 15 nm Final diameter of 160 nm	chitosan/PAA multilayer	cefradine	Layer-by-Layer (LBL) The drug molecules were entrapped inside the hollow spheres through diffusion process	pH responsive	Zhang et al., 2006
Fe₃O₄	Final diameter of >1 μm	sodium carboxy methyl cellulose and chitosan	------	self-assembly shell composed of layers of carboxy methyl cellulose and chitosan around the magnetic core	------------	Cui et al., 2011
Fe₃O₄	Core diameter of 8 nm Final diameter of of 107 nm	chitosan	cefradine	cross-linking the particles with glutaraldehyde and the drug is embedded in the polymer matrix	pH responsive	Li et al., 2007
Fe₃O₄	Core diameter of 5 nm Final diameter of 1–1.5cm	Alginate / chitosan	insulin	insulin encapsulation in alginate/chitosan beads. The beads containing insulin were prepared in triplicate by extrusion method.	Magnetic field	Finotelli et al., 2010

Type of magnetic nanoparticle	Particle size	Coating agent	Drug	Design matrix	Drug release mechanism	Ref
Fe_3O_4	Final diameter of 200 nm	multiwalled carbon nanotubes (MWNTs)	doxorubicin	The MWNT-hybrid nanocomposites provided an efficient way for the extraction and enrichment of doxorubicin via π–π stacking of DOX molecules onto the polyaromatic surface of MWNTs.	pH responsive	Shen et al., 2011
Fe_3O_4	Core diameter of 3 nm	CNTs	---------	Magnetic nanoparticles adsorb on the CNT ends	------	Panczyk et al., 2010
Fe_3O_4	Core diameter of 5–10 nm. CNTs average diameter of about 30–50 nm and average length of about 100–500 nm	CdTe QDs and CNTs	-------	CNT-SPIO-CdTe nanohybrids via LBL assembly	----------	Chen et al., 2010
γ-Fe_2O_3	Core diameter of 10 nm	CNT	Diaminophenothiazine (methylene blue)	monodisperse, inherently open-ended, multi-wall CNTs loaded with magnetic iron-based nanoparticles that are encapsulated within the tube graphitic walls		Vermisoglou et al., 2011
Fe_3O_4	Core diameter of 8–12 nm mACs had a mean diameter of about 30 nm MWNTs= 40-60 nm	(mMWNTs) and magnetic-activated carbon particles (mACs)	gemcitabine (GEM)	Fe_3O_4 nanoparticles are on the outer surface of the PAA functionalized MWNTs and the drug is adsorbed on the surface .		Yang et al., 2011
$CoFe_2O_4$ nanoparticles	Core diameter of 6 nm MWCNTs with an outer diameter of 10–30 nm and an average length of 0.5–2 μm	MWCNT/cobalt ferrite ($CoFe_2O_4$) magnetic hybrids	doxorubicin	cobalt ferrite is on the outer surface of the MWCNT	pH responsive	Wu et al., 2011
γ-Fe_2O_3	Core diameter of 5 nm Final diameter of 100 nm	DNA	fluorescein	Single-stranded DNA was immobilized onto the silica network, and the magnetic particles are loaded onto the network. The complementary DNA sequence was then attached to magnetic nanoparticles.	Temperature responsive	Ruiz-Hernandez et al., 2011

Type of magnetic nanoparticle	Particle size	Coating agent	Drug	Design matrix	Drug release mechanism	Ref
Fe₃O₄	Core diameter of of 8 nm Final diameter of 150 nm	PEG-functionalized porous silica shell	doxorubi-cin	DOZ conjugated magnetite particles are coated with silica to obtain core/shell nanoparticles and the whole composite is coated with PEG	the breaking of the bonding of the drug to the carrier or the swelling and degradation of the polymer.	Chen et al., 2010
α-Fe₂O₃	Core diameter of 13 nm micron-sized mesoporous molecular sieves (with 2.9-nm pores) MCM-41 and MCM-48 powders gave mean pore sizes of 3.7 and 3.5 nm, a size between 1 and 4 μm. and hollow silica microcapsules (pores of 2.7, average diameter being around 3 μm. and 15 nm. 250-nm wall thickness	hollow silica microcapsules	--------	Magnetic particles are encapsulated inside the hollow silica microcapsules	-----------	Arruebo et al., 2006
Fe₃O₄	Core diameter of 10 nm Final diameter of 100 nm with 20 nm silica shell	SiO₂@ Fe₃O₄ core–shell NPs		Silica-magnetite nanocomposites are emulsified and self-assembly of magnetic-mesoporous heteronanorods at the interface of water-in-oil droplets takes place.		Zhang et al., 2011
Fe₃O₄	Particles between 150nm and 4.5 μm	silica,arabic acid and cross-linked polysaccharide	antibody	particles with starch derivative or polymeric arabic acid as matrix material functionalized with an antibody	---	Sieben et al., 2001
Fe₃O₄	Final diameter if 202 nm	β-cyclodextrin and pluronic polymer (F-127)	curcumin	multi-layer polymer coating around the magnetic particle and the drug is encapsulated via diffusion into polymer matrix	The initial burst of release was due to immediate dissociation of surface bound curcumin molecules that	Yallapu et al., 2011

Type of magnetic nanoparticle	Particle size	Coating agent	Drug	Design matrix	Drug release mechanism	Ref
					exist on the CD or F127 polymer matrix. The remaining sustained drug release was due to the slow release of the drug entrapped inside CD and/or F127 polymer layers.	
Fe_3O_4	Core diameter of 14.8 nm	2-hydroxypropyl-cyclodextrin (HCD) onto the gum arabic modified magnetic nanoparticles (GAMNP)	ketoprofen	polymers grafted onto magnetic particles(Multilayer polymer matrix)	drug molecules are rapidly released from HCDGAMNP, whereas some remains associated to degredation of HCD-GAMNP	Banerjee & Chen, 2009
Fe_3O_4	Final diameter of 13 nm.	(3-aminopropyl) triethoxysilane coated (APTES-MNPs) with b-cyclodextrin (β-CD).	-------	layer-by-layer	---------	Cao et al., 2009
Fe_3O_4	Core diameter of 9.2 nm	Oleic acid, sodium dodecyl benzene sulfonate SDBS, bovine serum albumin (BSA)	---	Oleic acid capped magnetic nanoparticles are embedded in the SDBS micelle and BSA adsorbs onto the micellar entity.	----	Yang et al., 2009
Fe_3O_4	Final diameter of 300 nm	poly (N-isopropylacrylamide) PNIPAAm and poly(D,L-lactide-co-glycolide) PLGA	Bovine serum albumin (BSA) and curcumin	(MLNPs) with a magnetic core and two shells made up of temperature-sensitive polymers (PNIPAAm) were encapsulated with PLGA. BSA was first loaded into PNIPAAm magnetic nanoparticles. Second, curcumin was loaded to PLGA to form the multilayer nanoparticles	Temperature responsive	Koppolu et al., 2010
Fe_3O_4	Final diameter of 150 nm	dextran	fluorescein (Fluo) or TEXAS RED® (Texas) fluorescent dye	By oxidizing Ferumoxides (FE) (suspension consisting of dextran- coated SPION) hydroxyl groups on the dextran coating are oxidized to aldehyde groups. Lysine fixable fluorescein (Fluo) or TEXAS RED® (Texas) fluorescent dye (supplied as lysine fixable dextran conjugates) was reacted with aldehyde FE and the fluorescent dye is conjugated to FE SPION (FL FE).	----	Lee et al., 2008

Type of magnetic nanoparticle	Particle size	Coating agent	Drug	Design matrix	Drug release mechanism	Ref
Fe_3O_4	Core diameter of 5 5 nm Final diameter of 4 μm,	Fe_3O_4/ PAH	fluorescei n isothiocya nate (FITC)-Dextran	layer-by-layer (LbL) assembly FITC-dextran nanoparticle is coated with PSS polyelectrolyte which contains the magnetic particles forming a magnetic shell around the particle.	Magnetic field	Hu et al., 2008
Fe_3O_4	Core diameter of 12 nm	coated with starch, dextran, PEG or MPEG	----	Polymeric networks cover a large number of continuous magnetic monodomains.	----	Huong et al., 2009
magnetic fluids Carboxyde-xtran coated DDM128 P6 (dextran–magnetite) Aminosilane coated (aminosilane–magnetite) MFL AS	DDM128 P6: core diameter of 3 nm MFL AS: core diameter of 15 nm.	dextran- or aminosilane-coated	----		-----	Jordan et al., 2006
Fe_3O_4	Core diameter of 7 nm	PVA and starch		PVA coated particles as large clusters where starch coated ones are be densely dispersed in the polymeric matrix		Voit et al., 2001
Fe_3O_4	Final diameter of 110±22 nm	starch	------	Core-shell particles	-----	Chertok et al., 2008
Fe_3O_4	coated with starch (G100) particles final diameter of 110 (±22) nm gumarabic polysaccha-ride Matrix (Gara) particles final diameter of 189nm Final diameter 225 nm after PEI addition	Polyethyleneimine (PEI)	--------	Surface modification of carboxyl-bearing Gara nano particles with PEI	--------	Chertok et al., 2010
Fe_3O_4	Final diameter of (140-190 nm)	Aminated, cross-linked starch and aminosilane coated Fe_3O_4 modified with PEG		To ensure that cross-linked starch particles was functionally similar to aminosilane coated particles, starch particles were covalently strengthened and aminated with concentrated ammonia to form aminated-precursor (DN). PEG is then linked to aminated precursors, DN and aminosilane particles with N-Hydroxysuccinimide (NHS) chemistry.		Cole et al., 2011

Type of magnetic nanoparticle	Particle size	Coating agent	Drug	Design matrix	Drug release mechanism	Ref
Fe_3O_4	Core diameter of 4-10 nm	PVA and PVA with partially exchanged carboxyl groups.	----		-----	Lee et al., 1996
Fe_3O_4	Core diameter of 10 nm	PVA matrix	---	the films of 200 mm depth and different concentrations of iron oxide particles in the PVA matrix.	----	Novakova et al., 2003
Fe_3O_4	Core diameter of 5–10 nm. Final diameter of 108-155 nm	PVA	----	core-shell, all iron-oxide particles surrounded by a layer of PVA polymer.	----	Qui & Winnik, 2000
γ-Fe_2O_3	Core diameter of 14, 19 and 43 nm. Final particles are of diameter 43 nm	PNIPAM	doxorubicin	MNP cluster is coated with PNIPAM and the nanoparticl is dehydrated. Core shell morphology is achieved with dispersion free-radical polymerization	Thermoresponsive	Purushotham et al., 2009
Fe_3O_4	core diameter of 13 nm	PNIPAM	doxorubicin	Core shell morphology by dispersion polymerization where drug loaded PNIPAM shell contains magnetite clusters.	Thermoresponsive	Purushotha m et al., 2010
Fe_3O_4	Core diameter of 11.21 nm. Final particles are of diameter less than 250 μm	PMMA	fluorescein isothiocyanate (FITC)		Thermoresponsive	Urbina et al., 2008
γ-Fe_2O_3	Core diameter of 20 nm. Final particles are of diameter 400 nm	carbon	doxorubicin	Drug is released form the surface of on-coated or partially coated magnetic particles	released from the surface of our particles at a slow rate via desorption	Ibarra et al., 2007
Fe_3O_4	Final particles are of diameter ~10–20 nm	poly[aniline-co-sodium N-(1-onebutyric acid)] aniline (SPAnNa)	1,3-bis(2-chloroethyl)-1-nitrosourea	Microcapsule nanoparticles are encapsulated during the aggregation, forming the Fe_3O_4/SPAnH nanoparticles	Ultrasound and externally applied magnetic field.	Chen et al., 2010
Fe_3O_4	Core diameter of 8 nm. Final particles of diameter 5.2 μm	PEs: poly(styrene sulfonate) (PSS, Mw~70000) and poly(allylamine hydrochloride) (PAH, Mw~50000).		Melamine formaldehyde microparticle is coated with polyelectrolytes (PE) in a layer-by-layer (LbL) assembly by solvent controlled precipitation of PE. The core is then dissolved and nanoparticles are infiltrated into the capsule core.		Gaponik et al., 2004
Fe_3O_4	Final particle diameter of 300–1300 nm	polystyrene		Similar technique to abovementioned method.		Madani et al., 2011

Type of magnetic nanoparticle	Particle size	Coating agent	Drug	Design matrix	Drug release mechanism	Ref
Fe_3O_4	Core diameter of 13 nm Final particle diameter of 3 μm	poly(sodium 4-styrenesulfonate) (PSS) and poly(allylamine hydrochloride) (PAH)	Dye	Similar technique to abovementioned method.	Magnetic heating	Katagiri et al., 2010
Fe_3O_4	Core diameter of 20 nm Final particle diameter of 2.82 μm	(PDDA/PSS)2/PDDA	Dye	Similar technique to abovementioned method.	Magnetic heating	Katagiri et al., 2011
Fe_3O_4 and γ-Fe_2O_3	Fe_3O_4 and γ-Fe_2O_3 core diameters of 9.5 and 4.3 nm, respectively	Ca alginate beads	-----	The nanoparticles were entrapped in Ca alginate beads, "egg-box like" structure of Ca alginate	------	Finotelli et al., 2005
Fe_3O_4	Particle diameter of 58 nm	NP aggragates in humic acid (HA)	---	HA adsorbs onto magnetite particles	------	Hu et al., 2010
Fe_3O_4	Final particle diameter of 7.5 nm	amino silane(3-aminopropyl triethoxysilane)	---	nearly monolayer coating of amino silane on the magnetite particle surface	---	Ma et al., 2003
Fe_3O_4	Core particle diameter of 10–15 nm Final particle diameter of 400±80 nm	poly-L-lysine hydrochloride (PLL), poly-L-glutamic acid (PGA)	DNA	layer-by-layer (LbL) assembly on polycarbonate templates with subsequent removal of these templates. In the inner surface of polycarbonate templates, first poly-L-lysine hydrochloride (PLL) and poly-L-glutamic acid (PGA) are absorbed linking by electrostatic interactions as a polyelectrolyte layer. Then, multi polyelectrolyte layers are assembled on polycarbonate membrane and Fe_3O_4 nanoparticles are linked to PLL layer as Fe_3O_4/PLL bilayers.	----------	He et al., 2008
γ-Fe_2O_3	Core diameters of 12 nm. Final particle diameter of 35 nm (PEI) and 46 nm (PEI plus PEO-PGA)	Poly(ethylene imine) and Poly(ethylene oxide)-block-poly(glutamic acid)	---	MNPs stabilized with polymers in two layer-by-layer deposition steps.	----	Thunemann et al., 2006
Fe_3O_4	Core diameter of 12 nm	aminosilane coating	---	----	---	Maier-Hauff et al., 2011

Type of magnetic nanoparticle	Particle size	Coating agent	Drug	Design matrix	Drug release mechanism	Ref
Fe₃O₄ and γ-Fe₂O₃	Core diameters of 10 nm Final particle diameter of 96 ±15 nm	poly(ethylene glycol) (PEG)	doxorubic in	one-pot synthesis of colloids of SPION-DOX-PEG particles, PEG shell reduces the access of cellular enzymes to the drug-particle linkage and thus limits and/or delays the anticancer effect.	specific release mechanism for drug delivery is enzymatic cleavage, however the PEG shell seems to reduce the access of cellular enzymes to the drug-particle linkage and thus limits and/or delays the anticancer effect.	Shkilnyy et al., 2010

Table 1. Summary of magnetic nanomaterials used in drug delivery.

5. Conclusion

In this review, uses of magnetic nanoparticles in drug delivery are summarized. Magnetic nanoparticles gained a lot of interest due to their biocompatibility, low toxicity and their ability to be manipulated upon application of a magnetic field. These special properties allow them to be utilized as drug carrier vehicles, either by direct attachment of the drug onto the particle or often by using a natural or synthetic polymer to aid carry the drug and embedding the magnetic particles in the polymer matrix. Several types of drugs and coatings have been explored as drug carriers and a very limited selection is summarized in Table 1. The ease of surface modification of these particles opens the opportunity for targeting moieties to be attached onto particle surface, facilitating the targeting. Targeting with magnetic nanoparticles is predominantly carried out upon application of an external magnetic field, which act as an external force to localize the particles in the desired areas in the body. Applying an alternating magnetic field to magnetic particles once they are in the vicinity of a tumor, results in the temperature of the medium to rise up to 42 °C, which is the temperature required for hyperthermia, a complementary treatment along with chemotherapy and radiotherapy. We believe that these fascinating particles will find further potential applications along with more success in the present ones in the very near future.

Author details

Seyda Bucak and Banu Yavuztürk
Yeditepe University, Istanbul, Turkey

Ali Demir Sezer
Marmara University, Istanbul, Turkey

6. References

Alexiou, C.; Tietze, R.; Schreiber, E.; Jurgons, R.; Richter, H.; Trahms, L.; Rahn, H.; Odenbach, S. & Lyer, S. (2011). Cancer therapy with drug loaded magnetic nanoparticles—magnetic drug targeting, Journal of Magnetism and Magnetic Materials, Vol.323, pp.1404-1407.

Alphandéry, E.; Guyot, F. & Chebbi, I. (2012). Preparation of chains of magnetosomes, isolated from Magnetospirillum magneticum strain AMB-1 magnetotactic bacteria, yielding efficient treatment of tumors using magnetic hyperthermia, International Journal of Pharmaceutics, Vol.434, pp.444-452.

Arruebo, M.; Galan, M.; Navascues, N.; Tellez, C.; Marquina, C.; Ibarra, M.R. & Santamaria, J. (2006). Development of Magnetic Nanostructured Silica-Based Materials as Potential Vectors for Drug-Delivery Applications, Chemistry of Materials, Vol.18, pp.1911-1919.

Auffan, M.; Decome, L.; Ros,e J.; Orsiere, T.; De Meo, M. & Briois, V. (2006). In vitro interactions between DMSA-coated maghemite nanoparticles and human fibroblasts: a physicochemical and cyto-genotoxical study, Environmental Science & Technology, Vol.40, pp.4367-4373.

Baba, D.; Seiko, Y.; Nakanishi, T.; Zhang, H.; Arakaki, A.; Matsunaga, T. & Osaka, T. (2012). Effect of magnetite nanoparticles on living rate of MCF-7 human breast cancer cells, Colloids Surf B Biointerfaces, Vol.95, pp.254-257.

Bae, J.-E.; Huh, M.-I.; Ryu, B.-K.; Do, J.-Y.; Jin, S.-U.; Moon, M.-J.; Jung, J.-C.; Chang, Y.; Kim, E.; Chi, S.-G.; Lee, G.-H. & Chae, K.-S. (2011). The effect of static magnetic fields on the aggregation and cytotoxicity of magnetic nanoparticles, Biomaterials, Vol.32, pp.9401-9414.

Banerjee, S.S. & Chen D.-H. (2009). Cyclodextrin-conjugated nanocarrier for magnetically guided delivery of hydrophobic drugs, Journal of Nanoparticle Research, Vol.11, pp.2071-2078.

Berry, C.C.; Wells, S.; Charles, S. & Curtis, A.S. (2003). Dextran and albumin derivatised iron oxide nanoparticles: influence on fibroblasts in vitro, Biomaterials, Vol.24, pp.455-457.

Bolfarini, G.C.; Siqueira-Moura, M.P.; Demets, G.J.F.; Morais, P.C. & Tedesco, A.C. (2012). In vitro evaluation of combined hyperthermia and photodynamic effects using magnetoliposomes loaded with cucurbit[7]uril zinc phthalocyanine complex on melanoma, Journal of Photochemistry and Photobiology B: Biology, DOI:10.1016/j.jphotobiol.2012.05.009, impress.

Cao, H.; He, J.; Deng, L. & Gao, X. (2009). Fabrication of cyclodextrin-functionalized superparamagnetic Fe$_3$O$_4$/amino-silane core–shell nanoparticles via layer-by-layer method, Applied Surface Science, Vol.255, pp.7974-7980.

Caruntu, D.; Caruntu, G. & O'Connor, C.J. (2007). Magnetic properties of variable-sized Fe3O4 nanoparticles synthesized from non-aqueous homogeneous solutions of polyols, Journal of Physics D: Applied Physics, Vol.40, pp.5801-5809.

Chan, W.C.W.; Maxwell, D.J.; Gao, X.H.; Bailey, R.E.; Han, M.Y. & Nie, S.M. (2002). Luminescent QDs for multiplexed biological detection and imaging, Current Opinion in Biotechnology, Vol.13, pp.40-46.

Chang, E.; Alexander, H.R.; Libutti, S.K.; Hurst, R.; Zhai, S.; Figg, W.D. & Bartlett, D.L. (2001). Laparoscopic continuous hyperthermic peritoneal perfusion, Journal of the American College of Surgeons, Vol.193, pp.225–229.

Chen, A.-Z.; Lin, X.-F.; Wang, S.-B.; Li, L.; Liu, Y.-G.; Ye, L. & Wang, G.-Y. (2012). Biological evaluation of Fe3O4–poly(l-lactide)–poly(ethylene glycol)–poly(l-lactide) magnetic microspheres prepared in supercritical CO2, Toxicology Letters, Vol.212, pp.75-82.

Chen, B.; Zhang, H.; Zhai, C.; Du, N.; Sun, C.; Xue, J.; Yang, D.; Huang, H.; Zhang, B.; Xiec, Q. & Wu Y. (2010). Carbon nanotube-based magnetic-fluorescent nanohybrids as highly efficient contrast agents for multimodal cellular imaging, Journal of Materials Chemistry, Vol.20, pp.9895-9902.

Chen, D.; Jiang, M.; Li, N.; Gu, H.; Xu, Q.; Ge, J.; Xia, X. & Lu, J. (2010). Modification of magnetic silica/iron oxide nanocomposites with fluorescent polymethacrylic acid for cancer targeting and drug delivery, Journal of Materials Chemistry, Vol.20, pp.6422-6429.

Chen, F.-H.; Zhang, L.-M.; Chen, Q.-T.; Zhang, Y. & Zhang, Z.-J. (2010). Synthesis of a novel magnetic drug delivery system composed of doxorubicin-conjugated Fe3O4 nanoparticle cores and a PEG-functionalized porous silica Shell, Chemical Communications, Vol.46, pp.8633-8635.

Chen, P.-Y.; Liu, H.-L.; Hua, M.-Y.; Yang, H.-W.; Huang, C.-Y.; Chu, P.-C.; Lyu, L.-A.; Tseng, I-C.; Feng, L.-Y.; Tsai, H.-C.; Chen, S.-M.; Lu, Y.-J.; Wang, J.-J.; Yen, T.-C.; Ma, Y.-H.; Wu, T.; Chen, J.-P.; Chuang, J.-I.; Shin, J.-W.; Hsueh, C. & Wei, K.-C. (2010). Novel magnetic/ultrasound focusing system enhances nanoparticle drug delivery for glioma treatment, Neuro-Oncology, Vol.12, pp.1050-1060.

Chertok, B.; David, A.E. & Yang, V.C. (2010). Polyethyleneimine-modified iron oxide nanoparticles for brain tumor drug delivery using magnetic targeting and intra-carotid administration, Biomaterials, Vol.31, pp.6317-6324.

Chertok, B.; Moffat, B.A.; David, A.E.; Yu, F.; Bergemann, C.; Ross, B.D. & Yang, V.C. (2008). Iron Oxide Nanoparticles as a Drug Delivery Vehicle for MRI Monitored Magnetic Targeting of Brain Tumors, Biomaterials, Vol.29, pp.487-496.

Cole, A.J.; David, A.E.; Wang, J.; Galbán, C.J.; Hill, H.L. & Yang, V.C. (2011). Polyethylene glycol modified, cross-linked starch-coated iron oxide nanoparticles for enhanced magnetic tumor targeting, Biomaterials, Vol.32, pp.2183-2193.

Cole, A.J.; David, A.E.; Wang, J.; Galbán, C.J. & Yang, V.C. (2011). Magnetic brain tumor targeting and biodistribution of long-circulating PEG-modified, cross-linked starch-coated iron oxide nanoparticles, Biomaterials, Vol.32, pp.6291-6301.

Cole, A.J.; Yang, V.C. & David, A.E. (2011). Cancer theranostics: the rise of targeted magnetic nanoparticles, Trends in Biotechnology, Vol. 29, pp. 323-332.

Cui, M.; Wang, F.-J.; Shao, Z.-Q.; Lu, F.-S. & Wang, W.-J. (2011). Influence of DS of CMC on morphology and performance of magnetic microcapsules, Cellulose, Vol.18, pp.1265-1271.

De Châtel, P.F.; Nándori, I.; Hakl, J.; Mészáros, S. & Vad, K. (2009). Magnetic particle hyperthermia: Néel relaxation in magnetic nanoparticles under circularly polarized field, Journal of Physics: Condensed Matter, Vol.21, pp.124202-10.

Ding, J.; Tao, K.; Li, J.; Song, S. & Sun K. (2010). Cell-specific cytotoxicity of dextran-stabilized magnetite nanoparticles, Colloids and Surfaces B: Biointerfaces, Vol.79, pp.184–190.

Ding, G.; Guo, Y.; Lv, Y.; Liu, X.; Xu, L. & Zhang, X. (2012). A double-targeted magnetic nanocarrier with potential application in hydrophobic drug delivery, Colloids and Surfaces B: Biointerfaces, Vol.91, pp.68-76.

Dutz, S.; Kettering, M.; Hilger, I.; Müller, R. & Zeisberger, M. (2011). Magnetic multicore nanoparticles for hyperthermia--influence of particle immobilization in tumor tissue on magnetic properties, Nanotechnology, Vol.22, pp.265102-09.

Elsherbini, A.A.; Saber, M.; Aggag, M.; El-Shahawy, A. & Shokier, H.A. (2011). Magnetic nanoparticle-induced hyperthermia treatment under magnetic resonance imaging, Magnetic Resonance Imaging, Vol.29, pp.272–280.

Falk, M.H. & Issels, R.D. (2001). Hyperthermia in oncology, International Journal of Hyperthermia, Vol.17, pp.1–18.

Feldman, A.L.; Libutti, S.K.; Pingpank, J.F.; Bartlett, D.L.; Beresnev, T.H.; Mavroukakis, S.M.; Steinberg, S.M.; Liewehr, D.J.; Kleiner, D.E. & Alexander, H.R. (2003). Analysis of Factors Associated with Outcome in Patients with Malignant Peritoneal Mesothelioma Undergoing Surgical Debulking and Intraperitoneal Chemotherapy, Journal of Clinical Oncology, Vol.21, pp.4560-4567.

Finotelli, P.V.; Da Silva, D.; Sola-Penna, M.; Rossi, A.M.; Farina, M.; Andrade, L.R.; Takeuchi, A.Y. & Rocha-Leao, M.H. (2010). Microcapsules of alginate/chitosan containing magnetic nanoparticles for controlled release of insulin, Colloids and Surfaces B: Biointerfaces, Vol.81, pp.206-211.

Finotelli, P.V.; Sampaio, D.A.; Morales, M.A.; Rossi, A.M. & Rocha-Leão, M.H. (2005). Ca Alginate as Scaffold for Iron Oxide Nanoparticles Synthesis, 2nd Mercosur Congress on Chemical Engineering, 4th Mercosur Congress on Process Systems Engineering, Rio de Janeiro – Brazil.

Forbes, Z.G.; Yellen, B.B.; Barbee, K.A. & Friedman, G. (2003). An Approach to Targeted Drug Delivery Based on Uniform Magnetic Fields, IEEE Transactions on Magnetics, Vol.39, pp.3372-3377.

Gaponik, N.; Radtchenko, I.L.; Sukhorukov, G.B. & Rogach, A. L. (2004). Luminescent Polymer Microcapsules Addressable by a Magnetic Field, Langmuir, Vol.20, pp.1449-1452.

Gitter, K. & Odenbach, S. (2011). Experimental investigations on a branched tube model in magnetic drug targeting, Journal of Magnetism and Magnetic Materials, Vol. 323, pp.1413-1416.

Gitter, K. & Odenbach, S. (2011). Quantitative targeting maps based on experimental investigations for a branched tube model in magnetic drug targeting, Journal of Magnetism and Magnetic Materials, Vol.323, pp.3038-3042.

Glöckl, G.; Hergt, R.; Zeisberger, M.; Dutz, S.; Nagel, S. & Weitschies, W. (2006). The effect of field parameters, nanoparticle properties and immobilization on the specific heating power in magnetic particle hyperthermia, Journal of Physics: Condensed Matter, Vol.18, pp.S2935-S2949.

Gonzales-Weimuller, M.; Zeisberger, M. & Krishnan, K.M. (2009). Size-dependant heating rates of ironoxide nanoparticles for magnetic fluid hyperthermia, Journal of Magnetism and Magnetic Materials, Vol.321, pp.1947-1950.

Goya, G.F.; Lima, E.; Jr.; Arelaro, A.D.; Torres, T.; Rechenberg, H.R.; Rossi, L.; Marquina, C. & Ibarra, M.R. (2008). Magnetic Hyperthermia with Fe3O4 Nanoparticles: The Influence of Particle Size on Energy Absorption, IEEE Transactions on Magnetics, Vol.44, pp.4444-4447.

Häfeli, U.A.; Riffle, J.S.; Carmichael-Baranauskas, A.; Harris-Shekhawat, L.; Mark, F.; Dailey, J.P. & Bardenstein, D. (2009) Cell Uptake and in vitro Toxicity of Magnetic Nanoparticles Suitable for Drug Delivery, Molecular Pharmaceutics, Vol.6, pp.1417-1428.

Hayashi, K.; Maeda, K.; Moriya, M.; Sakamoto, W. & Yogo, T. (2012). In situ synthesis of cobalt ferrite nanoparticle / polymer hybrid from a mixed Fe–Co methacrylate for magnetic hyperthermia, Journal of Magnetism and Magnetic Materials, Vol.324, pp.3158-3164.

He, Q.; Tian, Y.; Cui, Y.; Möhwald H. & Li, J. (2008). Layer-by-layer assembly of magnetic polypeptide nanotubes as a DNA carrier, Journal of Materials Chemistry, Vol.18, pp.748-754.

Hergt, R. & Dutz, S. (2007). Magnetic particle hyperthermia—biophysical limitations of a visionary tumor therapy, Journal of Magnetism and Magnetic Materials, Vol.311, pp.187-192.

Hergt, R.; Dutz, S.; Müller, R. & Zeisberger, M. (2006). Magnetic particle hyperthermia: nanoparticle magnetism and materials development for cancer therapy, Journal of Physics: Condensed Matter, Vol.18, pp.S2919-S2934.

Hu, J.-D.; Zevi, Y.; Kou, X.-M.; Xiao, J.; Wang, X.-J. & Jin, Y. (2010). Effect of dissolved organic matter on the stability of magnetite nanoparticles under different pH and ionic strength conditions, Science of the Total Environment, Vol.408, pp.3477-3489.

Hu, S.-H.; Tsai, C.-H.; Liao, C.-F.; Liu, D.-M. & Chen, S.-Y. (2008). Controlled Rupture of Magnetic Polyelectrolyte Microcapsules for Drug Delivery, Langmuir, Vol.24, pp.11811-11818.

Hua, M.-Y.; Liu, H.-L.; Yang, H.-W.; Chen, P.-Y.; Tsai, R.-Y.; Huang, C.-Y.; Tseng, I.-C.; Lyu, L.-A.; Ma, C.-C.; Tang, H.-J.; Yen, T.-C. & Wei, K.-C. (2011). The effectiveness of a magnetic nanoparticle-based delivery system for BCNU in the treatment of gliomas, Biomaterials, Vol.32, pp.516-527.

Hua, M.Y.; Yang, H.W.; Liu, H.L.; Tsai, R.Y; Pang, S.T.; Chuang, K.L.; Chang, Y.S.; Hwang, T.L.; Chang Y.H.; Chuang, H.C. & Chuang, C.K. (2011). Superhigh-magnetization nanocarrier as a doxorubicin delivery platform for magnetic targeting therapy, Biomaterials, Vol.32, pp.8999-9010.

Huang, C.; Tang, Z.; Zhou, Y.; Zhou, X.; Jin, Y.; Li, D.; Yang, Y. & Zhou, S. (2012). Magnetic micelles as a potential platform for dual targeted drug delivery in cancer therapy, International Journal of Pharmaceutics, Vol.429, pp.113-22.

Huong, N.T.; Giang, L.T.K.; Binh, N.T. & Minh, L.Q. (2009). Surface modification of iron oxide nanoparticles and their conjunction with water soluble polymers for biomedical application, Journal of Physics: Conference Series, Vol.187, pp.012046-51.

Ibarra, M.R.; Fernandez-Pacheco, R.; Valdivia, J.G.; Marquina C. & Gutierrez, M. (2007). Magnetic Nanoparticle Complexes for Drug Delivery, and Implanted Magnets for Targeting, American Institute of Physics, Vol.898, pp.99-105.

Ichiyanagia, Y.; Shigeoka, D.; Hiroki, T.; Mashino, T.; Kimura, S.; Tomitaka, A.; Ueda, K. & Takemura, Y. (2012). Study on increase in temperature of Co–Ti ferrite nanoparticles for magnetic hyperthermia treatment, Thermochimica Acta, Vol.532, pp.123–126.

Jordan, A.; Scholz, R.; Maier-Hauff, K.; van Landeghem, F.K.H.; Waldoefner, N.; Teichgraeber, U.; Pinkernelle, J.; Bruhn, H.; Neumann, F.; Thiesen, B.; von Deimling, A. & Felix, R. (2006). The effect of thermotherapy using magnetic nanoparticles on rat malignant glioma, Journal of Neuro-Oncology, Vol.78, pp.7-14.

Jordan, A.; Wust, P.; Fähling, H;. John, W.; Hinz, A. & Felix, R. (1993). Inductive heating of ferrimagnetic particles and magnetic fluids: physical evaluation of their potential for hyperthermia, International Journal of Hyperthermia, Vol.9, pp.51-68.

Jung, C.W. & Jacobs, P. (1995). Physical and chemical properties of superparamagnetic iron oxide MR contrast agents: ferumoxides, ferumoxtran, ferumoxsil, Magnetic Resonance Imaging, Vol.13, pp.661-674.

Kallumadil, M.; Tada, M.; Nakagawa, T.; Abe, M.; Southern P. & Pankhurst, Q.A. (2009). Suitability of commercial colloids for magnetic hyperthermia, Journal of Magnetism and Magnetic Materials, Vol. 321, pp. 1509-1513.

Kappiyoor, R.; Liangruksa, M.; Ganguly, R. & Puri, I.K. (2010). The effects of magnetic nanoparticle properties on magnetic fluid Hyperthermia, Journal of Applied Physics, Vol.108, pp.094702-8.

Karlsson, H.L.; Cronholm, P.; Gustafsson, J. & Moller, L. (2008). Copper oxide nanoparticles are highly toxic: a comparison between metal oxide nanoparticles and carbon nanotubes, Chemical Research in Toxicology, Vol.21, pp.1726-1732.

Karlsson, H.L.; Gustafsson, J.; Cronholm, P. & Moller L. (2009). Size dependent toxicity of metal oxide particles--a comparison between nano- and micrometer size, Toxicology Letters, Vol.188, pp. 112-118.

Katagiri, K.; Imai, Y. & Koumoto, K. (2011). Variable on-demand release function of magnetoresponsive hybrid capsules, Journal of Colloid and Interface Science, Vol.361, pp.109-114.

Katagiri, K.; Nakamura, M. & Koumoto, K. (2010). Magnetoresponsive Smart Capsules Formed with Polyelectrolytes, Lipid Bilayers and Magnetic Nanoparticles, American Chemical Society, Vol. 2, pp.768-773.

Koppolu, B.; Rahimi, M.; Nattama, S.; Wadajkar, A. & Nguyen, K.T. (2010). Development of multiple-layer polymeric particles for targeted and controlled drug delivery, Nanomedicine: Nanotechnology, Biology, and Medicine, Vol.6 pp.355-361.

Krukemeyer, M.G.; Krenn, V.; Jakobs, M. & Wagner, W. (2012). Mitoxantrone-iron oxide biodistribution in blood, tumor, spleen and liver—magnetic nanoparticles in cancer treatment, Journal of Surgical Research, Vol.175, pp.35-43.

Krupskaya, Y.; Mahn, C.; Parameswaran, A.; Taylor, A.; Kramer, K.; Hampel, S.; Leonhardt, A.; Ritschel, M.; Büchner, B. & Klingeler, R. (2009). Magnetic study of iron-containing carbonnanotubes: Feasibility for Magnetic hyperthermia, Journal of Magnetism and Magnetic Materials, Vol.321, pp.4067-4071.

Kulshrestha, P.; Gogoa, M.; Bahadur, D. & Banerjee, R. (2012). *In vitro* application of paclitaxel loaded magnetoliposomes for combined chemotherapy and hyperthermia, Colloids and Surfaces B: Biointerfaces, Vol.96, pp.1-7.

Kumar, C.S.S.R. & Mohammad, F. (2011). Magnetic nanomaterials for hyperthermia-based therapy and controlled drug delivery, Advanced Drug Delivery Reviews, Vol.63, pp.789–808.

Kuznetsov, O.A.; Brusentsov, N.A.; Kuznetsov, A.A.; Yurchenko, N.Y.; Osipov, N.E. & Bayburtskiy, F.S. (1999). Correlation of the coagulation rates and toxicity of biocompatible ferromagnetic microparticles, Journal of Magnetism and Magnetic Materials, Vol.194, pp.83-89.

Le Renard, P.-E.; Jordan, O.; Faes, A.; Petri-Fink, A.; Hofmann, H.; Rüfenacht, D.; Bosman, F.; Buchegger, F. & Doelker, E. (2010). The *in vivo* performance of magnetic particle-loaded injectable, in situ gelling, carriers for the delivery of local hyperthermia, Biomaterials, Vol.31, pp.691–705.

Lee, E.-H.; Kim, C.-Y. & Choa, Y.-H. (2012). Magnetite nanoparticles dispersed within nanoporous aerogels for hyperthermia Application, Current Applied Physics, 2012, doi:10.1016/j.cap.2012.02.017, impress.

Lee, J.; Isobe, T. & Senna, M. (1996). Magnetic properties of ultrafine magnetite particles and their slurries prepared via in-situ precipitation, Colloids and Surfaces A: Physicochemical and Engineering Aspects, Vol.109, pp.121-127.

Lee, J.-H.; Schneider, B.; K. Jordan, E.; Liu, W. & Frank, J. A. (2008). Synthesis of complexable fluorescent superparamagnetic iron oxide nanoparticles (FL SPIONs) and its cell labeling for clinical application, Advanced Material, Vol.20, pp.2512-2516.

Lee, K.-J.; An, J.-H.; Shin, J.-S.; Kim, D.-H.; Yoo, H.-S. & Cho, C.-K. (2011). Biostability of γ-Fe_2O_3 nanoparticles Evaluated using an *in vitro* cytotoxicity assays on various tumor cell lines, Current Applied Physics, Vol.11, pp.467-471.

Li, L.; Chen, D.; Zhang, Y.; Deng, Z.; Ren, X.; Meng, X.; Tang, F.; Ren, J. & Zhang, L. (2007). Magnetic and fluorescent multifunctional chitosan nanoparticles as a smart drug delivery system, Nanotechnology, Vol.18, pp.405102-08.

Liao, C.; Sun, Q.; Liang, B.; Shen, J. & Shuai, X. (2011). Targeting EGFR-overexpressing tumor cells using cetuximab-immunomicelles loaded with doxorubicin and superparamagnetic iron oxide, European Journal of Radiology, Vol.80, pp.699-705.

Liu, R.-t.; Liu, J.; Tong, J.-q.; Tang, T.; Kong, W.-C.; Wang, X.-w.; Li, Y. & Tang, J.-t. (2012). Heating effect and biocompatibility of bacterial magnetosomes as potential materials used in magnetic fluid hyperthermia, Progress in NaturalScience: Materials International, Vol.22, pp.31-39.

Ma, J.; Chen, D.; Tian, Y. & Tao, K. (2000). Toxicity of Magnetic Albumin Microspheres Bearing Adriamycin, Journal of Tongji Medical University, Vol.202, pp.261-262.

Ma, M.; Zhang, Y.; Yu, W.; Shen, H.-y.; Zhang, H.-q. & Gu, N. (2003). Preparation and characterization of magnetite nanoparticles coated by amino silane, Colloids and Surfaces A: Physicochemical and Engineering Aspects, Vol.212, pp.219-226.

Madani, M.; Sharifi-Sanjani, N. & Faridi-Majidi, R. (2011). Magnetic polystyrene nanocapsules with core–shell morphology obtained by emulsifier-free miniemulsion polymerization, Polymer Science, Ser. A, Vol.53, pp.143-148.

Mahmoudi, M.; Sant, S.; Wang, B.; Laurent, S. & Sen, T. (2011). Superparamagnetic iron oxide nanoparticles (SPIONs): Development, surface modification and applications in chemotherapy, Advanced Drug Delivery Reviews, Vol.63, pp.24–46.

Mahmoudi, M.; Simchi, A.; Imani, M.; Milani, A.S. & Stroeve, P. (2009). An *in vitro* study of bare and poly(ethylene glycol)-co-fumarate coated superparamagnetic iron oxide nanoparticles: a new toxicity identification procedure, Nanotechnology, Vol.20, pp. 225104.

Mahmoudi, M.; Simchi, A.; Imani, M.; Shokrgozar, M.A.; Milani, A.S.; Häfeli, U.O. & Stroeve, P. (2010). A new approach for the *in vitro* identification of the cytotoxicity of superparamagnetic iron oxide nanoparticles, Colloids and Surfaces B: Biointerfaces, Vol.75, pp.300–309.

Mahmoudi, M.; Simchi, A.; Milani, A.S. & Stroeve, P. (2009). Cell toxicity of superparamagnetic iron oxide nanoparticles, Journal of Colloid and Interface Science, Vol.336, pp.510-518.

Maier-Hauff, K.; Ulrich, F.; Nestler, D.; Niehoff, H.; Wust, P.; Thiesen, B.; Orawa, H.; Budach, V. & Jordan, A. (2011). Efficacy and safety of intratumoral thermotherapy using magnetic iron-oxide nanoparticles combined with external beam radiotherapy on patients with recurrent glioblastoma multiforme, Journal of Neuro-Oncology, Vol.103, pp.317-324.

Mangual, J.O.; Aviles, M.O.; Ebner, A.D. & Ritter, J.A. (2011). *In vitro* study of magnetic nanoparticles as the implant for implant assisted magnetic drug targeting, Journal of Magnetism and Magnetic Materials, Vol.323, pp.1903-1908.

Martín-Saavedra, F.M.; Ruíz-Hernández, E.; Boré, A.; Arcos, D.; Vallet-Regí, M. & Vilaboa, N. (2010). Magnetic mesoporous silica spheres for hyperthermia therapy, Acta Biomaterialia, Vol.6, pp.4522-4531.

Meenach, S.A.; Hilt, J.Z. & Anderson, K.W. (2010). Poly(ethylene glycol)-based magnetic hydrogel nanocomposites for hyperthermia cancer therapy, Acta Biomaterialia, Vol.6, pp.1039-46.

Mishima, F.; Takeda, S.; Izumi, Y. & Nishijima, S. (2007). Development of Magnetic Field Control for Magnetically Targeted Drug Delivery System Using a Superconducting Magnet, IEEE Transactions on Applied Superconductivity, Vol.17, pp.2303-2306.

Miyazaki, T.; Miyaoka, A.; Ishida, E.; Li, Z.; Kawashita, M. & Hiraoka, M. (2012). Preparation of ferromagnetic microcapsules for hyperthermia using water/oil emulsion as a reaction field, Materials Science and Engineering C, Vol.32, pp.692-696.

Moroz, P.; Pardoe, H.; Jones, S.K.; St Pierre, T.G.; Song, S. & Gray, B.N. (2002). Arterial embolization hyperthermia: hepatic iron particle distribution and its potential determination by magnetic resonance imaging, Physics in Medicine and Biology, Vol.47, pp.1591-1602.

Muldoon, L.L.; Sandor, M.; Pinkston, K.E. & Neuwelt, E.A. (2005). Imaging, distribution, and toxicity of superparamagnetic iron oxide magnetic resonance nanoparticles in the rat brain and intracerebral tumor, Neurosurgery, Vol.57, pp.785-796.

Novakova, A.A.; Lanchinskaya, V.Yu.; Volkov, A.V.; Gendler, T.S.; Kiseleva, T.Yu.; Moskvina, M.A.& Zezin, S.B. (2003). Magnetic properties of polymer nanocomposites containing iron oxide nanoparticles, Journal of Magnetism and Magnetic Materials, Vol.258, pp.354-357.

Panczyk, T.; Warzocha, T.P. & Camp, P.J. (2010). A magnetically controlled molecular nanocontainer as a drug delivery system: The effects of carbon nanotube and magnetic nanoparticle parameters from monte carlo simulations, The Journal of Physical Chemistry C, Vol.114, pp.21299-21308.

Pardoe, H.; Clark, P.R.; St. Pierre, T.G.; Moroz, P. & Jones, S.K. (2003). A magnetic resonance imaging based method for measurement of tissue iron concentration in liver arterially embolized with ferromagnetic particles designed for magnetic hyperthermia treatment of tumors, Magnetic Resonance Imaging, Vol.21, pp.483-488.

Park, J.-H.; Im, K.-H.; Lee, S.-H.; Kim, D.-H.; Lee, D.-Y.; Lee, Y.-K.; Kim, K.-M. & Kim, K.-N. (2005). Preparation and characterization of magnetic chitosan particles for hyperthermia application, Journal of Magnetism and Magnetic Materials, Vol.293, pp.328–333.

Pisanic, T.R. 2nd; Blackwell, J.D.; Shubayev, V.I.; Finones, R.R. & Jin, S. (2007). Nanotoxicity of iron oxide nanoparticle internalization in growing neurons, Biomaterials, Vol.28, pp.2572–2581.

Pradhan, P.; Giri, J.; Rieken, F.; Koch, C.; Mykhaylyk, O.; Döblinger, M.; Banerjee, R.; Bahadur, D. & Plank, C. (2010). Targeted temperature sensitive magnetic liposomes for thermo-chemotherapy, Journal of Controlled Release, Vol.142, pp.108-121.

Purushotham, S.; Chang, P.E.J.; Rumpel, H.; Kee, I.H.C.; Ng, R.T.H.; Chow, P.K.H.; Tan, C.K. & Ramanujan, R.V. (2009). Thermoresponsive core–shell magnetic nanoparticles for combined modalities of cancer Therapy, Nanotechnology, Vol.20, pp.305101-12.

Purushotham, S. & Ramanujan, R.V. (2010). Thermoresponsive magnetic composite nanomaterials for multimodal cancer therapy, Acta Biomaterialia, Vol.6, pp.502-510.

Qui, X.-p. & Winnik, F. (2000). Preparation and characterization of PVA coated magnetic nanoparticles Chinese journal of polymer science, Vol.18, pp.535-539.

Raju, H.B.; Hu, Y.; Vedula, A.; Dubovy, S.R. & Goldberg, J.L. (2011). Evaluation of magnetic micro- and nanoparticle toxicity to ocular tissues, PLoS One, Vol.6, pp.e17452-63.

Raynal, I.; Prigent, P.; Peyramaure, S.; Najid, A.; Rebuzzi, C. & Corot, C. (2004). Macrophage endocytosis of superparamagnetic iron oxide nanoparticles: mechanisms and comparison of ferumoxides and ferumoxtran-10, Investigative Radiology, Vol.39, pp.56-63.

Rivera, G.P.; Huhn, D.; del Mercato, L.L.; Sasse, D. & Parak, W.J. (2010). Nanopharmacy: Inorganic nanoscale devices as vectors and active compounds, Pharmacological Research, Vol.62, pp.115-25.,

Ruiz-Hernandez, E.; Baeza, A. & Vallet-Regi, M. (2011). Smart Drug Delivery through DNA/Magnetic Nanoparticle Gates, American Chemical Society, Vol.5, pp.1259-1266.

Saavedra, F.M.; Ruíz-Hernández, E.; Boré, A.; Arcos, D.; Vallet-Regí, M. & Vilaboa, N. (2010). Magnetic mesoporous silica spheres for hyperthermia therapy, Acta Biomaterialia, Vol.6, pp.4522-4531.

Sahu, S.K.; Maiti, S.; Pramanik, A.; Ghosh, S.K. & Pramanik, P. (2012). Controlling the thickness of polymeric shell on magnetic nanoparticles loaded with doxorubicin for targeted delivery and MRI contrast agent, Carbohydrate Polymers, Vol.87, pp.2593-2604.

Salloum, M.; Ma, R. & Zhu, L. (2008). An in-vivo experimental study of temperature elevations in animal tissue during magnetic nanoparticle hyperthermia, International Journal of Hyperthermia, Vol.24, pp.589-601.

Salloum, M.; Ma, R. & Zhu, L. (2009). Enhancement in treatment planning for magnetic nanoparticle hyperthermia: optimization of the heat absorption pattern, International Journal of Hyperthermia, Vol.25, pp.309-321.

Schweiger, C.; Pietzonka, C.; Heverhagen, J. & Kissel, T. (2011). Novel magnetic iron oxide nanoparticles coated with poly(ethylene imine)-g-poly(ethylene glycol) for potential biomedical application: Synthesis, stability, cytotoxicity and MR imaging, International Journal of Pharmaceutics Vol.408, pp.130-137.

Sharifi, I.; Shokrollahi, H. & Amiri, S. (2012). Ferrite-based magnetic nanofluids used in hyperthermia applications, Journal of Magnetism and Magnetic Materials, Vol.324, pp.903–915.

Shen, S.; Ren, J.; Chen, J.; Lu, X.; Deng, C. & Jiang, X. (2011). Development of magnetic multiwalled carbon nanotubes combined with near-infrared radiation-assisted desorption for the determination of tissue distribution of doxorubicin liposome injects in rats, Journal of Chromatography A, Vol.1218, pp. 4619-4626.

Shkilnyy, A.; Munnier, E.; Herve, K.; Souce, M.; Benoit, R.; Cohen-Jonathan, S.; Limelette, P.; Saboungi, M.-L.; Dubois, P. & Chourpa, I. (2010). Synthesis and Evaluation of Novel Biocompatible Super-paramagnetic Iron Oxide Nanoparticles as Magnetic Anticancer Drug Carrier and Fluorescence Active Label, Journal of Physical Chemistry C, Vol.114, pp.5850-5858.

Shundo, C.; Zhang, H.; Nakanishi, T. & Osaka, T. (2012). Cytotoxicity evaluation of magnetite (Fe3O4) nanoparticles in mouse embryonic stem cells, Colloids and Surfaces B: Biointerfaces, Vol.97, pp.221-225.

Sieben, S.; Bergemann, C.; LuKbbe, A.; Brockmann, B. & Rescheleit, D. (2001). Comparison of different particles and methods for magnetic isolation of circulating tumor cells, Journal of Magnetism and Magnetic Materials, Vol.225, pp.175-179.

Simioni, A.R.; Primo, F.L.; Rodrigues, M.M.A.; Lacava, Z.G.M.; Morais, P.C. & Tedesco, A.C. (2007). Preparation, Characterization and in vitro Toxicity Test of Magnetic Nanoparticle-Based Drug Delivery System to Hyperthermia of Biological Tissues, IEEE Transactions on Magnetics, Vol.43, pp.2459-2461.

Singh, N.; Jenkins, G.J.S.; Nelson, B.C.; Marquis, B.J.; Maffeis, T.G.G.; Brown, A.P.; Williams,P.M.; Wright, C.J. & Doak, S.H. (2012). The role of iron redox state in the genotoxicity of ultrafine superparamagnetic iron oxide nanoparticles, Biomaterials, Vol.33, pp.163-170.

Skumiel, A. (2006). Suitability of water based magnetic fluid with CoFe2O4 particles in hyperthermia, Journal of Magnetism and Magnetic Materials, Vol.307, pp.85-90.

Su, W.; Wang, H.; Wang, S.; Liao, Z.; Kang, S.; Peng, Y.; Han, L. & Chang, J. (2012). PEG/RGD-modified magnetic polymeric liposomes for controlled drug release and tumor cell targeting, International Journal of Pharmaceutics, Vol.426, pp.170-181.

Sun, Y.; Chen, Z.; Yang, X.; Huang, P.; Zhou, X. & Du X. (2009). Magnetic chitosan nanoparticles as a drug delivery system for targeting photodynamic therapy, Nanotechnology, Vol.20, pp.135102-10.

Thunemann, A.F.; Schutt, D.; Kaufner, L.; Pison, U. & Mohwald, H. (2006). Maghemite Nanoparticles Protectively Coated with Poly(ethylene imine) and Poly(ethylene oxide)-block-poly(glutamic acid), Langmuir, Vol.22, pp.2351-2357.

Tung, W.L.; Hu, S.H. & Liu, D.M. (2011). Synthesis of nanocarriers with remote magnetic drug release control and enhanced drug delivery for intracellular targeting of cancer cells, Acta Biomaterialia, Vol.7, pp.2873-2882.

Urbina, M.C.; Zinoveva, S.; Miller, T.; Sabliov, C.M.; Monroe, W.T. & Kumar, C.S.S.R. (2008). Investigation of Magnetic Nanoparticle-Polymer Composites for Multiple-controlled Drug Delivery, The Journal of Physical Chemistry C, Vol.112, pp.11102–11108.

Van der Zee, J. (2002). Heating the patient: a promising approach?, Annals of Oncology, Vol.13, pp.1173–1184.

Veiseh, O.; Gunn, J.W. & Zhang M. (2010). Design and fabrication of magnetic nanoparticles for targeted drug delivery and imaging, Advanced Drug Delivery Reviews, Vol.62, pp.284–304.

Vermisoglou, E.C.; Pilatos, G.; Romanos, G.E.; Devlin, E.; Kanellopoulos, N.K. & Karanikolos, G.N. (2011). Magnetic carbon nanotubes with particle-free surfaces and high drug loading capacity, Nanotechnology, vol.22, pp.355602-12.

Voit, W.; Kim, D.K.; Zapka, W.; Muhammed, M. & Rao, K.V. (2001). Magnetic behavior of coated superparamagnetic iron oxide nanoparticles in ferrofluids, Materials Research Society Symposium Proceedings, Vol. 676, pp.Y7.8.1- Y7.8.6.

Wang, H.; Wang, S.; Liao, Z.; Zhao, P.; Su, W.; Niu, R. & Chang, J. (2012). Folate-targeting magnetic core–shell nanocarriers for selective drug release and imaging, International Journal of Pharmaceutics, Vol.430, pp.342-349.

Wang, L.; Neoh, K.G.; Kang, E.-T. & Shuter, B. (2011). Multifunctional polyglycerol-grafted Fe3O4@SiO2 nanoparticles for targeting ovarian cancer cells, Biomaterials, Vol.32, pp.2166-2173.

Winer, J.L.; Liu, C.Y. & Apuzzo, M.L.J. (2011). The Use of Nanoparticles as Contrast Media in Neuroimaging: A Statement on Toxicity, World Neurosurgery, DOI:10.1016/j.wneu.2011.08.013, impress.

Wu, H.; Liu, G.; Wang, X.; Zhang, J.; Chen, Y.; Shi, J.; Yang, H.; Hua, H. & Yang, S. (2011). Solvothermal synthesis of cobalt ferrite nanoparticles loaded on multiwalled carbon nanotubes for magnetic resonance imaging and drug delivery, Acta Biomaterialia, Vol.7, pp.3496-3504.

Wust, P.; Hildebrandt, B.; Sreenivasa, G.; Rau, B.; Gellermann, J.; Riess, H.; Felix, R. & Schlag, P.M. (2002). Hyperthermia in combined treatment of cancer, The Lancet Oncology, Vol.3, pp.487–497.

Wust, P.; Hildebrandt, B.; Sreenivasa, G.; Rau, B.; Gellermann, J.; Riess, H.; Felix, R. & Schlag, P.M. (2002). Hyperthermia in combined treatment of cancer. The Lancet Oncology Vol.3, pp.487–497.

Yallapu, M.M.; Othman, S.F.; Curtis, E.T.; Gupta, B.K.; Jaggi, M. & Chauhan, S.C. (2011). Multi-functional magnetic nanoparticles for magnetic resonance imaging and cancer therapy, Biomaterials, Vol.32, pp.1890-1905.

Yang, F.; Fu, D.L.; Long, J. & Ni, Q.X. (2008). Magnetic lymphatic targeting drug delivery system using carbon nanotubes, Medical Hypotheses, Vol.70, pp.765-767.

Yang, F.; Jin, C.; Yang, D.; Jiang, Y.; Li, J.; Di, Y.; Hu, J.; Wang, C.; Ni, Q. & Fu, D. (2011). Magnetic functionalised carbon nanotubes as drug vehicles for cancer lymph node metastasis treatment, European Journal of Cancer, Vol.47, pp.1873-1882.

Yang, J.; Lee, H.; Hyung, W.; Park, S.-B. & Haam, S. (2006). Magnetic PECA nanoparticles as drug carriers for targeted delivery: Synthesis and release characteristics, Journal of Microencapsulation, Vol.23, pp.203-212.

Yang, Q.; Liang, J. & Han, H. (2009). Probing the Interaction of Magnetic Iron Oxide Nanoparticles with Bovine Serum Albumin by Spectroscopic Techniques, The Journal of Physical Chemistry B, Vol. 113, pp.10454-10458.

Yang, X.; Hong, H.; Grailer, J.J.; Rowland, I.J.; Javadi, A.; Hurley, S.A.; Xiao, Y.; Yang, Y.; Zhang, Y.; Nickles, R.J.; Cai, W.; Steeber, D.A. & Gong, S. (2011). cRGD-functionalized, DOX-conjugated, and ^{64}Cu-labeled superparamagnetic iron oxide nanoparticles for targeted anticancer drug delivery and PET/MR imaging, Biomaterials, Vol.32, pp.4151-4160.

Yang, Y.; Jiang, J.S.; Du, B.; Gan, Z.F.; Qian, M. & Zhang, P. (2009). Preparation and properties of a novel drug delivery system with both magnetic and biomolecular targeting, Journal of Materials Science: Materials in Medicine, Vol.20, pp.301-307.

Yao, A.; Ai, F.; Wang, D.; Huang, W. & Zhang, X. (2009). Synthesis, characterization and in vitro cytotoxicity of self-regulating magnetic implant material for hyperthermia application, Materials Science and Engineering C, Vol.29, pp.2525-2529.

Yellen, B.B.; Forbes, Z.G.; Halverson, D.S.; Fridman, G.; Barbee, K.A.; Chorny, M.; Levy, R. & Friedman, G. (2005). Targeted drug delivery to magnetic implants for therapeutic applications, Journal of Magnetism and Magnetic Materials, Vol.293, pp.647-654.

Yildirimer, L.; Thanh, N.T.K.; Loizidou, M. & Seifalian, A.M. (2011). Toxicological considerations of clinically applicable Nanoparticles, Nano Today, Vol.6, pp.585-607.

Zefeng, X.; Guobin, W.; Kaixiong, T.; Jianxing, L. & Yuan, T. (2005). Preparation and acute toxicology of nano-magnetic ferrofluid, Journal of Huazhong University of Science and Technology -- Medical Sciences, Vol.25, pp.59-61.

Zhang, L.; Zhang, F.; Wang, Y.-S.; Sun, Y.-L.; Dong, W.-F.; Song, J.-F.; Huo, Q.-S. & Sun, H.-B. (2011). Magnetic colloidosomes fabricated by Fe_3O_4–SiO_2 hetero-nanorods, Soft Matter, Vol.7, pp. 7375-7381.

Zhang, Y.Q.; Li, L.L.; Tang, F. & Ren, J. (2006). Controlled Drug Delivery System Based on Magnetic Hollow Spheres/Polyelectrolyte Multilayer Core–Shell Structure, Journal of Nanoscience and Nanotechnology, Vol.6, pp.3210–3214.

Zhou, H.; Tao, K.; Ding, J.; Zhang, Z.; Sun, K. & Shi, W. (2011). A general approach for providing nanoparticles water-dispersibility by grinding with poly (ethylene glycol). Colloids and Surfaces A: Physicochemical and Engineering Aspects 2011; Vol.389, pp.18-26.

Chapter 9

Targeted Nanoparticles for Cancer Therapy

M.D. Blanco, C. Teijón, R.M. Olmo and J.M. Teijón

Additional information is available at the end of the chapter

1. Introduction

The World Health Organization (WHO) estimates that 84 million people will die of cancer between 2005-2015 [1]. According using the WHO mortality database it has been estimated the total number of cancer deaths in the European Union (EU) and in 2012 is predicted to be 1283101, of which 717398 men and 565703 women [2]. The most common types of cancer that will be diagnosed are lung (C33-C34), intestine (colon and rectum; C18-C21) and prostate (C61) for men, and breast (C50), intestine (C18-C21) and lung (C33-C34) for women.

Cancer is a group of diseases which cause an abnormal and uncontrolled cell division coupled with malignant behavior such as invasion and metastasis [3]. A tumor malignant is a neoplasm characterized by a failure in the regulation of tissue growth. The abnormal proliferation of tissues is caused by mutations of genes (oncogenes that promote cell growth and reproduction, and tumor suppressor genes that inhibit cell division and survival). Typically, changes in many genes are required to transform a normal cell into a cancer cell.

It is necessary to improve our knowledge of cancer physiopathology for effective cancer therapy, which will allow discover new anti-cancer drugs and develop novel biomedical technologies. The benefits of traditional chemotherapy are limited by the toxicity associated with anticancer drugs in healthy tissues. The common features of cancer and healthy cells make it difficult to achieve pharmacoselectivity of drugs at the target site.

The development of drug delivery systems that are able to modify the biodistribution, tissue uptake and pharmacokinetics of therapeutic agents is considered the great importance in biomedical research and the pharmaceutical industry. Controlled release in drug delivery can significance enhance the therapeutic effect of a drug. A constant concentration of a drug over an extended period of time keeping the drug concentration within the optimum range, or a pulsatile drug release in response to an environmental change, can be achieved with controlled drug delivery systems [4]. In these type of systems, the drug is protected from degradation following administration, the delivery system can be administered close to the tumoral cells, the drug is released with a specific patron and the action of the drug on tumoral cells can be direct.

Nanotechnology, refers to the understanding and control of matter at dimensions between approximately 1 and 100 nanometers in at least one dimension. Nanomaterials have a large surface area to volume ratio and their biological and physicochemical properties, such as friction and interaction with other molecules, are distinct from equivalent materials at a larger scale. These new properties open opportunities in a wide variety of areas of technology, ranging from intelligent nanoscale materials to medicine and biology, where first nanotechnology applications have demonstrated an enormous potential [5]. Thus, the term nanomedicine has been taking shape and has been defined as the applications of nanotechnology for treatment, diagnosis, monitoring and control of biological systems by the National Institutes of Health [6]. Nanomedicine attempts to use sophisticated approaches to either kill specific cells or repair them one cell at a time, offering new possibilities towards the development of personalized medicine [7] focused on certain diseases which are currently being investigated, especially cancer.

One of the most important and hopeful tools employed in nanomedicine are nanoparticles (NPs), which are solid, colloidal particles consisting of macromolecular substances that are being developed to: improve drug bioavailability, abrogate treatment-induced drug resistance, and reduce nonspecific toxicity in the field of medicine. Depending on the method of preparation NPs can be constructed to possess different properties and release characteristics for the best delivery or encapsulation of the therapeutic agent [8]. In all these types, drugs can be absorbed onto the surface, entrapped inside, or dissolved within the matrix of the NPs [9]. One advantage of NPs is their ability to overcome various biological barriers and to localize into the target tissue. The first generation of NPs comprises passive delivery systems that, in case of cancer, reach the tumor through the fenestrations in the adjacent neovasculature [10]. The unique mechanism of driving systems to the tumor site is the nanometer size of particles, not specific recognition of the tumor or neovascular targets.

In order to optimize the therapeutic index of antitumor drugs, decreasing their toxicity to normal tissues, a second generation of nanosystems includes additional functionalities that allow for molecular recognition of the target tissue or for active or triggered release of the payload at the disease site. Thus, the presence of reactive pendant groups in NPs make easy their vectorization forward specific cell motif by binding of ligands. These include various ligands [11-13] that bind to specific target cell surface markers or surfacemarkers expressed in the disease microenvironment. Responsive systems, such as pH-sensitive polymers, are also included in this category. Hence, over the past years, efforts have been focused on the development of nanomedicines such as NPs, liposomes, micelles or dendrimers for the specific delivery of anticancer drugs to tumor tissues [14].

2. Physiological characteristics of solid tumors

Tumors are characterized by poorly differentiated, highly chaotic arrangement of vessel which have endothelial cell-cell junctions and discontinuous basement membrane. Angiogenesis is not only a prerequisite for the transformation from a small, often dormant cluster of cancer cells to a solid tumor, but is also required for the spread of tumor. Microvascular network is absolutely essential for the development of solid tumors. Once a tumor cell cluster, whether in its initial stage as a primary tumor or in later stages when forming metastases, induces an angiogenic switch, its vasculature and microenvironment changes dramatically, and abnormal cellular organization, vessel structure, and physiology function develops (Figure 1). Angiogenesis is defined as the formation of new blood vessels from existing ones. For solid tumors of 1-2 mm^3, oxygen and nutrients can reach the center of the tumor by simple diffusion. Because of their non-functional or non-existent vasculature, non-angiogenic tumors are highly dependent on their microenvironment of oxygen and the supply nutrients. When tumor reaches 2 mm^3, a state of cellular hypoxia begins, initiating angiogenesis.

Angiogenesis is regulated by a fine balance of activators and inhibitors [15]. The vascular endothelial grown factor (VEGF), also called vascular permeability factor (VPF), plays an important role in regulating the process of tumor angiogenesis. VEGF has been shown to stimulate the proliferation, migration and invasion of endothelial by interacting with a family of tyrosine kinase receptor expressed on vascular endothelium. VEGF is also known to have the ability to enhance the permeability of microvessels, favoring the rapid and reversible increases in extravasation of plasma protein in tissue [16]. In the angiogenesis process, different phases can be distinguished: Dilation of existing vessels, endothelial cell activation, migration and proliferation, hyperpermeability of postcapillary venules and vessel destabilization, basement membrane degradation by proteases such as matrix metalloproteases, cathepsines, urokinase and plasmin, endothelial cell migration, vessel formation and angiogenic remodeling [17].

The new tumor vessels formed during angiogenesis differ markedly from those of normal tissues and the neovasculatures is characterized by an irregular shape, high density, and heterogeneity, and also have different oxygenation, perfusion, pH and metabolic states. The abnormal vascular architecture plays a mayor role for an EPR (Enhanced Permeability and Retention) effect [18]. Extensive angiogenesis and hypervasculature, lack of smooth-muscle layer, pericytes, defective vascular architecture: fenestrations, no constant blood flow and direction, inefficient lymphatic drainage that leads to enhanced retention in the interstitium of tumor and slow venous return that leads to accumulation from the interstitium of tumor.

Physiological changes in blood flow within the tumors and in transport properties of tumor vessels are consequences of these vascular abnormalities. The osmotic pressure in tumors is high [19]. The interstitial compartment of tumors is significantly different to that of normal tissues. Primarily, as a result of vessel leakiness and hyperpermeability with a concomitant bulk flow of free fluid into the interstitial space that cannot be removed effectively due to a lack of functional lymphatics, due to cancer cells compress lymphatic vessels causing their collapsed. The lymphatic network transports interstitial fluid and immune cells out of normal tissue and is essential for immune function and maintenance of fluid balance in tissue interstitium. In tumor cells the vessels are compressed by solid stresses. The function of lymphatic vessels depends on their localization, when they are at the periphery of the tumor or the periphery tumor interface possesses functionality, while those within the tumor are functionality defective. VEGF factors (VEGF-C and VEGF-D) and their corresponding receptors have been identified as specific lymphangiogenesis factors in several tumors, and have been implicated in increased lymphatic metastases in numerous tumors [20].

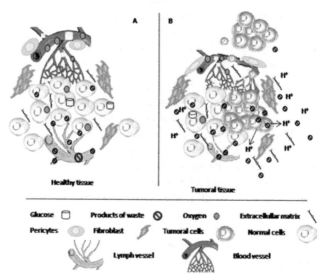

Figure 1. Differences between healthy and tumor tissues. A) Healthy tissue is characterized by a good flow in blood vessel. These vessels are supported by pericytes with a good physiological organization and structure. They provide adequate amounts of glucose and oxygen to normal cells. Collagen fibres, fibroblasts and macrophages are present in the extracellular matrix. Lymph vessels are present and allow the elimination of waste products. B) Tumoral tissue is characterized by vascular disorganization, with fenestrations and discontinuous basement membrane, that promotes the metastasis of abnormal cells to other tissues, inadequate supply of nutrients and poor lymphatic network that does not drain properly increasing the amount of waste products in these tissues and also increasing the protons concentration which decrease the physiological pH. Components of extracellular matrix (collagen fibres, fibroblasts and macrophages) in this type of tumor tissue are also increased

Leaky tumor vasculature and dysfunctional lymphatics in tumor interstitium result in undesirable accumulation of vascular contents in the tumor leading to interstitial hypertension [19]. In normal tissues the interstitial fluid pressure (IFP) is approximately 0 mm Hg, and the pressure in the capillary is around 1-3 mmHg, this gradient facilitates the transport of macromolecules. In tumor tissues the pressure gradient is contrary, consequently, interstitial hypertension results in reduce convection across the walls of tumor blood vessels. IFP tends to be higher at the center of solid tumors, diminishing toward the periphery, creating a mass flow movement of fluid away from the central region of tumor. The microvasculature pressure in tumors is also one to two orders of magnitude higher than in normal tissues.

Abnormal tumor vasculature reduces blood flow and limit delivery of oxygen throughout the tumor resulting in regions of hypoxia. There are different types of hypoxia: inadequate perfusion (ischemia), increased diffusion distance (chronic hypoxia), anemia and hypoxemia [20]. The hypoxic condition initiates signaling events that trigger the upregulation of multiple pro-angiogenic factors in the tumor lesion, another consequence, the lack of oxygen promotes an anaerobic metabolism of tumor cells and an extracellular acidosis in tumor tissues, primarily due to excessive production of lactic acid and CO_2 [20].

So, while the intracellular pH of cells within healthy tissues and tumors is similar, tumors exhibit a lower extracellular pH than normal tissues. Accordingly, although tumor pH may vary according to the tumor area, average extracellular tumor pH is between 6.0 and 7.0, whereas in normal tissues and blood the extracellular pH is around 7.4 [21-22]. Low pH and low pO_2 are intimately linked and a variety of insights now support their roles in the progression of tumor from in situ to invasive cancer [23]. The low extracellular tumor pH mostly arises from the high glycolysis rate in hypoxic cancer cells. However, ATP hydrolysis, glutaminolysis, and ketogenesis also contribute to this extracellular acidic pH.

Therefore, due to the cancer cell presents differences compared to normal cell including vascular abnormalities, interstitial pressure, oxygenation, pH, metabolic states, and abnormal lymphatics, a preferential accumulation of encapsulated drug at desired sites can be obtained either by passive or active targeting.

3. Targeted drug delivery nanoparticles

Targeted NP therapeutics have shown great potential for cancer therapy, as they provide enhanced efficacy and reduced side effects [24]. NP drug delivery can be either an active or passive process. Passive delivery refers to NP transport through leaky tumor capillary fenestrations into the tumor interstitium and cells by passive diffusion or convection [25]. Selective accumulation of NP and drug then occurs by the already mentioned characteristics of the tumor microenvironment (Figure 2).

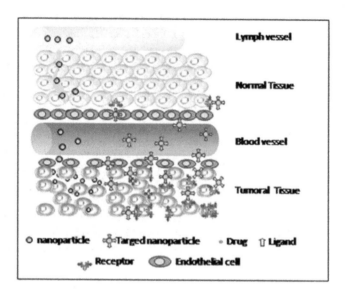

Figure 2. NPs are more able to reach tumor cells through passive targeting due to the characteristics of tumor tissue (vascular disorganization, fenestrations, discontinuous basement membrane, etc.). In normal tissues the lower amount of nanoparticles that able to reach it are removed by lymph vessels while, in tumor tissues, lymphatic network is too damaged to perform its function promoting the accumulation of nanoparticles in the tissue. The functionalized nanoparticles are internalized not only by passive targeting but also by active targeting. This active targeting is more effective in the tumor tissue due to tumor cells overexpress some receptors that allow them a better uptake of functionalized nanoparticles.

Active targeting involves drug delivery to a specific site based on molecular recognition. One such approach is to couple a ligand, such monoclonal antibodies, lectins, aptamers, folate, and peptides, to a NP so that the ligand can interact with its receptor at the target cell site (Figure 2). Depending on the type of ligand-receptor interaction, the rate of cellular internalization would differ. This is an important factor as rates of internalization could affect the accumulation of NP in tumor sites. The use of a targeting moiety also facilitates cellular uptake of the drug by receptor mediated endocytosis, which is an active process requiring a significantly lower concentration gradient across the plasma membrane than simple endocytosis. Thus there is plenty of room to improvise these systems to address the above-mentioned issues and different groups are working to improve the targeting properties of NPs and for the development of targeted therapeutics [26]. In table 1 are shown various nanocarriers evaluated to deliver therapeutic agents into cancer cells.

Ligand	Nanosystem	Drug	Cell/tumor model	Reference
AS1411 DNA apt	nucleolin /liposomes	cisplatin	MCF-7	[27]
	PEG-PLGA NPs	PTX	C6 glioma cells	[28]
Sgc8c apt	SWNTs	Dau	acute lymphoblastic leukemia T-cells (Molt-4).	[29]
Thrombin apt	Mesoporous silica NP	Dtxl	HeLA cells	[30]
EGF	SWNTs	Cisplatin	HNSCC	[31]
antiHER-2 ab: Trastuzamab	PLGA/MMT NPs	PTX	breast cancer	[32]
Tf	PLA-PEG NPs	PTX	BT4C rat glioma model	[33]
	PLGA–NPs	PTX	C6 glioma cells PC3 Prostate cancer cell	[34]
	G4 PAMAM dendrimers	Dox,	C6 glioma cells	[35]
FA	G5 PAMAM dendrimers	MTX	human KB tumor xenografts	[36]
	PEG liposomes	Dox	KB cells	[37]
	NIPA-NPAM-2AAECM	5-FU, TMX	T47D cells, HeLa cells	[38]
cRGD	PEG-PTMC micellar NPs	PTX	U87 MG cells	[39]
Antiαv integrin ab	HSA NPs	Dox	Melanoma cells	[40]

Table 1. Examples of nanocarriers used for active targeted drug delivery

3.1. Aptamers

Originally discovered in 1990, aptamers are short nucleic-acid-based single stranded ligands (DNA, RNA, oligonucleotide), whose size could vary from 20 to 80 nucleotides [27,41], that, through intramolecular interactions, fold into unique tertiary conformations capable of binding to target proteins with high affinity (K_D=10 pmol/l to 10 μmol/l) and specificity. This property makes them an attractive class of targeting molecules as they are also nonimmunogenic and exhibit remarkable stability. Aptamers can tolerate a moderate change in temperature, pH (4-9), and ionic strength, and can be processed with organic solvents without a lost of activity [13]. Aptamers are chemically synthesized and they possess additional advantages over natural antibodies [42] including a smaller size, and single-chain variable fragment antibodies what allows for more efficient penetration into biological compartments [43] and due to which they accumulate quickly within the tumor tissue. It is possible to chemically modify aptamers to facilitate covalent conjugation to nanomaterials, for example, with 50 or 30 amino or thiol groups. These properties in aptamers enable them to withstand the common production conditions encountered during NP preparation. However, due to this small size, aptamers can be cleared quickly by the kidneys. To delay their clearance, polyethylene glycol (PEG) or cholesterol can be added to aptamer NPs [44-45]. Aptamers that are internalized by cells can be used to study internalization pathways or used as drug targeting agents [24].

Traditionally, a number of compounds were assayed to isolate a ligand for the production of aptamers. However, development of a technique called 'in vitro selection' or Systematic Evolution of Ligands by Exponential Enrichment (SELEX) has allowed the rapid and selective production of aptamers. Briefly, the SELEX method starts with a random library of 1013–1016 single-stranded DNA or RNA and uses an iterative process that specifically amplifies sequences that have high binding affinity to the target molecules [46-47]. Although many complex forms of SELEX exist, there are two basic forms of SELEX (Cell-SELEX and Automated SELEX) [41].

Aptamers can be designed as targeting ligands, and can differentiate diseased cells from healthy cells, thus enabling the selective delivery of therapeutic compounds to target cells [41,47]. A large number of aptamers have been raised against cancer-associated antigens such us AS1411 aptamer for targeting nucleolin protein, which is highly expressed in the membrane of cancer cells [48-49], aptamers CPG 7909 and IMO 2055, that target Toll-like receptor 9 (TLR9), which is expressed by certain immune cells, TD05 aptamer, which was selected for the Burkitt's lymphoma Ramos cell line [47], Sgc8c aptamer which targets leukemia biomarker protein tyrosine kinase-7 (PTK7) [46,50] and can recognize target leukemia cells, DNA aptamers to leukemic lymphoid (CEM) cells [46], and fruoropyrimidine RNA aptamers which target Prostate-specific membrane antigen (PSMA) [51] for targeting prostate cancer. And also another aptamers against antigens such as pigpen [52] for targeting the tumor microvasculature, or mucin 1 (MUC1) [53] for targeting various epithelial neoplasms that upregulate MUC1, whose expression has been associated with carcinomas.

Aptamer-functionalized NPs have also been widely used for cancer cell specific drug delivery. Aptamers that were conjugated to NPs resulted in increased targeting and more efficient therapeutics, as well as more selective diagnostics. For instance, it has been synthesized NPs of poly(D,L-lactide-coglycolyde) [PLGA] and PEG triblock copolymer using aptamers as a targeting ligand for PSMA and Docetaxel (Dtxl)-encapsulated demonstrated that they bind and are taken up by LNCaP prostate ephitelial cells resulting in a significantly enhanced in vitro cellular toxicity as compared with nontargeted NP [24]. In the same way A10 aptamer is being explored for the targeted delivery of several anticancer agents, by including paclitaxel (PTX) and cisplatin in NPs [51,54]. Guo and coworkers conjugated DNA aptamers to a PEG-PLGA NP as a novel drug delivery system capable of targeting cancer cells and endothelia cells in angiogenic blood vessels [28]. In the tested C6 glioma cells, aptamer-nucleolin specific binding resulted in the cellular association of NPs and thereby enhanced the cytotoxicity of the PTX delivery. They suggested the potential of utilizing Ap-PTX-NP as therapeutic drug delivery platform for gliomas treatment [28].

Besides organic NPs, inorganic systems of Au-Ag nanorods (NRs) were synthesized to serve as a platform for binding several aptamer molecules. Thus, Au-Ag NRs have been conjugated with multiple anti-PTK7 aptamers, such as scg8 aptamer, for targeted cancer photothermal therapy [48,55]. By using Au-Ag NRs that can be conjugated around 80 aptamers, 26 times higher binding affinity was obtained compared to individual aptamer strands [48]. By functionalizing the surface of Au NPs with an RNA aptamer that binds to PSMA, NP–aptamer conjugates were used for targeted molecular computed tomography imaging and treatment of prostate cancer [56].Yin et al. reported a one-step method for the synthesis of DNA-aptamer templated fluorescent silver nanoclusters (AgNCs) [57]. The Sgc8c aptamer strands were immobilized onto AgNCs through cytosine-rich sequence, and the resulting Sgc8c-modified AgNCs showed specific targeting to CCRF-CEM cancer cell over control cells.

In addition to their ability to recognize a target molecule with high specificity, certain aptamers can also modulate the activities of proteins implicated in pathological conditions, making aptamers potentially useful as pharmaceutical agents. For instance, one of the most important success of aptamers so far has been the development of aptamers that are able to bind VEGF [58] such as Pegaptanib sodium aptamer (Macugen, Pfizer, and Eyetech). However, as aptamers are expensive to produce, it is more economical to use aptamers as targeting agents rather than as therapeutic agents. Another example is AS1411, that binds specifically to nucleolin, a bcl-2 mRNA binding protein involved in cell proliferation, which is found on the surface of many cancer cells. Once bound, the AS1411 aptamer is taken into the cancer cell, where it causes death by apoptosis [47,59].

Furthermore, antidotes for anticancer agent toxicities are of interest to regulate drug activity. Thus, aptamers can also be prepared as antidotes for anticancer drugs to modulate anticancer effects. In this way, cDNA aptamer was recently designed for inhibiting cisplatin activity. The multifunctional carrier system consisted of cisplatin as the anticancer agent, which was encapsulated within a liposomal system and conjugated to AS1411-derived aptamer. In the absence of cDNA, the targeted NP showed cell-specific targeting and an improved cytotoxicity. When de cDNA aptamer was administered, it inhibited the cytotoxic activity of cisplatin. However, the interval between the administration of cDNA and NP seemed to be critical [11,27].

3.2. Human epidermal receptor

The Human epidermal receptor (HER)-family tyrosine kinases play a central role in the proliferation, differentiation, and development of cells as they are known to mediate a cell signaling pathway for growth and proliferation in response to the binding of the growth factor ligand [60]. The family consists of four members: epidermal growth factor receptor (EGFR or HER1), HER2 (also known as ERBB2 or HER-2/neu), HER3 and HER4. Each of these receptors has an extracellular region, a single transmembrane region, and a cytoplasmic sequence containing a tyrosine kinase domain and a C-terminal tail [61].

EGFR has six known endogenous ligands: EGF, transforming growth factor-α (TGF-α), amphiregulin, betacellulin, heparin-binding EGF (HB-EGF), and epiregulin [60]. Using any of these ligands as targeting moieties offers a method for targeting the EGFR; especially

TGF-α and EGF as are the most commonly detected in humans. Ligand binding to EGFR results in activation of intracellular signaling cascades in cancer cell proliferation, apoptosis, migration, sensitivity to chemoradiation therapy, and tumor angiogenesis, and the complex is internalized for destruction and recycling [12, 62-63]. Over one-third of all solid tumors have been shown to express EGFR, and in many of these tumors, EGFR expression characterizes a more advanced disease stage [60]. The presence of EGFR corresponds directly to the metastatic capabilities in various types of cancer, such as colorectal [12]. Among the wide range of tumors that overexpress EGFR are breast, lung, colorectal, pancreatic cancers [63], glioblastomas [64], and brain cancers [65].

Hence EGF target delivery systems have been used in cancer molecular imaging diagnosis and therapy [63]. Thus, cisplatin and EGF were attached to single-wall carbon nanotubes (SWNTs) to target squamous cancer cells HNSCC which overexpress EGFR. Through Qdot luminescence and confocal microscopy, it was shown that SWNT–Qdot–EGF bioconjugates was rapidly internalized into the cancer cells, and HNSCC cells were selectively killed in vitro, while tumor growth was regressed in vivo [31]. A current cancer treatment that targets EGFR is the monoclonal antibody Cetuximab, which targets the extracellular domain of EGFR and small-molecule inhibitors of tyrosine kinase activity [66]. One study showed that boronated immunoliposomes with conjugated Fab' fragments of Cetuximab mAb delivered ~8 times more boron to EGFRpositive cells (F98EGFR) than non-targeted IgG immunoliposomes [67].

With regard to HER2, among tumor biomarkers the HER2 membrane receptor is one of the most promising targets for immunotherapy. The surface accessibility, the high level of expression in certain primary and metastatic tumors and the internalization of these antigens via receptor-mediated endocytosis [68] promote preferential intracellular accumulation of drug nanocarriers [69]. The gene encoding HER2 protein is present in normal cells as a single copy and is expressed at low levels in many normal epithelial cells. Amplified HER2 gene and its over-expressed protein product are found in many types of cancers, including breast, ovary, lung, pancreas [63,70], stomach and renal. The overexpression of HER2antigens (c-erbB-2, neu) in 20–30% of breast and ovarian cancers is correlated with a high occurrence of metastasis and angiogenesis processes, as well as with a poor prognosis [71]. The ligand binding to the extracellular domain of HERB2 causes the dimerization of the receptor and in this way the activation of many intracellular signaling proteins and physiological pathways, such as the mitogen-activated protein kinases (MAPK) pathway, phospahtidylinositol 3-kinase/AKT/mTOR pathway, and Src tyrosine kinase [61].

Thus, antibodies and antibody fragments, consisting of only the Fab binding regions, against the HER2 receptor are common examples of receptor targets. These antibodies generally exhibit strong interactions with corresponding receptors, with dissociation constants in the nanomolar range. The advantages of the antibody fragments is that they are smaller, and do not contain the Fc region of the antibody which can induce immunogenicity and antigenicity [72]. Antibody-labeled NP is one of the most coveted modes of active targeting of NPs. Blocking the activity of the upregulated receptor by binding it with a ligand, such as monoclonal antibody (mAb) represented on the nanovector, would ensure arrest of the signalling pathway(s).

Anti-Her2 mAbs (trastuzumab; Herceptin®), a humanized mAb designed to specifically antagonize HER2 function, was approved in 1998 for metastatic breast cancer overexpressing HER2 antigens [70]. Hence Herceptin® is used as a targeting moiety for various NP systems. For instance, incorporation of anti-HER2 antibodies onto the surfaces of PEGylated liposomes has indeed shown greater efficiency for drug delivery compared to non-targeted PEG-liposomes [73] and significantly higher intracellular accumulation was observed with targeted liposomes in xenografts of the HER2 overexpressing BT-474 tumors compared to MCF-7 tumors [69]. It has also been used PTX-loaded anti-HER2 immunonanoparticles (NPs-PTX-HER) which were prepared by the covalent coupling of humanized monoclonal anti-HER2 antibodies (trastuzumab, Herceptin®) to PTX-loaded poly (DL-lactic acid) NPs (NPs-PTX) for the active targeting of tumor cells that overexpress HER2 receptors [71]. NPs-PTX were thiolated and conjugated to activated anti-HER2 mAbs to obtain immunonanoparticles. The immunoreactivity and the *in vitro* efficacy of NPs-PTX-HER were tested on SKOV-3 ovarian cancer cells that overexpress HER2 antigens and it was demonstrated the greater cytotoxic effect of NPs-PTX-HER compared to other PTX formulations. Lyu and coworkers [74] used a single-chain Fv antibody (scFv23) targeting HER-2/neu to deliver tumor necrosis factor (TNF) to TNF-resistant pancreatic cancer cells and compared the cell responses to TNF alone, scFv23/TNF, herceptin, and combinations of scFv23/TNF with various chemotherapeutic agents including 5-Fluorouracil (5-FU), cisplatin, doxorubicin (Dox), gemcitabine, and etoposide. Their results indicated that delivery of TNF to HER2/neu-expressing pancreatic cancer cells using HER2/neu as a targeting molecule may be an effective therapy for pancreatic cancer especially when utilized in combination with 5-FU.

3.3. Transferrin receptor

Transferrin (Tf) (M_w=80 kDa) is the fourth most abundant serum nonheme iron-binding glycoprotein. It is synthesized by the liver and secreted to plasma, where it binds to endogenous iron, forming the iron-transferrin chelate which is an important physiological source of iron for cells in the body. It helps to transport iron to proliferating cells [75], which is required as a cofactor for DNA synthesis [76], and it also plays a pivotal role in the transportation of iron for the synthesis of hemoglobin. Based on these facts, Tf can be potentially utilized as a cell marker for tumor detection.

Normally at a cell, Tf offloads the iron onto a transferrin receptor (TfR). The natural ligand for TfR, Tf, binds to its receptor with a dissociation constant of around 40nM. TfR, also known as CD71, is a dimeric transmembrane glycoprotein (180 kDa) [77]. The receptor for Tf, referred to as TfR1, is ubiquitously expressed at low levels in most normal human tissues. A second member of the TfR family is TfR2, a protein that is homologous to TfR1 but whose expression is largely restricted to hepatocytes [76]. This receptor is an attractive molecule for the targeted therapy of cancer since it is upregulated on the surface of many cancer types and is efficiently internalized. Serving as the main port of entry for iron bound Tf into cells, TfR1 is a type-II receptor that resides on the cell membrane and cycles into acidic endosomes into the cell in a clathrin/dynamin dependent manner [78]. The low pH environment triggers dissociation of the iron and the iron-poor Tf is released out of the cell for recycling. As cancer cells rapidly proliferate, the TfR is overexpressed in the surface of malignant cells due to the increased requirement of iron [12]. In this sense, many studies have indicated that the expression level of TfR on tumor cells is much higher than that on normal cells [79], such as the surface of cerebral endothelium and brain tumor cells [80], breast cancer, prostate cancer, and squamous cell carcinomas [63]. This enhanced TfR expression, at levels correlating with the grade of malignancy [81], can be exploited for actively delivering anticancer agents specifically to tumor tissues. This receptor can be targeted in two ways: 1) for the delivery of therapeutic molecules into malignant cells or 2) to block the natural function of the receptor leading directly to cancer cell death [78].

A wide variety of therapeutic agents have been used for TfR-targeted cancer therapy. They include chemotherapeutic drugs, bacterial toxins, plant toxins, DNA, oligonucleotides, short inhibitory RNA (siRNA), and enzymes. Vast types of anti-cancer drugs that have been delivered into cancer cells employing a variety of receptor binding molecules including the use of its natural ligand Tf, anti-TfR antibodies, or TfR-binding peptides alone or in combination with carrier molecules including NPs and viruses [78].

With regard to NPs, Tf has a number of properties that allow it to be successfully incorporated as a targeting ligand in NP systems, such as its stability over a wide pH range (3.5-11) and that has shown to be unaffected by repeated freeze-thaw cycles; hence, it can be subjected to processing conditions commonly encountered during NP preparation [11]. Furthermore, Tf is available in recombinant version (Optiferrin) [82] and, as a human protein, has low immunogenicity [83]. Normally, Tf can be conjugated to NPs less than 100 nm in size to obtain an enhanced cytotoxic activity. If the NPs are greater than 100 nm, it may lead to poor accumulation of these NPs in the tumor cells, which results in moderate anticancer activity. To overcome this issue, the actively targeted system can be directly administered into the tumor tissue by intratumoral injection [84].

Tf-conjugated NPs have been explored in a number of studies for the delivery of anticancer agents. Thus, gold NPs were conjugated with Tf molecules for targeting, imaging and therapy of breast cancer cells (Hs578T, ATCC), showing that, the Tf–TfR-mediated cellular uptake of gold NPs is six times of that in the absence of this interaction [85].

It has also been [86] prepared PTX loaded NPs with shells formed of the biodegradable polymer, PLGA, conjugated to Tf via epoxy linkages. The Tf-conjugated NPs demonstrated greater cellular uptake and reduced exocytosis, yielding greater antiproliferative activity and more sustained effects compared to the free drug or unconjugated NPs. In a similar way, particulate nanodrugs consisting of PLGA loaded with PTX were conjugated to Tf (PTX–NPs–Tf) using an epoxy compound (Denacol-EX-521) [84]. These PTX–NPs–Tf showed a 70% in vitro inhibition of proliferation in human prostate cancer PC3 cells, while at the same concentration the NPs without ligand exhibited 25% inhibition, and PTX in solution resulted in a 35% [84]. Tf-conjugated lipid-coated PLGA NPs carrying the aromatase inhibitor, 7α-(4'-amino)phenylthio-1,4-androstadiene-3,17-dione (7α-APTADD), were synthesized and evaluated for aromatase inhibition efficiency in SKBR-3 breast cancer cells. PLGA NPs loaded with the 7α-APTADD were significantly more effective preventing proliferation of the human breast cancer cell line SK-BR-3 than non-targeted NPs. These results suggested that the aromatase inhibition activity of the Tf-NPs was enhanced relative to that of the non-targeted NPs, which was attributable to TfR mediated uptake [87]

Gan and coworkers observed that Tf-conjugated poly(lactide)-D-α-tocopheryl polyethylene glycol succinate diblock copolymer NPs loaded with Dtxl could be more efficient eliciting cytotoxicity against C6 glioma cells than other nontargeted formulations [88].

Transferrin–PEG–adamantane (Tf-PEG-AD) conjugates synthesized for NP modification have been used to target malignant tumors including Ewing's sarcoma [89-90]. Thus, several Tf-NPs have been successfully entered into clinical trials. CALA-01 [91] is one of the first clinically successful transferrin-conjugated nanoparticulate system. This system consists of a duplex of synthetic nonchemically modified siRNA, which self-assembles to a cationic copolymer containing cyclodextrin, AD-PEG as a stabilizing agent, and AD-PEG-Tf as the targeting moiety. After administration, the nanocomplex provides siRNA protection from nucleases in the serum, minimizes erythrocyte aggregation, and reduces complement fixation. At the tumor site, the Tf binds to the tumor cell TfR, which leads to preferential uptake of the complex within the tumor cell. In the cell, the polymer unpacks from the small interfering RNA allowing it to interfere with RNA resulting in reduced tumor growth [92].

Hydroxycamptothecin (HCPT)-loaded stealth niosomes(NS) modified with transferrin (Tf-PEG-NS) were prepared with poly(methoxy-polyethylene glycol cyanoacrylate-co-hexadecyl cyanoacrylate) (MePEG-PHDCA) as surface modification material [93]. Tf-PEG-NS demonstrated the strongest cytotoxicity to three carcinomatous cell lines (KB, K562 and S180 cells), the greatest intracellular uptake especially in nuclei, the highest drug concentration and largest area under the intratumoral HCPT concentration curve, as well as the most powerful anti-tumor activity compared with other niosomes. More reciently Tf modified stealth NPs (Tf-PEG-NP) encapsulating PEG-HCPT conjugate were prepared and was studied the possibility of combination of the functions of passive and active targeting by Tf-PEG-NP, as well as sustained drug release in tumor by PEGylated drug for most efficient tumor targeting and anti-tumor effects enhancement. The advantages of such system included prolonging drug residence time in circulation and increasing EPR effect by the sterically stabilising action of PEG-PHDCA NPs, active targeting function of transferrin by transferring receptor-mediated endocytosis, and sustained releasing drug in tumor by PEGylation of the drug. The prepared Tf-PEG-NP showed more sustained in vitro release profile. The pharmacokinetic and biodistribution studies found that Tf-PEG-NP demonstrated the longest retention time in blood, the highest tumor accumulation, as well as the most powerful anti-tumor activity with the inhibition rate up to 93% against S180 tumor in mice [94].

A pH-sensitive dual-targeting drug carrier (G4-Dox-PEG-Tf-TMX) was synthesized with Tf conjugated on the exterior and Tamoxifen (TMX) in the interior of the fourth generation (G4) Poly(amido amine))(PAMAM) dendrimers for enhancing the blood brain barrier (BBB) [35].

The pH-triggered Dox release was 32% at pH 4.5 and 6% at pH 7.4, indicating a comparatively fast drug release at weak acidic condition and stable state of the carrier at physiological environment. MDR proteins, such as P-glycoprotein (P-gp), MRP4 (ABCC4), and breast cancer resistance protein (BCRP), are over expressed on the BBB and glioma cells, thus causing the block of overcoming the BBB and low uptake of drugs by the tumor cells [95]. The in vitro assay of the drug transport across the BBB model showed that G4-Dox-PEG-Tf-TMX exhibited higher BBB transportation ability. The carrier was internalized into C6 glioma cells upon crossing the BBB model by the coactions of TfR-mediated endocytosis and the inhibition effect of TMX to the drug efflux transports. Moreover, it also displayed the in vitro accumulation of DOX in the avascular C6 glioma spheroids made the tumor volume effectively reduced.

But, besides of its natural ligand, Tf, it have also been used other ligands conjugated to NPs. Thus, antibodies and antibody fragments against the TfR are common examples of receptor targets [72]. Among these are the mAbs A24 [96], Rat anti-murine TfR RI7 217 and YE1/9.9, Murine anti-human TfR Antibody HB21(also known as 5E9), Antibody 454A12, Antibody B3/25, Antibody OKT9, R17217 and OX26 mAb [95,97-99].

For instance the R17217, a rat IgG2a antibody against the mouse TfR which binds to this receptor on mouse cells [99], and the OX26, a murine Ab to the rat TfR, which is used for the delivery of peptides across the BBB [100], have been used in NP systems. Hence, it has been developed human serum albumin (HSA) NPs to which Tf was coupled, and was evaluated the potential of these NPs to deliver drugs across the BBB and, in addition, the possibility of achieving similar results by the coupling of the above-mentioned mAbs against the TfR receptor to the NPs was investigated. The analgesic Loperamide was chosen as the model drug since it does not cross the BBB [101]. HSA NPs coupled to Tf or TfR-mAb are enabling a significant loperamide transport across the BBB into the brain. The loperamide-loaded, Tf- or TfR-mAb-coupled HSA NPs achieved strong antinociceptive effects, whereas IgG2a-modified HSA NPs were not able to transport this drug across the BBB [80]. Therefore, these novel NPs with attached Tf or TfR-mAb represent very useful carriers for the transport of drugs into the brain. It have also been used fluorescein labeled Chitosan (CS) nanospheres conjugated with PEG obtained with the PRINT (Particle Replication In Non-wetting Templates) technology that were bioconjugated either with the OKT9 murine anti-human TfR antibody (NPs–OKT9) or with human Tf (NPs–hTf) [102]. In both cases greater than 80% uptake was observed in several human tumor cell lines (HeLa, Ramos, H460, SKOV-3, HepG2, and LNCaP) compared to bovine Tf conjugated NPs (NPs–bTf) or control IgG1 (NPs–IgG1). The targeting efficiency was dependent on nanocarrier concentration, ligand density, dosing time, and level of cell surface receptor expression. For these cells a strong correlation was found between the viability and the amount of ligand (OKT-9 or hTf) that can be conjugated to the surface of the NPs, with lower cell viability associated with higher percentage of ligand conjugate, suggesting that the polyvalency of the moiety targeting TfR plays a role in the toxicity in some malignancies [102].

3.4. Folate receptor

Folic acid (FA) or folate, a member of the B complex group of vitamins with small-molecular weight (441 Da), is required by eukaryotic cells as is an important co-factor in one-carbon transfer reactions for biosynthesis of nucleotide bases (purines and pyrimidines) and plays a key role in DNA and RNA synthesis, epigenetic processes, cellular proliferation, and survival [103-104]. Since folic acid is required for essential cell function, the cargo attached the ligand is retained within an endocytic vesicle or released into the cytoplasm. FA conjugates have the ability to deliver a variety of drugs or imaging agents to pathological cells without causing harm to normal tissues. Furthermore FA targeting is an interesting approach for cancer therapy because it offers several advantages over the use of monoclonal antibodies. Thus, FA is known to be stable, inexpensive, non-toxic, non-immunogenic, easy to conjugate to carriers [105], and FA-conjugated drugs or NPs are rapidly internalized via receptor-mediated endocytosis.

Distinct transporters mediate cellular FA uptake. Among them, the FA transporter named as the folate receptor (FR) [9]. Three FR isoforms (FR-α, FR-β and FR-γ) have been identified in human tissues and tumors. FA can be internalized in cells by a low-affinity (K_D of approximately 1-5 μmol/l) membrane-spanning protein, which transports reduced FAs directly into the cytosol or it can be endocytosed by a high-affinity glycoprotein (K_D of approximately 100 pmol/l). FR, often referred to as the high affinity folate-binding protein, is a 38 kDa cell surface glycosyl-phophatidylinositol (GPI)-anchored glycopeptides that characteristically binds folic acid and transports it by a nonclassical endocytic mechanism [106]. The receptor-mediated uptake of FA conjugates proceeds through a series of distinct steps [107]. The process begins with the conjugate binding to FRs on the cell surface. The plasma membrane then invaginates and eventually forms a distinct intracellular compartment. The endocytic vesicles become acidified, and then lysozymes are activated allowing the FR to release the FA conjugates. The membrane-bound FRs recycle back to the cell surface, allowing them to mediate the delivery of additional FA conjugates. Concurrently, the FA conjugates released from FRs escape the endosome, resulting in drug deposition in the cytoplasm. Functional FRs are largely localized to the apical surfaces of polarized epithelia [105]. Normal tissues express insignificant level of FR-α and low level of FR-β (such as liver), and FR-γ is only found in haematopoietic cells. However, FR-α and FR-β are vastly overexpressed in many human tumors such as uterus, colon, lung, prostate, ovaries, mammary glands, nose, throat and brain [11,107-108] which makes it a rational target for drug delivery to tumor tissues. At the tumor site, FA has a very high affinity for tumor cell surface FR and the complex is rapidly internalized into tumor cells (3×10^5 FA molecules/h) [109]. Studies have shown a significant correlation between FR-α expression and the grade and differentiation status of the tumor, thus poorly differentiated and aggressive tumors express high levels of FR-α [110]. However, immunochemistry studies have shown the overexpression of FA receptors in normal tissues like placenta and kidneys [13].

A wide range of chemical conjugates of FA, antifolate drugs, and immunological agents have been used for developing therapeutic and imaging agents for various diseases. Thus, it is not surprising that FA targeted NPs have shown to be effective in a number of tumors. A range of polymers with an improved biocompatibility have been used for the development of FR-targeted NPs [11]. In a typical FR-targeted NP, the anticancer agent is encapsulated in a stabilizing polymer and the FA is conjugated on the surface of the polymer. PEG is often used as a polymer in a FR-targeted nanoparticulate system to enhance its circulation time and also to improve the association of the targeted NP with the tumor cells [111]. The surface density and length of PEG chains should be optimal to maintain the system targeting and stealth properties [72]. The mole fraction of FA added to a NP system is also thought to affect the cytotoxic capability of the system. It is presumed that higher ligand content would give an enhanced targeting ability. However, when excessive FA molecules are present on the surface of the NPs, they can self-assemble to form dimers, trimers or tubular quartets, which cannot interact with FR (only one molecule of FA can bind to FR) [112]. FA-PEG-liposome loaded with Dox showed a 45-fold higher uptake in FR-rich KB cells compared to nontargeted liposomal-doxorubicin and 86-fold greater cytotoxicity. In mice bearing KB cell tumor xenografts, treatment with FA-targeted liposomal Dox produced a 31% inhibition of tumor growth [37].

Similar to PEG, PLGA NPs can be coated with FA to target the FR to further enhance accumulation of these NPs into tumor cells [113]. Copolymeric nanohydrogels based on N-isopropylacrylamide (NIPA), N-(pyridin-4-ylmethyl)acrylamide (NPAM) and tert-butyl-2-acrylamidoethyl carbamate (2AAECM), as well as FA-conjugate copolymeric nanogels, were synthesized and evaluated for antitumor therapy by loading them with TMX and 5-FU. Nanohydrogels were assayed as TMX and 5-FU delivery systems in vitro. Cell culture experiments were performed using MCF7, T47D and HeLa cells which have different degrees of FR expression. FA-targeted nanohydrogels showed a larger uptake into T47D and HeLa cells due to the fact that these cells are FR-positive. Furthermore, TMX-loaded and 5-FU-loaded nanohydrogels showed effective elimination of carcinoma cells [38]. Loaded with the same drugs, it have also been synthesized FA-conjugate poly[(p-nitrophenyl acrylate)-co-(N-isopropylacrylamide)] systems. TMX and 5-FU-loaded folate-systems present effective elimination of both MCF7 and HeLa cellular lines, and the presence of folate in the particles enhances their internalization, especially in HeLa cells [114-115].

A natural polymer (poly(3-hydroxybutyrate-co-3-hydroxyhexanoate), PHBHHX) was used as a base matrix for the production of a novel nanotherapeutic including antineoplastic agent, etoposide and attached FA as a ligand on the NPs. In the cytotoxicity tests, etoposide loaded and folic acid attached PHBHHX NPs were observed as more effective on HeLa cells than etoposide loaded PHBHHX NPs without attached folic acid. Furthermore the cytotoxicity of folic acid conjugated PHBHHX NPs to cancer cells was found to be much higher than that of normal fibroblast cells, demonstrating that the FA conjugated NPs has the ability to selectively target to cancer cells [116].

CS NPs have also been conjugated to FA to target contrast dye to tumor tissues. The mucoadhesive property of CS provides sustained interaction with the target cells and the FR-mediated uptake leads to an enhanced imaging effect [117]. The cytotoxic activity of CS NP conjugated to FA has also been explored to show a higher cellular cytotoxicity due to enhanced uptake by receptor-mediated endocytosis complemented with a depot effect, which leads to sustained drug release providing grater apoptosis and enhanced cell cycle arrest [118]. An alginate-complexed FA CS NP has been reported for photodynamic early detection of colorectal carcinoma. These NPs are readily engulfed by the cancer cells through FR-mediated endocytosis, furthermore an improved release in the cellular lysosome was observed when they are loaded with 5-aminolevulinic acid (5-ALA) [119].

In other system, FA was coupled with HSA NPs through carbodiimide reaction resulting in the formation of HSA-NPs spheres. The cellular binding and uptake was studied in normal foreskin fibroblasts (HFF), human neuroblastoma cells UKF-NB3, and in rat glioblastoma cell lines. An inceased NP uptake was observed in cancer cells, but not in normal HFFs [9].

3.5. Integrin

Integrins are heterodimeric cell-surface receptors that consist of α- and β-subunits, such as integrins $\alpha_v\beta_3$ and $\alpha_v\beta_5$, and which are barely detectable or entirely absent from normal blood vessels but are abundantly expressed on tumor-associated endothelial cells [120-121]. Furthermore the $\alpha_v\beta_3$ integrin is important in the calcium-dependent signaling pathway leading to endothelial cell migration [122]. Endothelial cells undergoing angiogenesis experience at least three cellular alterations, including an increase in proliferation, increase in locomotion, and endothelial cell interaction with the ECM. These alterations are directly related to the adhesion processes of the $\alpha_v\beta_3$ integrin [122]. Thus, integrins represent potential pharmacological targets for antiangiogenic therapy. Several antibodies and peptides capable of functionally blocking the $\alpha_v\beta_3$ and $\alpha_v\beta_5$ integrins have been demonstrated to inhibit neovascularization in tumor-bearing mice. The targeting scheme for the $\alpha_v\beta_3$ integrin has centered upon the three amino acid sequence RGD. An important characteristic of the $\alpha_v\beta_3$ integrin is that it is intrinsically associated with VEGFR-2 signaling. Upon $\alpha_v\beta_3$ integrin binding to the components that harbor the RGD sequence, there is an upregulation of VEGF signaling in cell cultures. By blocking $\alpha_v\beta_3$ integrin binding, there would be a reduction in VEGF signaling, proving the use of $\alpha_v\beta_3$ blocking agents for anti-angiogenesis [120]. Targeting the $\alpha_v\beta_3$ integrin with an active targeting NP system increases the effectiveness of anti-angiogenic treatments by the downregulation of VEGF.

Park and coworkers [123] reported the development of self-assembled hydrogel NPs capable of imbibing a peptide sequence that specifically binds to $\alpha_v\beta_3$ integrin. The authors observed that NPs made of hydrophobically modified CS could release the peptide in a sustained manner, and showed that they might be useful for monitoring or destroying angiogenic vessels. Peptides that contain RGD domains can preferentially bind cells in tumor microvasculature that express the $\alpha_v\beta_3$ integrin [13]. However, RGD sequences also act as adhesive molecules and can non-specifically bind tissues that also express its integrin complement. Integrin receptors are also expressed on the cell membrane of macrophages [124] and it is shown that RGD bioconjugates aggregate in spleen and liver tissues due to macrophage clearance [125].

Using an RGD-targeted stealth system, NPs carrying Dox were found to accumulate faster and in higher concentrations in the liver and the spleen [126]. The ligands are incorporated as RGD-PEG-lipid conjugates, which indicates their extension from the NP surface as a consequence of the brush-like state. A report showed that short peptide-targeted NPs exhibited lower cell-bindings abilities when higher mol% of PEG$_{2000}$ was included into the formulation [127-128]. As a sufficient PEG coating is essential for avoiding recognition by the RES, ligands should be extended away from NP surfaces, to avoid shielding by the polymer chains. Another study reported the targeting and imaging of MDA-MB-231 human breast cancer cells using RGD peptide-labeled Fluorescent silica NPs (FSiNPs). The FSiNPs exhibited high target binding to $\alpha_v\beta_3$ integrin receptor (ABIR)-positive MDA-MB-231 breast cancer cells in vitro [129].

Peptide-labeled NPs may also be used for targeted gene silencing. A study shows that RGD-CS-NP is a highly selective delivery system for siRNA with the potential for broad applications in human disease [130]. Binding of RGD-CS-NP with $\alpha_v\beta_3$ integrin and antitumor efficacy were examined, resulted in significant inhibition of tumor growth compared with controls. The targeted RGD non-peptide mimetic coupled to NPs were coupled to cDNA encoding ATPµ-Raf tagged with the FLAG epitope [131] and were proven to cause tumor regression in M21-L melanomas. Peptides harboring RGD sequences have also shown high efficiencies in targeting SLK tumor endothelial cells derived from Kaposi's sarcoma. A cyclic RGD pentapeptide was conjugated to the surface of Dox-loaded micelles at different densities. A higher density of RGD sequences led to a higher level of cellular internalization of the micelles over the range of RGD densities. A 30-fold enhancement in micelle internalization was achieved with 76% RGD-functionalized Dox-loaded micelles as compared to the non-targeted micelles [132].

There are studies with other ligands. Thus, integrin-targeted C16Y peptide-modified liposomes (C16Y-L) were prepared to enhance the intracellular uptake of drugs and genes specifically into tumor tissues [133]. The C16Y peptide is a 12-amino acid modified C16 synthetic peptide (DFKLFAVYIKYR-GGC), which is derived from the laminin γ1 chain, and binds to integrins $\alpha_v\beta_3$ and $\alpha_5\beta_1$ [134]. The cellular uptake of C16Y-L by both endothelial cells and cancer cells was higher than uptake of the un-labeled and scramble peptide-modified liposomes. Moreover, to evaluate whether the uptake depended on an integrin–ligand interaction, they examined the inhibition of C16Y-L uptake using recombinant integrin $\alpha_v\beta_3$ and found that the cellular uptake of C16Y-L treated with $\alpha_v\beta_3$ integrin decreased. This result suggests that C16Y-L can selectively target cells that highly express integrin $\alpha_v\beta_3$.

Finally, a new strategy is to use a multi-targeting NP systems. For instance, PTX-loaded NPs based on Herein, an hyperbranched amphiphilic poly[(amine-ester)-co-(D,L-lactide)]/1,2-dipalmitoyl-sn-glycero-3-phosphoethanolamine copolymer (HPAE-co-PLA/DPPE), which was modified with two targeting ligands, RGD and Tf were synthesized [135]. Thus, these dual-targeting NPs may achieve more accumulation and improved lethality of the PTX-loaded NPs in tumors. Active tumors targeting can be achieved in two steps: the ligand RGD enhances the targeting migration and accumulation of NPs to the $\alpha_v\beta_3$ integrin-expressing tumor vasculature and Tf then improves the cellular uptake of NPs by TfR-expressing tumor cells. In addition, a heterobifunctional cross-linker, p-maleimidophenyl isocyanate (PMPI), used for hydroxyl to sulfhydryl coupling was introduced to the HPAE-co-PLA/DPPE copolymer for the successful modification of targeting ligands [136-137]. Results showed the cytotoxicity and cellular uptake of PTX-loaded NPs against human cervical carcinoma (HeLa) cells for their tumor-targeting effects [135].

4. Tumor cell targeting

Cancer cells express different targets on their surface, some of them specific of each type of cancer. Active targeting of nanosystems for cancer treatment has been usually associated with a type of cancer and so with a specific target.

While chemotherapy has been the standard of care for patients with different types of cancer, efforts have shifted toward evaluating novel targeted agents in an attempt to improve outcome. These targeted agents are directed towards key components in several signaling pathways. The potential of targeted therapies has stimulated the study of targeted nanocarriers that can allow synergistically act by binding and inhibiting cancer pathways while delivering therapeutic payloads. Tumor cell targeting involves many targets associated with the uncontrolled cell proliferation and the angiogenesis and others specifics for the different types of cancer (Table 2)

CANCER TYPE	TARGET	AGENT	REFERENCE
Lung cancer (NSCLC)	VEGFR	Axitinib (Pfizer Inc., USA)	[138]
		Cediranib (Recentin®, AstraZeneca plc, UK)	[139]
	EGFR	Cetuximab (Erbiux®, ImClone/Bristol-Myer Squibb, USA)	[140]
		Erlotinib (Tarceva®, Genentech/Roche, Switzerland)	[141]
	IGF-1R	Figitumumab (CP-751871, Pfizer, USA)	[142]
Colorectal cancer	VEGF-A	Bevacizumab (Avastin®, Roche-Pharma AG, Germany)	[143-145]
	EGFR	Cetuximab (Erbiux®, ImClone/Bristol-Myer Squibb, USA)	[146]
		Panitumumab (Amgen Inc; Thousand Oaks, USA)	[147]
Breast cancer	HER2	Transtuzumab (Herceptin®, Genentech)	[148]
		Transtuzumab-DM1 (T-DM1; Genetech Inc/Roche)	[149]
		Pertuzumab (Omnitarg®; Genentech/Roche)	[150]
	PARP	Olaparib (AZD2281; AstraZeneca)	[151]
Prostate cancer	17-α-hydroxylase	Abiraterone acetate (Zytiga, Cougar Biotechnology)	[152]
	AR	MDV3100	[153]
	EGFR	Cetuximab (Erbiux®, ImClone/Bristol-Myer Squibb, USA)	[154]
	HER2	Transtuzumab (Herceptin®, Genentech)	[155]
	HER3	MM-121 (humanized antibody)	[156]
	PSMA	J591 (monoclonal antibody)	[157]

Table 2. Examples of targets for different types of cancer

4.1. Lung cancer

Non-small cell lung cancer (NSCLC) involves signaling pathways that influence angiogenesis, tumorigenesis and tumor growth, and different targeted agents have been used towards vascular endothelial growth factor receptor (VEGFR), platelet-derived growth factor receptor (PDGFR), EGFR and insulin-like growth factor 1 receptor (IGF-1R) [158-159]. Furthermore, there is an increasing interest in using combinations of targeted agents to inhibit more than one pathway.

Among agents that target VEGFR in the treatment of advanced NSCLC, axitinib [138] has resulted to be a potent selective inhibitor of these types of receptors; also cediranib [139] has been assayed in combination with carboplatin and PTX in the treatment of this kind of cancer.

Over-expression of EGFR has been associated with angiogenesis and poor prognosis in NSCLC [160]. Cetuximab (Erbiux®, ImClone/Bristol-Myer Squibb, USA) is a chimeric mAb that targets the EGFR pathway by binding to the extracellular domain of the receptor and in this way inhibiting the receptor-associated tyrosine kinase (TK) activity [140]. Furthermore, inhibitors of TK activity of EGFR have been used for targeting the receptor pathway. Small-molecule, such as erlotinib (Tarceva®, Genentech/Roche, Switzerland) and gefitinib (Iressa®, AstraZeneca plc, UK), compete reversibly with ATP to bind to the intracellular catalytic domain of EGFR TK and, thus, inhibit EGFR autophosphorylation and downstream signaling [161].

IGF-1R is a key signaling pathway that leads to the growth and survival of tumor cells [162] and is commonly overexpressed in lung cancer cells. Figitumumab (CP-751,871, Pfizer, USA) is a fully human monoclonal antibody that is a specific and potent inhibitor of IGF-1R. In combination with carboplatin/PTX, figitumumab has shown to be a promising antitumor agent as first line treatment of NSCLC [142]. Several other anti-IGF-1R mAbs are being investigated in the treatment of advanced NSCLC, among them IMC-A12 (cixutumumab; fully human IgG1 monoclonal antibody), MK0646 (dalotizumab; a humanized IgG1 monoclonal antibody) and R1507 (fully humanized monoclonal antibody) [163].

Lung cancer is a heterogeneous disease with multiple mutations, and it is unlikely that any single signaling pathway drives the oncogenic behaviour of all tumors. In fact, multilevel cross-stimulation among the targets of the new biological agents can contribute to the relative failure of some target therapies. In this way, combining targeted therapies is a promising research approach to the treatment of NSCL, and an exhaustive review has been recently published by Custodio and coworkers [163]

4.2. Colorectal cancer

The systemic treatment of metastatic colorectal cancer (mCRC) involves the use of active cytotoxic drugs and biological agents either in combination or as single agents.

Initial chemotherapy of mCRC is based on using several cytotoxic regimens [164]. These clinical trials are based on the results of key phase III studies conducted over the past decade. The IFL regimen [irinotecan (I), 5-FU and leucovorin (LV)] has been extensively used [143]. Furthermore, combination of oxaliplatin and 5-FU/LV (FOLFOX4) [165] has improved the overall survival of mCRC patients.

A significant percentage of patients with CRC receive a biological agent targeting the vascular endothelial growth factor A (VEGF-A) or EGFR over their treatment course. The currently available anti-VEGF-A agent is bevacizumab (Avastin®, Roche-Pharma AG, Germany), a humanized mAb. Different key clinical trials incorporating bevacizumab have been carried out. In the AVF2107 trial [144] the combination of IFL and bevacizumab improved the progression-free survival and the overall survival. The trial of bevacizumab plus oxaliplatin-based chemotherapy (FOLFOX4) or plus capecitabine/oxaliplation (XELOX) [143,145] showed a significantly increase in the progression-free survival, mainly with XELOX.

The anti-EGFR mAbs indicated for mCRC treatment are cetuximab (Erbiux®, ImClone/Bristol-Myer Squibb, USA; a chimeric monoclonal antibody) and panitumumab (Amgen Inc; Thousand Oaks, USA; a fully human monoclonal antibody). Both of them are efficacy in the treatment of patients whose mCRC tumors express wild-type KRAS. Different clinical trials combining anti-EGFR agents and chemotherapy have been carried out. Thus, mCRC therapy (wild-type KRAS patients) based on cetuximab and FOLFIRY (CRYSTAL trial) [146] showed a significantly improved progression-free survival and overall survival. In a similar way, the combination of panitumumab and FOLFOX4 (PRIME trial) had a very positive impact on survival parameters in wild-type KRAS patients [147].

4.3. Breast cancer

Breast cancer is the most common cancer affecting females and one of the main causes of mortality of women. This disease shows a high heterogeneous nature in terms of genetic features, molecular profiles and clinical behaviour. The high mortality caused by breast cancer can be attributed to the development of metastatic breast cancer [166]. The discovery of "genetic signatures" in breast cancers can provide key insights into the mechanisms underlying tumorigenesis and can be proven useful for the design of targeted therapeutic approaches [167-168].

The HER2 is over-expressed 15-30% of invasive breast carcinomas [167]. Extracellular domain of HER2 has been the target of several monoclonal antibodies created in order to inhibit the proliferation of human cancer cells. Transtuzumab, a recombinant humanized anti-HER2 monoclonal antibody was approved by the FDA for immunotherapy of women with metastatic HER2 over-expressing breast carcinoma. This antibody provokes cell cycle arrest during G1 phase [148]. Transtuzumab has been extensively used to target different drug-loaded nanocarriers to breast cancer cells [169-170].

Many hormone receptor positive breast cancers are resistant to hormone therapies. Thus, clinical trials have been developed combining therapies with biological and targeted agents (anti EGFR and HER2) for the treatment of estrogen receptor (ER) positive breast cancer.

Combination of geftinib, an EGFR TK inhibitor, with anastrozole [171] or TMX [172] has conducted to a light prolongation of progression-free survival of patients. Clinical trials based on combination of transtuzumab and letrozole (Femara), an oral non-steroidal aromatase inhibitor for the treatment of hormonally-responsive breast cancer, in patients with ER+/HER2+ metastatic breast cancer have demonstrated clinical benefit [173]. A large proportion of HER2+ cancers have developed resistance to HER2-targeted therapeutics, including resistance of tumor cells to trastuzumab. Several agents have been developed to overcome resistance to this monoclonal antibody. The conjugation of maytansinoid DM1 with transtuzumab has generated transtuzumab-DM1 (T-DM1; Genetech Inc/Roche), that is active on HER2 overexpressing breast cancer and also transtuzumab-refractory tumors [149]. Another innovative targeted agent, which belongs, to the class of HER2-dimerization inhibitors, is pertuzumab (Omnitarg; Genentech/Roche), a recombinant humanized monoclonal antibody. Pertuzumab is directed against the highly conserved dimerization domain of HER2 [150]. The efficacy of adding pertuzumab to trastuzumab plus Dtxl for the first-line treatment of HER2-positive metastatic breast cancer was demonstrated in the randomized, double-blind, multinational, phase III CLEOPATRA trial [174].

Basal like breast cancers are the result of specific mutations. DNA lesions such as single-stand breaks (SSBs) and double-strand breaks (DSBs) are common in the normal cellular metabolism, and can be repaired by specific DNA repair mechanisms. In one of these DNA repair mechanisms, poly-(adenosine diphosphate ribose) polymerase 1 (PARP1) is an important key of the pathway. PARP1-inhibitors (PARP1-I) have been developed for the treatment of advanced breast cancer. Olaparib (AZD2281; AstraZeneca)), a PARP1-I has been evaluated in BRCA (a tumor suppressor protein) mutated patients [151]. Also iniparib (BSI 201; 4-iodo-3-nitrobenzamide; Sanofi-Aventis), an irreversible PARP1-I, is under study in patients with metastatic triple-negative breast cancer [175]. However, studies carried our by Liu and coworkers [176] shown that Iniparib nonselectively modifies cysteine-containing proteins in tumor cells, and the primary mechanism of action for iniparib is likely not via inhibition of PARP activity.

4.4. Prostate cancer

The current standard treatment of localized prostate cancer consists of prostatectomy and radiation therapy, sometimes supplemented with hormonal therapies to prevent testosterone production, which include anti-androgens and luteinizing hormone-releasing hormone (LH-RH) agonists. In locally advanced or widespread prostate cancer, the disease gradually transforms to a metastatic hormone-refractory state. Despite castrate levels of testosterone, the tumor will finally become independent of androgens resulting in death within a few years from diagnosis. In fact, the mortality rate of metastatic prostate cancer is extremely high. Thus, novel therapies [177-178] are on demand for the treatment of the malignant forms of prostate cancer that recur after initial therapies, including hormone refractory (HRPC) and castration resistant prostate cancer (CRCP).

Different molecules have been assayed as androgen and androgen receptor inhibitors. In this way, abiraterone acetate (Zytiga, Cougar Biotechnology) in combination with prednisone has been recently approved by FDA for the treatment of CRCP in men who have received prior Dtxl chemotherapy [152]. Arbiraterone inhibits 17-α-hydroxylase, an enzyme of the testosterone biosynthesis pathway, decreasing circulating levels of the hormone. This enzyme is expressed in testicular, adrenal and prostate tumors. Regarding of androgen receptor inhibitors (AR-I), MDV3100 is an oral androgen receptor antagonist [153], which irreversibly binds to this intracellular receptor and causes no transcription of the gen.

The EGFR family (EGFR/HER) receptors have long been implicated in prostate cancer initiation and progression. EGFR is overexpressed in 18-37% prostate cancers [179], and a direct correlation of HER2 overexpression with the risk of death and recurrence in prostate cancer has been reported [180]. Thus, monoclonal antibodies have been studied as treatment options for prostate cancer. The efficacy of combining cetuximab with mitoxantrone plus prednisolone have been analyzed in a phase II clinical trial in men with CRCP after receiving Dtxl, but the time to progression and overall survival did not improve with the addition of cetuximab [154]. In order to evaluate whether dual inhibition of EGFR and HER2 would prolong the effectiveness of androgen withdrawal therapy (AWT) treatment in prostate cancer, studies using EGFR inhibitors (erlotinib and AG1478) and HER2 inhibitors (trastuzumab and AG879) were realized [155]. Results indicate that dual EGFR/HER2 inhibition, administered together with AWT, sensitize prostate cancer cells to apoptosis during AWT. In general, studies using inhibitors of EGFR/HER1 and HER2 show that these molecules fared poorly in prostate cancer clinical trials.

Recent research suggests that another family member HER3 (ErbB3) abets emergence of the castration resistant phenotype. The prostate cancer, in comparison to the normal tissue, overexpresses HER3 protein, which indicate poor prognosis. Antibody-based therapy that prevents ligand binding to ErbB3 appears promising and fully-humanized antibodies that inhibit ligand-induced phosphorylation of HER3 (ErbB3) are currently in early development [181]. HER3's signaling functions depend upon ligand binding to its extracellular domain and inhibitors are generated to disrupt this interaction. A recently-characterized, HER3-specific humanized antibody MM-121 blocked ligand-dependent HER3 activation induced by the HER1, HER2 or MET receptors [156].

The IGF-R signaling pathway plays a role in prostate cancer. In fact, an increase risk of prostate cancer has been directly correlated with the circulating IGF-1 (one ligand of the IGF-R) levels [182]. An inhibitor de the IGF pathway is the anti-IGF-R mAb cixutumumab (IMC-A12; ImClone Systems), which was effective in both androgen-dependent and androgen-independent human prostate cancer in animal models [183].

PSMA has been identified as an ideal antigenic target in prostate cancer. PSMA is the most well-established, highly restricted prostate cancer cell surface antigen. It is expressed at high density on the cell membrane of all prostate cancers, and after antibody binding, the PSMA-antibody complex is rapidly internalized along with any payload carried by the antibody. J591 is the first IgG mAb developed to target the extracellular domain of PSMA, and it has been deimmunized (humanized) to allow repeated dosing in patients. Three phase I studies have been carried out, two using the β-emitting radiometals yttrium 90 and lutetium 177

(177Lu), and a third using a cytotoxin (DM1) linked to J591 [157]. A phase II clinical trial (NCT00859781) to test the effectiveness of the radiolabel monoclonal antibody, 177Lu-J591 in combination with ketoconazole and hydrocortisone against prostate cancer is in progress.

5. Conclusion

The development of drug delivery systems that are able to modify the biodistribution, tissue uptake and pharmacokinetics of therapeutic agents is considered of great importance in biomedical research. Controlled release in drug delivery can significantly enhance the therapeutic effect of a drug. Among drug delivery systems, nanocarriers are the smallest devices for transport of drugs, and they comprises a variety of the type of nanoparticles developed for cancer, including liposomes, nanoshells, nanocapsules, dendrimers, polymer-drug conjugates, polymeric nanogels and micelles, and polynucleotide nanoparticles. The attractive properties of nanomedicines include their ability of controlled release of drugs, the targeting of specific tissues and the biocompatibility. Because of their size, nanocarriers can be taken up, in many cases, very efficiently by cells, internalized and stored into cytoplasm or different organelles. Nanocarrier uptake into a cell depends on the cell-type, since some cells are more susceptible to include nonfunctionalized systems via their design. The unique attributes of tumors support extravasation of polymeric nanomedicines through large pores on the endotheliallayer and via the disordered neoplastic tissue architecture. Thus, nanoparticles target the tumor passively via the EPR effect if their size is smaller than 100nm. Therefore, current research involves novel strategies to attach targeting ligands with high affinity for receptors overexpressed on tumors or ways to utilize the tumor's own microenvironment as a stimulus for drug release. An active targeting strategy can improve the efficacy of the therapy and diminish side effects associated with drugs, since not all nanocarriers can overcome the cell membrane barrier without a targeting motif. Nanoparticle systems are able to target various portions of the tumor using specific targeting moieties and evade the problems associated with multi-drug resistance. Thus, to increase the delivery of a given drug to a specific target site, targeting ligands are conjugated to carriers. The presence of reactive pendant groups in nanogels make easy their vectorization forward specific cell motif by binding of ligands. Furthermore, it is an important fact that targeting ligands lead to macrophage recognition and faster clearance compared to the non-targeted nanoparticles. Various molecules, that include folates, transferrin, antibody and antibody fragments, peptides, aptamers, small molecules, and carbohydrates, have been used to target nanocarriers to specific receptors on tumoral cell surfaces. In many cases, ligand-targeted nanoparticles demonstrate better internalization by cancer cells and more effective intracellular drug delivery than other preparatios. The search for more molecular targets will advance the ability to improve delivery at the tumor level while decreasing toxicity to normal tissue. As a result, moieties-targeted drug-loaded nanoparticles, searching for new tumor targets, novel ligands, new strategies for targeting, and particle stabilization, are generally considered as promising candidates for cancer chemotherapy and we can expect their extensive clinical evaluation in the near future.

Nomenclature

2AAECM: *tert*-butyl-2-acrylamidoethyl carbamate
5-ALA: 5-aminolevulinic acid
5-FU: 5-Fluorouracil
7α-APTADD: 7α-(4′-amino)phenylthio-1,4-androstadiene-3,17-dione)
ABIR: $\alpha_v\beta_3$ integrin receptor
AD: adamantane
Apt: aptamer
AR-I: androgen receptor inhibitor
AWT: androgen withdrawal therapy
BBB: blood brain barrier
BCRP: breast cancer resistance protein
CEM: leukemic lymphoid cells
CRCP: castration resistant prostate cancer
CS: Chitosan
Dox: doxorubicin
DSBs: double-strand breaks
Dtxl: Docetaxel
ECM: extracellular matrix
EGF: epidermal growth factor
EGFR (or HER1): epidermal growth factor receptor 1
EPR: Enhanced Permeability and Retention
ER: estrogen receptor
EU: European Union
FA: Folic acid or folate
FDA: Food and Drug Administration
FR: folate receptor
FSiNPs: Fluorescent silica nanoparticles
GPI: glycosyl-phophatidylinositol
HB-EGF: heparin-binding epidermal growth factor
HCPT: Hydroxycamptothecin
HER: Human epidermal receptor
HER2: epidermal growth factor receptor 2
HER3: epidermal growth factor receptor 3
HFF: Human foreskin fibroblasts
HNSCC: Head and neck squamous cell carcinoma
HPAE-co-PLA/DPPE: hyperbranched amphiphilic poly[(amine-ester)-co-(D,L-lactide)]/1,2-dipalmitoyl-sn-glycero-3-phosphoethanolamine copolymer
HRPC: hormone refractory prostate cancer
HSA: human serum albumin
I: irinotecan
IFL regimen: irinotecan + 5-FU + leucovorin
IFP: interstitial fluid pressure
IGF: insulin-like growth factor

IGF-1R: insulin-like growth factor 1 receptor
LH-RH: luteinizing hormone-releasing hormone
LV: leucovorin
mAb: monoclonal antibody
MAPK: mitogen-activated protein kinases
mCRC: metastatic colorectal cancer
MePEG-PHDCA: poly(methoxy-polyethylene glycol cyanoacrylate-co-hexadecyl cyanoacrylate)
MTX: Methotrexate
MUC1: mucin 1
NCs: nanoclusters
NIPA: N-isopropylacrylamide
NPAM: N-(pyridin-4-ylmethyl)acrylamide
NPs: nanoparticles
NRs: nanorods
NS: niosomes
NSCLC: Non-small cell lung cancer
PAMAM: Poly(amido amine)
PARP1: poly-(adenosine diphosphate ribose) polymerase 1
PARP1-I: poly-(adenosine diphosphate ribose) polymerase 1 -inhibitors
PDGFR: platelet-derived growth factor receptor
PEG: polyethylene glycol
P-gp: P-glycoprotein
PHBHHX: poly(3-hydroxybutyrate-co-3-hydroxyhexanoate)
PLGA: poly(D,L-lactide-coglycolyde)
PMPI: p-maleimidophenyl isocyanate
PRINT technology: Particle Replication In Non-wetting Templates technology
PSMA: Prostate-specific membrane antigen
PTK7: protein tyrosine kinase-7
PTX: Paclitaxel
RES: reticuloendothelial system
RGD: tripeptide arginine–glycine–aspartic acid
SELEX: Systematic Evolution of Ligands by Exponential Enrichment
siRNA: short inhibitory RNA
SSBs: single-stand breaks
SWNTs: single-wall carbon nanotubes
Tf: Transferrin
TfR: Transferrin receptor
TGF-α: transforming growth factor-α
TK: tyrosine kinase
TLR9: Toll-like receptor 9
TMX: Tamoxifen
TNF: tumor necrosis factor
VEGF: vascular endothelial grown factor
VEGFR: vascular endothelial grown factor receptor

VPF: vascular permeability factor
WHO: World Health Organization

Author details

M.D. Blanco, R.M. Olmo and J.M. Teijón
Departamento de Bioquímica y Biología Molecular,
Facultad de Medicina, Universidad Complutense de Madrid, Spain

C. Teijón
Departamento de Enfermería, E.U. Enfermería,
Fisioterapia y Podología, Universidad Complutense de Madrid, Spain

Acknowledgement

The financial support of the Ministerio de Ciencia e Innovación of Spain (FIS PS09/01513 and MAT2010-21509-C03-03), and Universidad Complutense de Madrid-CAM for Consolidated Research Groups (Group 920613) are gratefully acknowledged.

6. References

[1] Danhier F, Feron O, Préat V. To exploit the tumor microenvironment: Passive and active tumor targeting of nanocarriers for anti-cancer drug delivery. J Control Release 2010;148:135-46.

[2] Malvezzi M, Bertuccio P, Levi F, La Vecchia C, Negri E. European cancer mortality predictions for the year 2012. Ann Oncol 2012; 23(4):1044-52.

[3] Djojosubroto MW, Choi YS, Lee HW, Rudolph KL. Telomeres and telomerase in aging, regeneration and cancer. Mol. Cell 2003;15:164-75.

[4] Prokop A, Davidson JM. Nanovehicular intracellular delivery systems. J Pharm Sci 2008;97:3518–3590.

[5] Tibbals HF. 2010. Medical Nanotechnology and Nanomedicine, CRC Press, 978-1-4398-0876-4, USA

[6] Moghimi SM, Hunter AC, Murray JC. Nanomedicine: current status and future prospects. FASEB J 2005; 19(3): 311-30.

[7] Gurwitz D, Livshits G. Personalized medicine Europe: health, genes and society: Tel-Aviv University, Tel-Aviv, Israel, June 19-21, 2005. Eur J Hum Genet 2006; 14(3):376-80.

[8] Barratt GM. Therapeutic applications of colloidal drug carriers. Pharm Sci Technol Today 2000; 3(5):163-71.

[9] Ranganathan R, Madanmoham S, Kesavan A, Baskar G, Krishnamoorthy YR, Santosham R, et al. Nanomedicine: towards development of patient-friendly drug-delivery systems for oncological applications. Int J Nanomed 2012;7:1043-60.

[10] Romberg B, Hennink WE, Storm G. Sheddable coatings for long-circulating nanoparticles. Pharm Res 2008; 25(1):55-71.

[11] Talekar M, Kendall J, Denny W, Garg S. Targeting of nanoparticles in cancer: drug delivery and diagnostics. Anti-Cancer Drugs 2011;22(10):949-62.

[12] Byrne JD, Betancourt T, Brannon-Peppas L. Active targeting schemes for nanoparticle systems in cancer therapeutics. Adv Drug Deliv Rev 2008;60:1615-26.

[13] Alexis F, Rhee JW, Richie JP, Radovic-Moreno AF, Langer R, Farokhzad OC. New frontiers in nanotechnology for cancer treatment. Urol Oncol-Semin Orig Investig 2008;26:74-85.

[14] Cho K, Wang X, Nie S, Chen Z, Shin DM. Therapeutic nanoparticles for drug delivery in cancer. Clin. Cancer Res. 2008;14:1310-6.

[15] Bergers G, Benjamin LE. Tumorigenesis and the angiogenic switch. Nat. Rev. Cancer 2003;3:401-10.

[16] Bae KH, Chung HJ, Park TG. Nanomaterials for Cancer Therapy and Imaging. Mol. Cells 2011;31:295-302.

[17] Carmeliet P. Mechanisms of angiogenesis and arteriogenesis. Nat. Med. 2000;6:389-95.

[18] Maeda H, Bharate GY, Daruwalla J. Polymeric drugs for efficient tumortargeted drug delivery based on EPR-effect. Eur. J. Pharm. Biopharm. 2009;71:409-19.

[19] Jain RK. Transport of molecules in the tumor interstitium: a review. Cancer Res. 1987;47:3039-51.

[20] Danquah MK, Zhang XA, Mahato RI. Extravasation of polymeric nanomedicines across tumor vasculature. Adv Drug Deliv Rev 2011;63:623-39.

[21] Vaupel P, Schaefer C, Okunieff P. Intracellular acidosis in murine fibrosarcomas coincides with ATP depletion, hypoxia, and high levels of lactate and total Pi. NMR Biomed. 1994;7:128-36.

[22] Cardone RA, Casavola V, Reshkin SJ. The role of disturbed pH dynamics and the Na+/H+exchanger in metastasis. Nat. Rev. Cancer 2005;5:786-95.

[23] Fang JS, Gillies RD, Gatenby RA. Adaptation to hypoxia and acidosis in carcinogenesis and tumor progression. Semin. Cancer Biol. 2008;18:330-7.

[24] Farokhzad OC, Cheng J, Teply BA, Sherifi I, Jon S, Kantoff PW et al. Targeted nanoparticleaptamer bioconjugates for cancer chemotherapy in vivo. Proc Natl Acad Sci USA 2006;103:6315-20.

[25] Haley B, Frenkel E. Nanoparticles for drug delivery in cancer treatment. Urol Oncol-Semin Orig Investig 2008;26:57-64.

[26] Gantert M, Lewrick F, Adrian JE, Rossler J, Steenpass T, Schubert R et al. Receptor-specific targeting with liposomes in vitro based on sterol-PEG(1300) anchors. Pharm Res 2009;26:529-38.

[27] Cao ZH, Tong R, Mishra A, Xu WC, Wong GCL, Cheng JJ, et al. Reversible cell-specific drug delivery with aptamer-functionalized liposomes. Angew Chem Int Ed 2009; 48:6494-98.

[28] Guo JW, Gao XL, Su LN, Xia HM, Gu GZ, Pang ZQ, et al. Aptamer-functionalized PEG-PLGA nanoparticles for enhanced anti-glioma drug delivery. Biomaterials 2011;32:8010-20.

[29] Taghdisi SM, Lavaee P, Ramezani M, Abnous K. Reversible Targeting and controlled release delivery of daunorubicin to cancer cells by aptamer-wrapped carbon nanotubes. Eur J Pharm Biopharm 2011;77:200-6.

[30] Gao L, Cui Y, He Q, Yang Y, Fei JB, Li JB. Selective recognition of co-assembled thrombin aptamer and docetaxel on mesoporous silica nanoparticles against tumor cell proliferation. Chem Eur J 2011; 17:13170-74.

[31] Bhirde AA, Patel V, Gavard J, Zhang G, Sousa AA, Masedunskas A, et al. Targeted killing of cancer cells in Vivo and in Vitro with EGF-directed carbon nanotube-based drug delivery. ACS Nano 2009;3: 307–16.

[32] Sun B, Ranganathan B, Feng SS. Multifunctional poly(D,L-lactide-coglycolide)/montmorillonite (PLGA/MMT) nanoparticles decorated by Trastuzumab for targeted chemotherapy of breast cancer. Biomaterials 2008; 29(4):475–86.

[33] Pulkkinen M, Pikkarainen J, Wirth T, Tarvainen T, Haapa-aho V, Korhonen H, et al. Three-step tumor targeting of paclitaxel using biotinylated PLA–PEG nanoparticles and avidin–biotin technology: formulation development and in vitro anticancer activity. Eur J Pharm Biopharm 2008;70:66-74.

[34] Shah N, Chaudhari K, Dantuluri P, Murthy RS, Das S. Paclitaxel-loaded PLGA nanoparticles surface modified with transferrin and Pluronic((R))P85, an in vitro cell line and in vivo biodistribution studies on rat model. J Drug Target 2009; 17: 533-42.

[35] Li Y, He H, Jia X, Lu WL, Lou J, Wei Y. A dual-targeting nanocarrier based on poly(amidoamine) dendrimers conjugated with transferrin and tamoxifen for treating brain gliomas. Biomaterials 2012;33:3899-908.

[36] Kukowska-Latallo JF, Candido KA, Cao Z, Nigavekar SS, Majoros IJ, Thomas TP, et al. Nanoparticle targeting of anticancer drug improves therapeutic response in animal model of human epithelial cancer. Cancer Res 2005; 65(12):5317-24.

[37] Lee RJ, Low PS. Folate-mediated tumor cell targeting of liposomeentrapped doxorubicin in vitro. Biochim Biophys Acta. 1995;1233:134-44.

[38] Blanco MD, Benito M, Olmo R, Teijón C, Pérez E, Katime I, et al. Synthesis and in vitro biological evaluation as antitumour drug carriers of folate-targeted N-isopropylacrylamide-based nanohydrogels. Polym Int 2012; 61:1202-12.

[39] Jiang X, Sha X, Xin H, Chen L, Gao X, Wang X, et al. Self-aggregated pegylated poly (trimethylene carbonate) nanoparticles decorated with c(RGDyK) peptide for targeted paclitaxel delivery to integrin-rich tumors. Biomaterials 2011; 32: 9457-94.

[40] Wagner S, Rothweiler F, Anhorn MG, Sauer D, Riemann I, Weiss EC, et al. Enhanced drug targeting by attachment of an anti αv integrin antibody to doxorubicin loaded human serum albumin nanoparticles. Biomaterials 2010; 31: 2388–98.

[41] Levy-Nissenbaum E, Radovic-Moreno AF, Wang AZ, Langer R, Farokhzad OC. Nanotechnology and aptamers: applications in drug delivery. Trends Biotechnol 2008;26(8):442-9.

[42] Famulok M. Hartig JS, Mayer G. Functional aptamers and aptazymes in biotechnology, diagnostics, and therapy. Chem. Rev. 2007;107:3715–43.

[43] Bouchard PR, Hutabarat RM, Thompson KM. Discovery and Development of Therapeutic Aptamers. Annu. Rev. Pharmacol. Toxicol. 2010;50:237–57.

[44] Nimjee SM, Rusconi CP, Sullenger BA. Aptamers: An emerging class of therapeutics. Ann Rev Med 2005;56:555-83.

[45] Hicke BJ, Stephens AW, Gould T, Chang YF, Lynott CK, Heil J, et al Tumor targeting by an aptamer. J Nucl Med 2006;47:668-78.

[46] Shangguan D, Li Y, Tang Z, Cao ZC, Chen HW, Mallikaratchy P, et al. Aptamers evolved from live cells as effective molecular probes for cancer study. Proc Natl Acad Sci USA 2006;103:11838-43.

[47] Tan W, Wang H, Chen Y, Zhang X, Zhu H, Yang C, et al. Molecular aptamers for drug delivery. Trends Biotechnol 2011;29(12):634-40.

[48] Huang YF, Chang HT, Tan W. Cancer cell targeting using multiple aptamers conjugated on nanorods. Anal. Chem. 2008;80:567-72.

[49] Ko HY, Choi KJ, Lee CH, Kim S. A multimodal nanoparticle-based cancer imaging probe simultaneously targeting nucleolin, integrin alphavbeta3 and tenascin-C proteins. Biomaterials 2011;32:1130-8.

[50] Xiao Z, Shangguan D, Cao Z, Fang X, Tan W, Cell-specific internalization study of an aptamer from whole cell selection. Chem-Eur J 2008;14:1769-75.

[51] Farokhaz OC, Jon SY, Khademhosseini A, Tran, TNT, LaVan DA, Langer, R. Nanoparticle–aptamer bioconjugates: a new approach for targeting prostate cancer cells. Cancer Res. 2004;64:7668-72.

[52] Blank M, Weinschenk T, Priemer M, Schluesener H. Systematic evolution of a DNA aptamer binding to rat brain tumor microvessels. selective targeting of endothelial regulatory protein pigpen. J Biol Chem 2001;276:16464-68.

[53] Ferreira CS, Matthews CS, Missailidis S. DNA aptamers that bind to MUC1 tumour marker: design and characterization of MUC1-binding single-stranded DNA aptamers. Tumor Biol. 2006; 27:289-301.

[54] InVitria. Cellastim. 2009 [cited; available from: http://www.invitria.com/ products-and-services/details/17/6/albumin/cellastim.html

[55] Huang YF, Sefah K, Bamrungsap S, Chang HT, Tan W. Selective photothermal therapy for mixed cancer cells using aptamer-conjugated nanorods. Langmuir 2008;24:11860-5.

[56] Kim D, Jeong YY, Jon S. A drug-loaded aptamer-gold nanoparticle bioconjugate for combined CT imaging and therapy of prostate cancer. ACS Nano 2010;4:3689-96.

[57] Yin JJ, He XX, Wang KM, Qing ZH, Wu X, Shi H, et al. One-step engineering of silver nanoclusters-aptamer assemblies as luminescent labels to target tumor cells. Nanoscale 2012;4:110-2.

[58] Green LS, Jellinek, D, Bell C, Beebe LA, Feistner BD, Gill SC, et al. Nuclease-Resistant nucleic acid ligands to vascular permeability factor/vascular endothelial growth factor. Chem. Biol. 1995;2:683-95.

[59] Bates PJ, Laber D, Miller DM, Thomas SD, Trent JO. Discovery and development of the G-rich oligonucleotide AS1411 as a novel treatment for cancer. Exp. Mol. Path. 2009;86:151-64.

[60] Laskin JJ, Sandler AB. Epidermal growth factor receptor: a promising target in solid tumours. Cancer Treat. Rev. 2004;30(1):1-17.

[61] Wieduwilt MJ, Moasser MM. The epidermal growth factor receptor family: biology driving targeted therapeutics. Cell Mol Life Sci 2008;65:1566-84.

[62] Agarwal A, Saraf S, Asthana A, Gupta U, Gajbhiye V, Jain NK. Ligand based dendritic systems for tumor targeting, Int. J. Pharm. 2008;350(1–2):3–13.

[63] Yu X, Zhang Y, Chen C, Yao Q, Li M. Targeted drug delivery in pancreatic cancer. Biochim Biophys Acta 2010;1805:97-104.

[64] Schwechheimer K, Huang S, Cavenee WK. EGFR gene amplification–rearrangement in human glioblastomas. Int. J. Cancer 1995;62(2):145–8.

[65] Laskin JJ, Sandler AB. Epidermal growth factor receptor inhibitors in lung cancer therapy. Semin. Respir. Crit. Care Med. 2004;25(Suppl 1):17–27.

[66] Mendelsohn J, Baselga J. Status of epidermal growth factor receptor antagonists in the biology and treatment of cancer. J. Clin. Oncol. 2003;21(14):2787–99.

[67] Pan X, Wu G, Yang W, Barth RF, Tjarks W, Lee RJ. Synthesis of cetuximabimmunoliposomes via a cholesterol-based membrane anchor for targeting of EGFR. Bioconjug. Chem. 2007;18(1):101–8.

[68] Nahta R, Esteva FJ. Herceptin: mechanisms of action and resistance. Cancer Lett. 2006;232:123–38.

[69] Kirpotin DB, Drummond DC, Shao Y, Shalaby MR, Hong K, Nielsen UB, et al. Antibody targeting of long-circulating lipidic nanoparticles does not increase tumor localization but does increase internalization in animal models. Cancer Res. 2006;66(13):6732–40.

[70] Harries M, Smith I. The development and clinical use of trastuzumab (Herceptin). Endocr. Relat. Cancer 2002;9(2):75–85.

[71] Cirstoiu-Hapca A, Buchegger F, Bossy L, Kosinski M, Gurny R, Delie F. Nanomedicnes for active targeting: Physico-chemical characterization of paclitaxel-loaded anti-HER2 immunonanoparticles and in vitro functional studies on target cells. Eur J Pharm Sci 2009;38:230-7.

[72] Wang M, Thanou M. Targeting nanoparticles to cancer. Pharmacol Res 2010;62:90-9.

[73] Park JW, Hong K, Kirpotin DB, Colbern G, Shalaby R, Baselga J, et al. Anti-HER2 immunoliposomes: enhanced efficacy attributable to targeted delivery. Clin. Cancer Res. 2002;8:1172–81.

[74] Lyu MA, Kurzrock R, Rosenblum MG. The immunocytokine scFv23/TNF targeting HER-2/neu induces synergistic cytotoxic effects with 5-fluorouracil in TNF-resistant pancreatic cancer cell lines. Biochem. Pharmacol. 2008;75:836–46.

[75] Singh M. Transferrin as a targeting ligand for liposomes and anticancer drugs. Curr. Pharm. Des. 1999;5(6):443–51.

[76] Daniels TR, Delgado T, Rodriguez JA, Helguera G, Penichet ML. The transferrin receptor part I: biology and targeting with cytotoxic antibodies for the treatment of cancer. Clin. Immunol. 2006;121: 144–58.

[77] Yang X, Koh CG, Liu S, Pan X, Santhanam R, Yu B, et al. Transferrin receptor-targeted lipid nanoparticles for delivery of an antisense oligodeoxyribonucleotide against Bcl-2. Mol. Pharm. 2009;6:221–30.

[78] Daniels TR, Bernabeu E, Rodríguez JA, Patel S, Kozman M, Chiappetta DA, et al. The transferrin receptor and the targeted delivery of therapeutic agents. Biochim Biophys Acta 2012;1820:291-317.

[79] Yoon DJ, Chu DSH, Ng CW, Pham EA, Mason AB, Hudson DM, et al. Genetically engineering transferrin to improve its in vitro ability to deliver cytotoxins. J Control Release 2009;133:178-84.

[80] Ulbrich K, Hekmatara T, Herbert E, Kreuter J. Transferrin- and transferrin-receptor-antibody-modified nanoparticles enable drug delivery across the blood-brain barrier (BBB). Eur J Pharm Biopharm 2009;71:251-6

[81] Elliott RL, Elliott MC, Wang F, Head JF. Breast carcinoma and the role of iron metabolism. A cytochemical, tissue culture, and ultrastructural study. Ann NY Acad Sci 1993;698:159–66.

[82] InVitria. Optoferrin. 2010 [cited; Available from: http://www.invitria.com/images/pdf/Optoferrin/7.2.6%20optoferrin%20guidelines%20for%20use.pdf]

[83] Ali SA, Joao HC, Hammerschmid F, Eder J, Steinkasserer A. An antigenic HIV-1 peptide sequence engineered into the surface structure of transferrin does not elicit an antibody response. FEBS Lett. 1999; 459:230–32.

[84] Sahoo SK, Ma W, Labhasetwar V. Efficacy of transferrin-conjugated paclitaxel-loaded nanoparticles in a murine model of prostate cancer. Int J Cancer 2004;112:335-40.

[85] Li JL, Wang L, Liu XY, Zhang ZP, Guo HC, Liu WM, et al. In vitro cancer cell imaging and therapy using transferrin-conjugated gold nanoparticles. Cancer Lett 2009;274:319-26.

[86] Sahoo SK, Labhasetwar V. Enhanced antiproliferative activity of transferrin-conjugated paclitaxel-loaded nanoparticles is mediated via sustained intracellular drug retention. Mol. Pharm. 2005;2(5):373–83.

[87] Zheng Y, Yu B, Weecharangsan W, Piao L, Darby M, Mao Y, et al. Transferrin-conjugated lipid-coated PLGA nanoparticles for targeted delivery of aromatase inhibitor 7α-APTADD to breast cancer cells. Int J Pharm 2010;390:234-41.

[88] Gan CW, Feng SS. Transferrin-conjugated nanoparticles of poly(lactide)-D-alpha-tocopheryl polyethylene glycol succinate diblock copolymer for targeted drug delivery across the blood–brain barrier. Biomaterials 2010;31:7748–57.

[89] Bellocq NC, Pun SH, Jensen GS, Davis ME. Transferrin-containing, cyclodextrin polymer-based particles for tumor-targeted gene delivery. Bioconjug. Chem. 2003;14(6):1122–32.

[90] Hu-Lieskovan S, Heidel JD, Bartlett DW, Davis ME, T.J. Triche TJ. Sequence specific knockdown of EWS-FLI1 by targeted, nonviral delivery of small interfering RNA inhibits tumor growth in a murine model of metastatic Ewing's sarcoma. Cancer Res. 2005;65(19):8984–92.

[91] Bartlett DW, Davis ME. Physicochemical and biological characterization of targeted, nucleic acid-containing nanoparticles. Bioconjugate Chem 2007;18:456-68.

[92] Heidel JD, Yu Z, Liu JYC, Rele SM, Liang Y, Zeidan RK, et al. Administration in non-human primates of escalating intravenous doses of targeted nanoparticles containing ribonucleotide reductase subunit M2 siRNA. Proc Natl Acad Sci USA 2007;104:5715-21.

[93] Hong MH, Zhu SJ, Jiang YY, Tang GT, Pei YY. Efficient tumor targeting of hydroxycamptothecin loaded PEGylated niosomes modified with transferrin. J Control Release 2009;133(2):96-102.

[94] Hong M, Zhu S, Jiang Y, Tang G, Sun C, Fang C, et al. Novel anti-tumor strategy: PEG-hydroxycamptothecin conjugate loaded transferrin-PEG-nanoparticles. J Control Release 2010;141:22-9.

[95] Aktas Y, Yemisci M, Andrieux K, Gursoy RN, Alonso MJ, Fernandez-Megia E, et al. Development and brain delivery of chitosan-PEG nanoparticles functionalized with the monoclonal antibody OX26, Bioconjug. Chem. 2005;16:1503–11.

[96] Callens C, Moura IC, Lepelletier Y, Coulon S, Renand A, Dussiot M, et al. Recent advances in adult T-cell leukemia therapy: focus on a new anti-transferrin receptor monoclonal antibody. Leukemia 2008;22:42–8.

[97] Boado RJ, Tsukamoto H, Pardridge WM. Drug delivery of antisense molecules to the brain for treatment of Alzheimer's disease and cerebral AIDS. J. Pharm. Sci. 1998;87:1308–15.

[98] Rivest V, Phivilay A, Julien C, Belanger S, Tremblay C, Emond V, et al. Novel liposomal formulation for targeted gene delivery. Pharm. Res. 2007;24:981–90.

[99] Lesley J, Schulte R, Woods J. Modulation of transferrin receptor expression and function by anti-transferrin receptor antibodies and antibody fragments. Exp. Cell Res. 1989;182:215–33.

[100] Bickel U, Yoshikawa T, Landaw EM, Faull KF, Pardridge WM. Pharmacologic effects in vivo in brain by vector-mediated peptide drug delivery. Proc. Natl. Acad. Sci. USA 1993; 90:2618–22.

[101] Berthold A, Cremer K, Kreuter J. Preparation and characterization of chitosan microspheres as drug carrier for prednisolone sodium phosphate as model for anti-inflammatory drugs. J Control Release 1996;39:17–25.

[102] Wang J, Tian S, Petros RA, Napier ME, Desimone JM. The complex role of multivalency in nanoparticles targeting the transferrin receptor for cancer therapies. J. Am. Chem. Soc. 2010;132:11306–13.

[103] Hilgenbrink AR, Low PS. Folate receptor-mediated drug targeting from therapeutics to diagnostics. J Pharmaceut Sci 2005;94:2135-46.

[104] Zhao XB, Muthusamy N, Lee RJ, Byrd JC. Chapter 33. Folate Receptor-Targeted Liposomes for Cancer Therapy. In: Amiji M, editor. Nanotechnology for cancer therapy. Boca Raton, Florida, USA: CRC Press; 2007.

[105] Low PS, Antony AC. Folate receptor-targeted drugs for cancer and inflammatory diseases. Adv. Drug Deliv. Rev. 2004;56(8):1055–58.

[106] Salazar MD, Ratnam M. The folate receptor: what does it promise in tissue-targeted therapeutics? Cancer Metastasis Rev. 2007;26:141–52.

[107] Park JH, Lee S, Kim JH, Park K, Kim K, Kwon IC. Polymeric nanomedicine for cancer therapy. Prog Polym Sci. 2008;33:113-37.

[108] Mathew ME, Mohan JC, Manzoor K, Nair SV, Tamura H, Jayakumar R. Folate conjugated carboxymethyl chitosan-manganese doped zinc sulphide nanoparticles for targeted drug delivery and imaging of cancer cells. Carbohydr. Polym. 2010;80(2):442-8.

[109] Xing H, Wong NY, Xiang Y, Lu Y. DNA aptamer functionalized nanomaterials for intracellular analysis, cancer cell imaging and drug delivery. Curr. Opin. Chem. Biol. http://dx.doi.org/10.1016/j.cbpa.2012.03.016

[110] Mathias CJ, Hubers D, Low PS, Green MA. Synthesis of [(99 m) Tc]DTPA-folate and its evaluation as a folate-receptor-targeted radiopharmaceutical. Bioconjugate Chem. 2000;11:253–57.

[111] Yu B, Tai HC, Xue W, Lee LJ, Lee RJ. Receptor-targeted nanocarriers for therapeutic delivery to cancer. Mol Membrane Biol 2010;27:286-98.

[112] Ohguchi Y, Kawano K, Hattori Y, Maitani Y. Selective delivery of folate-PEG-linked, nanoemulsion-loaded aclacinomycin A to KB nasopharyngeal cells and xenograft: effect of chain length and amount of folate-Peg linker. J Drug Target 2008;16:660-7.

[113] Ebrahimnejad P, Dinarvand R, Sajadi A, Jaafari MR, Nomani AR, Azizi E, et al. Preparation and in vitro evaluation of actively targetable nanoparticles for SN-38 delivery against HT-29 cell lines. Nanomed Nanotechnol Biol Med 2010;6(3):478-85.

[114] Blanco MD, Guerrero S, Benito M, Teijón C, Olmo R, Muñiz E, et al. Tamoxifen-loaded folate-conjugate poly[(p-nitrophenylacrylate)-co-(N-isopropylacrylamide)] sub-microgel as antitumoral drug delivery system. J Biomed Mat Res A 2010; 95A(4): 1028-40.

[115] Blanco MD, Guerrero S, Benito M, Fernández A, Teijón C, Olmo R, et al. In Vitro and In Vivo evaluation of a folate-targeted copolymeric submicrohydrogel based on N-Isopropylacrylamide as 5-fluorouracil delivery system. Polymers 2011; 3: 1107-25.

[116] Kılıçay E, Demirbilek M, Turk M, Guven E, Hazer B, Denkbas EB. Preparation and characterization of poly(3-hydroxybutyrate-co-3-hydroxyhexanoate) (PHBHHX) based nanoparticles for targeted cancer therapy. Eur. J. Pharm. Sci. 2011;44:310-20.

[117] Yang SJ, Chen JW, Lin FH, Young TH, Lou PJ, Shieh MJ. Colorectal cancer cell detection by folic acid-conjugated chitosan nanoparticles. Biomed Eng Appl Basis Comm 2010;22:9-17.

[118] Parveen S, Sahoo SK. Evaluation of cytotoxicity and mechanism of apoptosis of doxorubicin using folate-decorated chitosan nanoparticles for targeted delivery to retinoblastoma. Cancer Nanotechnol 2010; 1(1-6):47-62.

[119] Yang SJ, Lin FH, Tsai HM, Lin CF, Chin HC, Wong JM, et al. Alginate-folic acid-modified chitosan nanoparticles for photodynamic detection of intestinal neoplasms. Biomaterials. 2011;32:2174–82.

[120] Ruoslahti E. Specialization of tumour vasculature. Nat. Rev. Cancer 2002;2(2):83–90.

[121] Brannon-Peppas L, Blanchette JO. Nanoparticle and targeted systems for cancer therapy. Adv Drug Deliv Rev 2004;56:1649–59.

[122] Nisato RE, Tille JC, Jonczyk A, Goodman SL, Pepper MS. alphav beta 3 and alphav beta 5 integrin antagonists inhibit angiogenesis in vitro. Angiogenesis 2003;6(2):105–19.

[123] Park JH, Kwon S, Nam JO, Park RW, Chung H, Seo SB, et al. Self-assembled nanoparticles based on glycol chitosan bearing 5beta-cholanic acid for RGD peptide delivery. J Control Release 2004;95:579-88.

[124] Savill J, Dransfield I, Hogg N, Haslett C. Vitronectin receptor-mediated phagocytosis of cells undergoing apoptosis. Nature 1990;343:170–3.

[125] Xiong XB, Huang Y, Lu WL, Zhang X, Zhang H, Nagai T, et al. Intracellular delivery of doxorubicin with RGD-modified sterically stabilized liposomes for an improved antitumor efficacy: In vitro and in vivo. J Pharm. Sci. 2005;94:1782–93.

[126] Xiong XB, Huang Y, Lu WL, Zhang X, Zhang H, Nagai T et al. Enhanced intracellular delivery and improved antitumor efficacy of doxorubicin by sterically stabilized liposomes modified with a synthetic RGD mimetic. J Control Release 2005;107(2):262–75.

[127] Demirgoz D, Garg A, Kokkoli E. PR b-targeted PEGylated liposomes for prostate cancer therapy. Langmuir 2008;24:13518–24.

[128] Garg A, Tisdale AW, Haidari E, Kokkoli E. Targeting colon cancer cells using PEGylated liposomes modified with a fibronectin-mimetic peptide. Int J Pharm 2009;366:201–10.

[129] Wu P, He X, Wang K, Tan W, Ma D, Yang W, et al. Imaging breast cancer cells and tissues using peptide-labeled fluorescent silica nanoparticles. J Nanosci Nanotechnol 2008;8:2483–7.

[130] Han HD, Mangala LS, Lee JW, Shahzad MMK, Kim HS, Shen D et al. Targeted gene silencing using RGD-labeled chitosan nanoparticles. Clin Cancer Res. 2010;16(15):3910–22.

[131] Hood JD, Bednarski M, Frausto R, Guccione S, Reisfeld RA, Xiang R et al. Tumor regression by targeted gene delivery to the neovasculature. Science 2002;296(5577):2404–7.

[132] Nasongkla N, Shuai X, Ai H, Weinberg BD, Pink J, Boothman DA et al. cRGDfunctionalized polymer micelles for targeted doxorubicin delivery. Angew. Chem. Int. Ed. Engl. 2004;43(46):6323–7

[133] Hamano N, Negishi Y, Fujisawa A, Manandhar M, Sato H, Katagiri F et al. Modification of the C16Y peptide on nanoparticles is an effective approach to target endothelial and cancer cells via the integrin receptor. Int. J. Pharm. 2012;428:114-7.

[134] Ponce ML, Hibino S, Lebioda AM, Mochizuki M, Nomizu M, Kleinman HK. Identification of a potent peptide antagonist to an active laminin-1 sequence that blocks angiogenesis and tumor growth. Cancer Res. 2003;63:5060–4.

[135] Qing Xu Q, Liu Y, Su S, Li W, Chen C, Wu Y. Anti-tumor activity of paclitaxel through dual-targeting carrier of cyclic RGD and transferrin conjugated hyperbranched copolymer nanoparticles Biomaterials 2012;33:1627-39.

[136] Levesque SG, Shoichet MS. Synthesis of enzyme-degradable, peptide-crosslinked dextran hydrogels. Bioconjug Chem 2007;18:874-85.

[137] Annunziato ME, Patel US, Ranade M, Palumbo PS. p-Maleimidophenyl isocyanate: a novel heterobifunctional linker for hydroxyl to thiol coupling. Bioconjug Chem 1993;4:212-8

[138] Schiller JH, Larson T, Ou SI, Limentani A, Sandler AB, Vokes EE et al. Efficacy and safety of axitinib (AG-013736; AG) in patients (pts) with advanced non-small cell lung cancer (NSCLC): a phase II trial. J Clin Oncol 2007;25(18S) [abstr 7507].

[139] Goss GD, Arnold A, Shepherd FA, Dediu M. Ciuleanu TE, Fenton D, et al. Randomized, double-blind trial of carboplatin and paclitaxel with either daily oral cediranib or placebo in advanced non-small-cell lung cancer: NCIC clinical trials group BR24 study. J Clin Oncol 2010;28(1):49–55.

[140] Hirsch FR, Varella-Garcia M, Bunn Jr PA, Di Maria MV, Veve R, Bremnes RM, et al. Epidermal growth factor receptor in non-small-cell lung carcinomas: correlation between gene copy number and protein expression and impact on prognosis. J Clin Oncol 2003;21(20):3798–807.

[141] Moore MJ, Goldstein D, Hamm J, Figer A, Hecht JR, Gallinger S, et al. Erlotinib Plus Gemcitabine Compared With Gemcitabine Alone in Patients With Advanced Pancreatic Cancer: A Phase III Trial of the National Cancer Institute of Canada Clinical Trials Group. J Clin Oncol 2007; 20:1960-66.

[142] Karp DD, Paz-Ares LG, Novello S, Haluska P, Garland L, Cardenal F, et al. Phase II study of the anti-insulin-like growth factor type 1 receptor antibody CP-751, 871 in combination with paclitaxel and carboplatin in previously untreated, locally advanced or metastatic non-small-cell lung cancer. J Clin Oncol 2009;27(15):2516–22.

[143] Saltz LB, Clarke S, Diaz-Rubio E, Scheithauer W, Figer A, Wong R, et al. Bevacizumab in combination with oxaliplatin-based chemotherapy as first-line therapy in metastatic colorectal cancer: a randomized phase III study. J Clin Oncol 2008;26(12):2013–9.

[144] Hurwitz H, Fehrenbacher L, Novotny W, Cartwright T, Hainsworth J, Heim W, et al. Bevacizumab plus irinotecan, fluorouracil, and leucovorin for metastatic colorectal cancer. N Engl J Med 2004; 350(23):2335-42.

[145] Cassidy J, Clarke S, Diaz-Rubio E, Scheithauer W, Figer A, Wong R, et al. Randomized phase III study of capecitabine plus oxaliplatin compared with fluorouracil/folinic acid plus oxaliplatin as first-line therapy for metastatic colorectal cancer. J Clin Oncol 2008; 26(12):2006-12.

[146] Van Cutsem E, Köhne C-H, Láng I, Folprecht G, Nowacki MP, Cascinu S, et al. Cetuximab plus irinotecan, fluorouracil, and leucovorin as first-line treatment for metastatic colorectal cancer: updated analysis of overall survival according to tumor KRAS and BRAF mutation status. J Clin Oncol 2011; 29(15):2011-9.

[147] Douillard J-Y, Siena S, Cassidy J, Tabernero J, Burkes R, Barugel M et al. Randomized, phase III trial of panitumumab with infusional fluorouracil, leucovorin, and oxaliplatin (FOLFOX4) versus FOLFOX4 alone as first-line treatment in patients with previously untreated metastatic colorectal cancer: the PRIME study. J Clin Oncol 2010; 28(31):4697-705.

[148] Clifford A, Hudis MD. Trastuzumab—mechanism of action and use in clinical practice. N Engl J Med 2007;357:39–51.

[149] Krop IE, Beeram M, Modi S, Jones SF, Holden SN, Yu W, et al. Phase I study of trastuzumab-DM1, an HER2 antibody-drug conjugate, given every 3 weeks to patients with HER2-positive metastatic breast cancer. J Clin Oncol 2010;28:2698–704.

[150] Keating GM. Pertuzumab: in the first-line treatment of HER2-positive metastatic breast cancer. Drugs 2012;72 (3):353-60

[151] Tutt A, Robson M, Garber JE, Domchek SM, Audeh MW, Weitzel JN, et al. Oral poly(ADP-ribose) polymerase inhibitor olaparib in patients with BRCA1 or BRCA2 mutations and advanced breast cancer: a proof-of-concept trial. Lancet 2010;376(9737):235–44.

[152] de Bono JS, Logothetis CJ, Molina A, Fizazi K, North S, Chu L, et al. Abiraterone and increased survival in metastatic prostate cancer. N. Engl. J. Med. 2011;364:1995–2005.

[153] Scher HI, Beer TM, Higano CS, Anand A, Taplin ME, Efstathiou E, et al. Antitumour activity of MDV3100 in castration-resistant prostate cancer: a phase 1–2 study, Lancet 2010;375:1437–46.

[154] Fleming MT, Sonpavde G, Kolodziej M, Awasthi S, Martincic D, Rastogi A, et al. Association of Rash With Outcomes in a Randomized Phase II Trial Evaluating Cetuximab in Combination With Mitoxantrone Plus Prednisone After Docetaxel for Metastatic Castration-resistant Prostate Cancer. Clin Genitourin Cancer 2012;10:6-14.

[155] Chen LQ, Mooso BA, Jathal MK, Madhav A, Johnson SD, van Spyk E, et al. Dual EGFR/HER2 Inhibition Sensitizes Prostate Cancer Cells to Androgen Withdrawal by Suppressing ErbB3. Clin Cancer Res 2011;17:6218-28.

[156] Schoeberl B, Faber AC, Li D, Liang MC, Crosby K, Onsum M, et al. An ErbB3 antibody, MM-121, is active in cancers with ligand-dependent activation. Cancer Res. 2010;70:2485–94.

[157] Bander NH, Nanus DM, Milowsky M I, Kostakoglu L, Vallabahajosula S, Goldsmith SJ. Targeted systemic therapy of prostate cancer with a monoclonal antibody to prostate-specific membrane antigen. Semin Oncol 2003;30:667–76.

[158] Pallis AG, Serfass L, Dziadziuszko R, van Meerbeeck JP, Fennell D, Lacombe D, et al. Targeted therapies in the treatment of advanced/metastatic NSCLC. Eur J Cancer 2009;45:2473-87.

[159] Belani CP, Goss G, Blumenschein Jr G. Recent clinical developments and rationale for combining targeted agents in non-small cell lung cancer (NSCLC). Cancer Treat Rev 2012;38:173-84

[160] Pirker R, Pereira JR, Szczesna A, von Pawel J, Krzakowski M, Ramlau R, et al. Cetuximab plus chemotherapy in patients with advanced non-small-cell lung cancer (FLEX): an open-label randomised phase III trial. Lancet 2009;373(9674):1525–31.

[161] Ciardiello F, Tortora G. EGFR Antagonists in Cancer Treatment. N Engl J Med 2008; 358: 1160-74.

[162] Ryan PD, Goss PE. The emerging role of the insulin-like growth factor pathway as a therapeutic target in cancer. Oncologist 2008;13:16–24.

[163] Custodio A, Méndez M, Provencio M. Targeted therapies for advanced non-small-cell lung cancer: Current status and future implications. Cancer Treat Rev 2012;38:36-53

[164] Cartwright TH. Treatment Decisions After Diagnosis of Metastatic Colorectal Cancer. Clin. Colorectal Canc. 2011 (doi: 10.1016/j.clcc.2011.11.001)

[165] Goldberg RM, Sargent DJ, Morton RF, Fuchs CS, Ramanathan RK, Williamson SK, et al. Randomized controlled trial of reduced-dose bolus fluorouracil plus leucovorin and irinotecan or infused fluorouracil plus leucovorin and oxaliplatin in patients with previously untreated metastatic colorectal cancer: a North American Intergroup Trial. J Clin Oncol 2006;24(21):3347-53.

[166] Gold J, Winer EP. Chemotherapy for metastatic breast cancer. In: Bland KI, Copeland EM, editors. The Breast: Comprehensive Management of Benign and Malignant Disease. Philadelphia: Saunders Elsevier; 2009. p. 1233–61.

[167] Hayat MA. Breast Carcinoma: an introduction. In: Hayat MA editor. Handbook of Immunochemistry and in situ Hybridization of Human Carcinomas. Vol 1: Molecular Genetics; Lung and Breast Carcinomas. Elsevier (USA) 2009. p. 233-48

[168] Sotiriou C, Pusztai L. Gene-expression signatures in breast cancer. N Engl J Med 2009;360:790–800.

[169] Colombo M, Corsi F Foschi D, Mazzantini E, Mazzucchelli S, Morasso C, et al. HER2 targeting as a two-sided strategy for breast cancer diagnosis and treatment: Outlook and recent implications in nanomedical approaches. Pharmacol. Res. 2010;62:150–65.

[170] Corsi F, Fiandra L, De Palma C, Colombo M, Mazzucchelli S, Verderio P, et al. HER2 Expression in Breast Cancer Cells Is Downregulated Upon Active Targeting by Antibody-Engineered Multifunctional Nanoparticles in Mice. ACSNano 2011;5:6383–93

[171] Polychronis A, Sinnet HD, Hadjiminas D, Singhal H, Mansi JL, Shivapatham D, et al. Pre-operative gefitinib versus gefitinib and anastrozole in postmenopausal patients with oestrogen-receptor positive and epidermal growth factor receptor positive primary breast cancer: a double blind placebo-controlled phase II randomised trial. Lancet Oncol 2005;6(6):383–91.

[172] Osborne CK, Neven P, Dirix L, Mackey J, Robert J, Underhill C, et al. Randomized Phase II study of gefitinib (IRESSA) or placebo in combination with tamoxifen in patients with hormone receptor positive metastatic breast cancer. Breast Cancer Res Treat 2007;106(Suppl.1):S107 [Abstract 2067].

[173] Marcom PK, Isaacs C, Harris L, Wong ZW, Kommarreddy A, Novielli N, et al. The combination of letrozole and trastuzumab as first or second-line biological therapy produces durable responses in a subset of HER2 positive and ER positive advanced breast cancers. Breast Cancer Res Treat 2007;102(1):43–9.

[174] Baselga J, Cortés J, Kim SB, Im SA, Hegg R, Im YH, et al. CLEOPATRA Study Group. Pertuzumab plus trastuzumab plus docetaxel for metastatic breast cancer. N Engl J Med; 2012;366(2):109-19.

[175] O'Shaughnessy J, Osborne C, Pippen JE, Yoffe M, Patt D, Rocha C, et al. Iniparib plus chemotherapy in metastatic triple-negative breast cancer. N Engl J Med 2011;364(3):205–14.

[176] Liu X, Shi Y, Maag DX, Palma JP, Patterson MJ, Ellis PA, et al. Iniparib Nonselectively Modifies Cysteine-Containing Proteins in Tumor Cells and Is Not a Bona Fide PARP Inhibitor. Clin Cancer Res 2012;18:510-23.

[177] Stavridi F, Karapanagiotou EM, Syrigos KN. Targeted therapeutic approaches for hormone-refractory prostate cancer. Cancer Treat Rev 2010; 36:122–30.

[178] Fu W, Madan E, Yee M, Zhang H. Progress of molecular targeted therapies for prostate cancers. Biochim Biophys Acta 2012;1825:140–52.

[179] de Muga S, Hernandez S, Agell L, Salido M, Juanpere N, Lorenzo M, et al. Molecular alterations of EGFR and PTEN in prostate cancer: association with high-grade and advanced-stage carcinomas. Mod. Pathol. 2010;23:703–12.

[180] Neto AS, Tobias-Machado M, Wroclawski ML, Fonseca FL, Teixeira GK, Amarante RD, et al. Her-2/neu expression in prostate adenocarcinoma: a systematic review and meta-analysis. J. Urol. 2010;184: 842–50.

[181] Jatha MK, Chen L, Mudryj M, Ghosh PM. Targeting ErbB3: the New RTK(id) on the Prostate Cancer Block. Immunol Endocr Metab Agents Med Chem. 2011;11(2):131–49.

[182] Kojima S, Inahara M, Suzuki H, Ichikawa T, Furuya Y. Implications of insulinlike growth factor-I for prostate cancer therapies. Int. J. Urol. 2009;16:161–67.

[183] Wu JD, Haugk K, Coleman I, Woodke L, Vessella R, Nelson P, et al. Combined in vivo effect of A12, a type 1 insulinlike growth factor receptor antibody, and docetaxel against prostate cancer tumors, Clin. Cancer Res. 2006;12:6153–60.

Permissions

The contributors of this book come from diverse backgrounds, making this book a truly international effort. This book will bring forth new frontiers with its revolutionizing research information and detailed analysis of the nascent developments around the world.

We would like to thank Ali Demir Sezer, for lending his expertise to make the book truly unique. He has played a crucial role in the development of this book. Without his invaluable contribution this book wouldn't have been possible. He has made vital efforts to compile up to date information on the varied aspects of this subject to make this book a valuable addition to the collection of many professionals and students.

This book was conceptualized with the vision of imparting up-to-date information and advanced data in this field. To ensure the same, a matchless editorial board was set up. Every individual on the board went through rigorous rounds of assessment to prove their worth. After which they invested a large part of their time researching and compiling the most relevant data for our readers. Conferences and sessions were held from time to time between the editorial board and the contributing authors to present the data in the most comprehensible form. The editorial team has worked tirelessly to provide valuable and valid information to help people across the globe.

Every chapter published in this book has been scrutinized by our experts. Their significance has been extensively debated. The topics covered herein carry significant findings which will fuel the growth of the discipline. They may even be implemented as practical applications or may be referred to as a beginning point for another development. Chapters in this book were first published by InTech; hereby published with permission under the Creative Commons Attribution License or equivalent.

The editorial board has been involved in producing this book since its inception. They have spent rigorous hours researching and exploring the diverse topics which have resulted in the successful publishing of this book. They have passed on their knowledge of decades through this book. To expedite this challenging task, the publisher supported the team at every step. A small team of assistant editors was also appointed to further simplify the editing procedure and attain best results for the readers.

Our editorial team has been hand-picked from every corner of the world. Their multi-ethnicity adds dynamic inputs to the discussions which result in innovative outcomes. These outcomes are then further discussed with the researchers and contributors who give their valuable feedback and opinion regarding the same. The feedback is then collaborated with the researches and they are edited in a comprehensive manner to aid the understanding of the subject.

Apart from the editorial board, the designing team has also invested a significant amount of their time in understanding the subject and creating the most relevant covers. They scrutinized every image to scout for the most suitable representation of the subject and create an appropriate cover for the book.

The publishing team has been involved in this book since its early stages. They were actively engaged in every process, be it collecting the data, connecting with the contributors or procuring relevant information. The team has been an ardent support to the editorial, designing and production team. Their endless efforts to recruit the best for this project, has resulted in the accomplishment of this book. They are a veteran in the field of academics and their pool of knowledge is as vast as their experience in printing. Their expertise and guidance has proved useful at every step. Their uncompromising quality standards have made this book an exceptional effort. Their encouragement from time to time has been an inspiration for everyone.

The publisher and the editorial board hope that this book will prove to be a valuable piece of knowledge for researchers, students, practitioners and scholars across the globe.

List of Contributors

Paola Russo, Antonietta Santoro, Lucia Prota, Mariateresa Stigliani and Rita P. Aquino
Department of Pharmaceutical and Biomedical Sciences, University of Salerno, Fisciano, Italy

Hamed Hamishehkar
Pharmaceutical Technology Laboratory, Drug Applied Research Center, Tabriz University of Medical Sciences, Tabriz, Iran

Yahya Rahimpour
Student Research Committee and Faculty of Pharmacy, Tabriz University of Medical Sciences, Tabriz, Iran

Yousef Javadzadeh
Biotechnology Research Center and Faculty of Pharmacy, Tabriz University of Medical Sciences, Tabriz, Iran

Mohammed Maniruzzaman, Dennis Douroumis, Joshua S. Boateng and Martin J. Snowden
School of Science, University of Greenwich, Central Avenue, Chatham Maritime, Chatham, Kent, ME4 4TB, UK

Martins Ochubiojo Emeje
Centre for Nanomedicine and Biophysical Drug Delivery, National Institute for Pharmaceutical Research and Development, Nigeria

Ifeoma Chinwude Obidike
National Institute for Pharmaceutical Research and Development, Nigeria

Ekaete Ibanga Akpabio
University of Uyo, Akwa-Ibom State, Nigeria

Sabinus Ifianyi Ofoefule
University of Nigeria, Nsukka, Nigeria

Yahya Rahimpour
Biotechnology Research Center and Student Research Committee, Tabriz University of Medical Sciences, Tabriz, Iran

Hamed Hamishehkar
Pharmaceutical Technology Laboratory, Drug Applied Research Center, Tabriz University of Medical Sciences, Tabriz, Iran

Anthony A. Attama and Mumuni A. Momoh
Department of Pharmaceutics, Faculty of Pharmaceutical Sciences, University of Nigeria, Nsukka, Enugu State, Nigeria

Philip F. Builders
Department of Pharmaceutical Technology and Raw Material Development, National Institute for Pharmaceutical Research and Development, Idu, Abuja, Nigeria

José Juan Escobar-Chávez
Unidad de Investigación Multidisciplinaria, Laboratorio 12: Sistemas Transdérmicos y Materiales Nanoestructurados, Facultad de Estudios Superiores Cuautitlán-Universidad Nacional Autónoma de México, Estado de México

Isabel Marlen Rodríguez-Cruz
Departamento de Enseñanza e Investigación, Hospital Regional de Alta Especialidad de Zumpango, Zumpango, Estado de México

Clara Luisa Domínguez-Delgado
Departamento de Ingeniería y Tecnología, Sección de Tecnología Farmacéutica, Facultad de Estudios
Superiores Cuautitlán-Universidad Nacional Autónoma de México, Estado de México

Roberto Díaz- Torres
Unidad de Investigación Multidisciplinari,. Laboratorio 9: Toxicología y genética, Facultad de Estudios Superiores Cuautitlán-Universidad Nacional Autónoma de México, Estado de México

Alma Luisa Revilla-Vázquez
Laboratorio de Desarrollo de Métodos Analíticos, Facultad de Estudios Superiores Cuautitlán-Universidad Nacional Autónoma de México, Cuautitlán Izcalli, Estado de México

Norma Casas Aléncaster
Laboratorio de Propiedades Reológicas de Alimentos, Facultad de Estudios Superiores Cuautitlán-Universidad Nacional Autónoma de México, Cuautitlán Izcalli, Estado de México

Seyda Bucak and Banu Yavuztürk
Yeditepe University, Istanbul, Turkey

Ali Demir Sezer
Marmara University, Istanbul, Turkey

M.D. Blanco, R.M. Olmo and J.M. Teijón
Departamento de Bioquímica y Biología Molecular, Facultad de Medicina, Universidad Complutense de Madrid, Spain

C. Teijón
Departamento de Enfermería, E.U. Enfermería, Fisioterapia y Podología, Universidad Complutense de Madrid, Spain

Printed in the USA
CPSIA information can be obtained
at www.ICGtesting.com
JSHW011457221024
72173JS00005B/1106

9 781632 423979